BODY ENCYCLOPEDIA

BODY ENCYCLOPEDIA

A Guide to the Psychological Functions of the Muscular System

Lisbeth Marcher and Sonja Fich

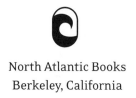

North Atlantic Books
Berkeley, California

Published by

North Atlantic Books   Cover art by Marina Winkel
P.O. Box 12327   Cover and book design by Suzanne Albertson
Berkeley, California 94712   Printed in the United States of America

The anatomical illustrations have been reproduced with kind permission from Feneis, H., *Anatomisches Bildwörterbuch der Internationalen Nomenklatur (Anatomical Picture Dictionary),* Georg Thieme Verlag. Stuttgart, 1988, illustrations by G. Spitzer. In Danish by Jørn Egeberg/2nd Edition, Munksgaard Publishers, Copenhagen.

All Bodymaps and illustrations for the Ego Functions and Character Structures, the descriptions of the various Character Structures, the table of the Character Structures in the Bodynamic System, and the circle-shaped figure showing the Elements of Coding have been reproduced with kind permission from Bodynamic International ApS.

Body Encyclopedia: A Guide to the Psychological Functions of the Muscular System is sponsored by the Society for the Study of Native Arts and Sciences, a nonprofit educational corporation whose goals are to develop an educational and cross-cultural perspective linking various scientific, social, and artistic fields; to nurture a holistic view of arts, sciences, humanities, and healing; and to publish and distribute literature on the relationship of mind, body, and nature.

North Atlantic Books' publications are available through most bookstores. For further information, visit our website at www.northatlanticbooks.com or call 800-733-3000.

Library of Congress Cataloging-in-Publication Data

Marcher, Lisbeth, 1940–
    Body encyclopedia: a guide to the psychological functions of the muscular system /
    Lisbeth Marcher and Sonja Fich.
        p.; cm.
    Includes bibliographical references and index.
    Summary: "An important contribution to the field of somatic psychology, Body Encyclopedia presents a unique, cutting-edge system based on extensive research that has practical applications for psychotherapists, body therapists, and other health practitioners"—Provided by publisher.
    ISBN 978-1-55643-940-7 (alk. paper)
    1. Mind and body therapies. 2. Psychotherapy. I. Fich, Sonja, 1942- II. Title.
    [DNLM: 1. Mind-Body Relations (Metaphysics) 2. Musculoskeletal System. 3. Psychosomatic Medicine—methods. WE 100 M316b 2010
    RC489.M53M37 2010
    616.89'14—dc22
                                                                        2010001946

2 3 4 5 6 7 8 9 UNITED 15 14 13 12 11

Dedication

We want to dedicate *Body Encyclopedia* to our families, to everyone who has participated in developing the Bodynamic System, and to everyone who has contributed to
the birth of this book.

Contents

Preface xv

SECTION 1: Introduction to the Bodynamic System 1

Definitions in the Bodynamic System	3
Ego Formation through the Coding Elements	9
Examples of Formation of Coding	17
Using This Book	25
Anatomical Terms	27

SECTION 2: The Bodynamic Psycho-Motor Anatomy 29

Descriptions of Muscles and Connective Tissue		31
Bodymap of the Front of the Body		34
Bodymap of the Back of the Body		35
Muscles and Connective Tissue*		37
*	Connective tissue of the back level with thoracic vertebrae 3-5	37
1a	Erector spinae	39
1b	Erector spinae at spinous processes-rotators	43
2a, b, c	Trapezius	45
3a, b	Rhomboids minor and major	49
4	Serratus posterior superior	51
5	Teres major	53
6	Teres minor	55
7a, b	Infraspinatus	57
8a, b, c	Serratus anterior	59
9a, b	Latissimus dorsi	61
10	Serratus posterior inferior	63
11	Quadratus lumborum	65
12	Iliac crest	67
13	Sacrum	69
14	Gluteus maximus	71
15	Gluteus medius	73

*Numbers refer to muscles and connective tissue that are tested and marked on the bodymap. Asterisks refer to muscles and connective tissue that are not tested nor marked on the bodymap because they are difficult or impossible to palpate, though they have been included because they do impact both motion and psychology.

16	Gluteus minimus	75
17	Piriformis	77
18	Gemelli and obturator internus	79
19	Quadratus femoris	81
20	Obturator internus	83
*	Pelvic floor	85
21	Sacrotuberous ligament	87
22	Tensor fascia lata	89
23	Iliotibial tract	91
24a, b, c, d	Biceps femoris (lateral hamstring)	93
25	Semitendinosus (medial hamstring)	97
26	Semimembranosus (medial hamstring)	99
27	Plantaris	101
28a, b	Gastrocnemius	103
29	Popliteus	105
30a, b	Soleus	107
31	Flexor hallucis longus	109
32	Flexor digitorum longus	111
*	Lumbricals	113
*	Quadratus plantae	115
33	Plantar aponeurosis	117
*	Insertions of abductor, flexors, and extensors on the proximal phalanx of the little toe	119
34	Abductor digiti minimi and flexor digiti minimi brevis	121
35	Flexor digitorum brevis	123
36	Abductor hallucis	125
37	Flexor hallucis brevis	127
38	Extensor digitorum brevis and extensor hallucis brevis	129
39	Tibialis anterior	131
40	Extensor digitorum longus	133
41	Extensor hallucis longus	135
*	Tibialis posterior	137
42a, b	Peroneus longus and brevis	139
43a	Rectus femoris	141
43b	Vastus lateralis	143
43c	Vastus intermedius	145
43d	Vastus medialis	147
44a, b	Sartorius	149
45	Pectineus	151
46	Adductor longus	153
47	Adductor brevis	155
48	Adductor magnus	157

49	Gracilis	159
*	Connective tissue around knee and ankle	161
*	Connective tissue of medial and lateral rotators of the hip joint	163
50	Inguinal ligament	165
*	Origin of iliacus	167
*	Insertion of iliopsoas	169
51a	Iliacus	171
51b	Iliopsoas	173
51c	Transversus abdominis	175
52	Obliquus externus and internus	177
53	Rectus abdominis	179
*	Pyramidalis	181
54	Umbilicus	183
55	Psoas major	185
56	Costal curve	187
57	Diaphragm	189
58	Transversus thoracis	191
59	Origin of pectoralis major-sternal head	193
60	Sternal fascia	195
61	Intercostals	197
62a, b, c	Pectoralis major	199
63	Pectoralis minor	203
64	Subclavius	205
65	Deltoid, anterior	207
66a, b	Biceps brachii	209
67	Coracobrachialis	211
68	Brachialis	213
69	Subscapularis	215
*	Connective tissue of medial and lateral rotators of the shoulder joint	217
*	Connective tissue around elbow and wrist	219
70	Pronator teres	221
71	Flexor carpi radialis	223
72	Flexor carpi ulnaris	225
73	Flexor digitorum superficialis	227
74	Flexor pollicis longus	229
75	Flexor digitorum profundus	231
*	Lumbricals	233
76	Palmar aponeurosis	235
77	Abductor pollicis brevis	237
78	Flexor pollicis brevis	239

79	Adductor pollicis	241
80	Opponens pollicis	243
*	Insertions of flexors and extensors on the proximal phalanx of the little finger	245
81	Abductor digiti minimi	247
82	Flexor digiti minimi brevis	249
83	Opponens digiti minimi	251
84a, b	Deltoid	253
85a, b, c	Triceps brachii	255
86	Anconeus	257
87	Brachioradialis	259
88	Extensor carpi radialis longus and brevis	261
89	Extensor carpi ulnaris	263
90	Extensor digitorum	265
91	Supinator	267
92	Extensor digiti minimi	269
93	Extensor indicis	271
94	Extensor pollicis brevis and abductor pollicis longus	273
*	Connective tissue on top of the shoulder (shoulder plexus)	275
95	Supraspinatus	277
96	Levator scapulae	279
97	Scalenus posterior	281
98	Semispinalis capitis	283
99	Splenius capitis	285
*	Splenius cervicis	287
100	Suboccipitals	289
101a	Galea aponeurotica (a spot on top of the head)	291
101b	Galea aponeurotica (half circle around the top of the head)	293
101c	Galea aponeurotica	295
102	Occipitofrontalis–venter occipitalis	297
103	Platysma	299
104	Scalenus anterior	301
105	Scalenus medius	303
106a, b	Sternocleidomastoid	305
107	Omohyoid	309
108	Mylohyoid	311
109	Digastricus, posterior belly	313
110	Longus capitis and longus colli	315
111	Occipitofrontalis–venter frontalis	317
112	"Third eye"	319
113a, b	Orbicularis oculi	321
114	Procerus	323

115	Corrugator supercilii	325
116	Nasalis	327
117	Tip of the nose	329
118	Temporalis	331
119	Zygomaticus	333
120	Buccinator	335
*	Risorius	337
121	Orbicularis oris	339
122	Mentalis	341
123	Medial pterygoid	343
124	Depressor anguli oris	345
*	Depressor labii	347
*	Depressor septi	349
125	Masseter	351

SECTION 3: **The Bodynamic Character Structure System** 353

The Character Structures in the Bodynamic System	355
A Table of the Character Structures in the Bodynamic System	357
A Theory of Personality Based on Psychomotor Development	359
Prenatal and Perinatal	361
Model of the Stages of Birth	362
The Muscles Marked on a Bodymap	364
All the Muscles and Connective Tissue in This Age Span	365
Some Essential Patterns of Movement in This Age Span	367
The Character Structure EXISTENCE: 2nd Trimester–3 Months	369
Character Positions	369
The Muscles Marked on a Bodymap	372
All the Muscles and Connective Tissue in This Age Span	373
The Location of Some of the Muscles and Connective Tissue in the Body	374
Some Essential Patterns of Movement in This Age Span	375
The Character Structure NEED: 1 Month–1½ Years	379
Character Positions	379
The Muscles Marked on a Bodymap	382
All the Muscles and Connective Tissue in This Age Span	383
The Location of Some of the Muscles in the Body	386
Some Essential Patterns of Movement in This Age Span	387
The Character Structure AUTONOMY: 8 Months–2½ Years	391
Character Positions	391
The Muscles Marked on a Bodymap	394
All the Muscles and Connective Tissue in This Age Span	395

The Location of Some of the Muscles in the Body 396
Some Essential Patterns of Movement in This Age Span 397

The Character Structure WILL: 2-4 Years 401
Character Positions 401
The Muscles Marked on a Bodymap 406
All the Muscles and Connective Tissue in This Age Span 407
The Location of Some of the Muscles in the Body 408
Some Essential Patterns of Movement in This Age Span 409

The Character Structure LOVE/SEXUALITY: 3-6 Years 415
Character Positions 415
The Muscles Marked on a Bodymap 418
All the Muscles and Connective Tissue in This Age Span 419
The Location of Some of the Muscles in the Body 420
Some Essential Patterns of Movement in This Age Span 421

The Character Structure OPINIONS: 5-9 Years 425
Character Positions 425
The Muscles Marked on a Bodymap 428
All the Muscles and Connective Tissue in This Age Span 429
The Location of Some of the Muscles in the Body 430
Some Essential Patterns of Movement in This Age Span 431

The Character Structure SOLIDARITY/PERFORMANCE: 7-12 Years 435
Character Positions 435
The Muscles Marked on a Bodymap 438
All the Muscles and Connective Tissue in This Age Span 439
The Location of Some of the Muscles in the Body 440
Some Essential Patterns of Movement in This Age Span 441

PUBERTY: 11-19 Years 445
The Muscles Marked on a Bodymap 446
All the Muscles and Connective Tissue in This Age Span 447
Some Essential Patterns of Movement in This Age Span 449

SECTION 4: The Bodynamic Ego Function System 451

The Ego Functions in the Bodynamic System 453
Overview of the Ego Functions and Their Subfunctions 454
The Eleven Ego Functions and Their Embodiment 455
I. The Ego Function CONNECTEDNESS 457
The Location of Some of the Muscles and Connective Tissue in the Body 458
All the Muscles and Connective Tissue in Each Subfunction 459
The Muscles Marked on a Bodymap 460
The Ego Function Connectedness 461

II. The Ego Function POSITIONING   463
    The Location of Some of the Muscles and Connective Tissue in the Body   464
    All the Muscles and Connective Tissue in Each Subfunction   465
    The Muscles Marked on a Bodymap   466
    The Ego Function Positioning   467

III. The Ego Function CENTERING   469
    The Location of Some of the Muscles and Connective Tissue in the Body   470
    All the Muscles and Connective Tissue in Each Subfunction   471
    The Muscles Marked on a Bodymap   472
    The Ego Function Centering   473

IV. The Ego Function BOUNDARIES   475
    The Location of Some of the Muscles and Connective Tissue in the Body   476
    All the Muscles and Connective Tissue in Each Subfunction   477
    The Muscles Marked on a Bodymap   478
    The Ego Function Boundaries   479

V. The Ego Function GROUNDING AND REALITY TESTING   481
    The Location of Some of the Muscles and Connective Tissue in the Body   482
    All the Muscles and Connective Tissue in Each Subfunction   483
    The Muscles Marked on a Bodymap   484
    The Ego Function Grounding and Reality Testing   485

VI. The Ego Function SOCIAL BALANCE   487
    The Location of Some of the Muscles and Connective Tissue in the Body   488
    All the Muscles and Connective Tissue in Each Subfunction   489
    The Muscles Marked on a Bodymap   490
    The Ego Function Social Balance   491

VII. The Ego Function COGNITIVE SKILLS   493
    The Location of Some of the Muscles and Connective Tissue in the Body   494
    All the Muscles and Connective Tissue in Each Subfunction   495
    The Muscles Marked on a Bodymap   498
    The Ego Function Cognitive Skills   499

VIII. The Ego Function MANAGEMENT OF ENERGY   501
    The Location of Some of the Muscles and Connective Tissue in the Body   502
    All the Muscles and Connective Tissue in Each Subfunction   503
    The Muscles Marked on a Bodymap   506
    The Ego Function Management of Energy   507

IX. The Ego Function SELF-ASSERTION   509
    The Location of Some of the Muscles and Connective Tissue in the Body   510
    All the Muscles and Connective Tissue in Each Subfunction   511
    The Muscles Marked on a Bodymap   512
    The Ego Function Self-Assertion   513

X. The Ego Function PATTERNS OF INTERPERSONAL SKILLS   515
    The Location of Some of the Muscles and Connective Tissue in the Body   516
    All the Muscles and Connective Tissue in Each Subfunction   517
    The Muscles Marked on a Bodymap   520
    The Ego Function Patterns of Interpersonal Skills   521

XI. The Ego Function GENDER SKILLS   523
    The Location of Some of the Muscles and Connective Tissue in the Body   524
    All the Muscles and Connective Tissue in Each Subfunction   525
    The Muscles Marked on a Bodymap   528
    The Ego Function Gender Skills   529

Indications of Shock and Post-Traumatic Stress Disorder (PTSD)   531
    The Muscles Marked on a Bodymap   532
    All the Muscles in Shock and PTSD   533

Bibliography 535

List of Muscles and Connective Tissue 539

About the Authors 545

Preface

Body Encyclopedia is a guide to 154 human muscles and related tissues. In addition to anatomical features, this book also describes how these muscles are linked to motor development and to the psychological themes and functions we have found in our research. This forms the basis of how we—in the Bodynamic System—include and integrate the body in our psychotherapeutic work.

Toward the end of the 1960s, I (Lisbeth Marcher) completed my education in Relaxation Pedagogy (now called Psycho-Motor Education). As a student I already had a strong interest in psychological defense mechanisms and how they are established, how the ego is formed, and what the connections are between psychological and physical features in human beings. My major sources of inspiration at that time included Lev Vygotsky; Erik Erikson; several ethologists and animal psychologists, especially Konrad Lorenz; and different anthropologists. During my education I was also inspired by Trygve Braatøy, a Norwegian neurophysiologist, psychiatrist, and psychoanalyst whose principal work, *De Nervøse Sinn (The Nervous Minds,* 1947) already described a long list of parallels between psychological and neuromuscular-neurophysiological conditions and processes.

The seeds of this book were planted when I started as primary teacher of the Individual Treatment course at the Afspændingspædagogisk Institut (Institute for Relaxation Education). In the early 1970s I started a more systematic collection of material describing the psychological aspects attached to the specific muscles.

Lillemor Johnsen, a Norwegian physical therapist with whom I had trained previously, had already developed a muscle testing system in which she tested a combination of muscle and connective tissue. In her system she found that muscles behaved in both hypertonic and hypotonic ways (Lillemor Johnsen 1970, 1975). Lillemor Johnsen tested muscles in terms of respiration response. I developed a very different testing system that evaluates the response of a muscle to a specific type of stimulus: a manual pull in the direction of the muscle fibers. My testing parameters involve the degree of the tenseness and elasticity of muscle response. Besides muscles, Bodynamic also tests a few fasciae and muscle tendons.

As the primary teacher of Individual Treatment, I taught my students to carry out the muscle testing I devised and to use it as a tool in their relaxation treatments. Their work gave me the opportunity to collect further information about relationships between motor development and psychological development as well as the specific muscles involved in both.

I also developed a graphic chart for recording the results of testing, which was later named the Bodymap in the Bodynamic System. The Bodymap offers a convenient tool as it clearly shows the client's resources and weaknesses. Furthermore, the Bodymap provides a fine tool for working out a prognosis.

With help from my students, I collected and then analyzed three types of data:

1. Observations of the psychological themes that emerged or were activated in a client each time a specific muscle was physically stimulated during treatment. Later on we started calling those themes Ego Functions.
2. Observations of the age level that was evoked in the client each time a specific muscle was physically stimulated during treatment. This was the beginning of the Character Structure Model.
3. Observations concerning the specific muscles that started to react each time the client talked about specific psychological themes. The phrase *started to react* means that the client was able to sense or feel those muscles and was also able to move them.

Another possibility of the method developed at that time was that the therapist could watch or palpate a muscle to see or sense changes in the muscles—and could give this as feedback to the client. That helped the client to expand his body awareness and to be able to sense these changes.

From the mid-1970s on I systematically collected such data from all the students. When they were in the role of therapist, they all delivered written reports of actual treatment sessions, focusing on the three types of observations indicated above. At the same time I received clients' reports with their side of the same observations. During a period of five years I received about 15,000 reports.

Along the way, I connected the data from the three types of observations with motor and psychological development—and was thrilled by the uniformity and precision of the information that emerged from the investigation. Every year I revised the handouts I passed out to my students to reflect the additional experience gained collectively during the year.

This whole procedure was research, but in a format where empirically collected data is mixed with a method that is most like "action research." This research method has the ambition to investigate and explore praxis in relationship with practitioners in order to create developmental action abilities and possibilities as well as professional action possibilities. The researcher must at the same time generate new knowledge based on the results that are being produced during the research process. During that five-year process at the Afspændingspædagogisk Institut, all teachers took part in the discussions and debates about the findings and the ways they should be employed to fine-tune the hypothesis.

The collection of data also incorporated methodical observations of children of different ages. An important set of information that emerged from these particular observations concerns the age when specific muscles or parts of muscles are first activated voluntarily in new movements serving important new motor functions such as rolling over, sitting up, creeping and crawling, standing and walking, etc. This investigation was followed up later at the Bodynamic Institute with a project in which Bodynamic analysts tested a number of well-functioning children in order to verify the theory that every muscle or part of a muscle is associated with a specific age level, as confirmed by muscle testing. The results of this project showed distinct connections with our previous findings at the Afspændingspædagogisk Institut.

So I would like to thank all the teachers at the school, especially Ruth Ryborg, who was principal; psychology teachers Niels Hoffmeyer and Jan Ivanouw; Ellen Ollars, who taught individual treatment; and Åse Hauch, who taught childhood development. I would also like to thank all the students for their reports, and even more so for the questions they came up with, which enabled me to be more precise in all details.

Bodynamic Institute was established in December 1982 by Lisbeth Marcher, Erik Jarlnaes, and Steen Joergensen with the purpose of teaching and researching the content of the Bodynamic System. In 1983 a group of ten colleagues worked together more systematically in order to create the first Danish-developed psychotherapy program. In 1985 we started our first Danish four-year psychotherapy training program. At the same time we started our foundation training in California, and slowly our programs began to spread out to other countries as well. In 2000 the Bodynamic System and all its activities were managed from Bodynamic International ApS. The name change reflected the slow but steady spread of the system. Today we have ongoing training in ten countries and workshops in seventeen countries.

A Decisive Turning Point

It was difficult to teach the different stages of development without having some "big boxes" to put the material into. By now I had read Freud, Reich, and Lowen, but their way of looking at character structure did not fit the material I had gathered in the investigations described above. My results came close to the development phases—age levels proposed by Erik Erikson, because he described two positions in each age level—although in his theories he had made no attempt to include the body.

Then one day in about 1982 or 1983 my colleague Steen Joergensen, a psychologist and relaxation educator, came to me with two articles. One was part of the 1,100-page *Clinical Theology* by English theologian and psychiatrist Frank Lake. The book described his theories and observations from his work with psychiatric patients. Lake described two different positions that he observed in the early age levels. The other article was "Stress and Character Structure" by David Boadella (1974), who was and still is one of the greatest European body-psychotherapists and authors. He employed the "two position" understanding of Frank Lake together with the Reich-Lowen model in an attempt to develop a new, expanded model.

This gave us a decisive push to develop our Character Structure model, which I elaborated together with Steen Joergensen over the years 1984 and 1985. The first Character Structure workshop had its inauguration in 1985 with our staff and with outside experts invited specially to the event as participants.

The unique and distinguishing feature of our Character Structure Model is that we propose three positions in each structure or age level: an early position (hyporesponsive), a late position (hyperresponsive), and a neutral position (neutral response). A key feature of the model is that these positions directly correlate to the responses obtained in muscle testing.

All the teachers at the Bodynamic Institute helped refine and define both the Character Structure Model and the Ego Function Model (whose themes include Boundaries, Centering, Energy Management, and several more). We had developed that material over time in response to a real need. Working with psychotherapy clients, we needed to be able to evaluate the client's progress in relation to the issue or issues that he or she wanted to work on. The two models developed gradually as an increasingly well-organized and detailed frame of reference for such evaluation.

For the birth of this book I would like to express my special thanks to many people:

Ellen Ollars, Bodynamic analyst, psychotherapist, and relaxation educator, for her cooperation with Sonja Fich in describing how individual muscles are tested. Furthermore for her important work in her precise reading and feedback on each page with muscle content.

Lennart Ollars, psychologist, Bodynamic analyst, psychotherapist, and relaxation educator. In the early 1970s we organized a series of workshops on personal development that included the body called "Body Awareness, Identity, and Relationships," and he has continued to be my sparring partner since then. In this book he has worked on the section around the individual Ego Functions, which he handed to me just before his untimely death in 2004.

Steen Joergensen, psychologist, Bodynamic analyst, psychotherapist, and relaxation educator, for having developed the Character Structures with me and for his drawings of our "muscle men," the images that show what muscles are associated with each Character Structure and Ego Function.

Niels Thorball, internist, our anatomy expert, and instructor, who also drew the image of the pelvic floor and its muscles.

Erik Jarlnaes, Bodynamic analyst, psychotherapist, relaxation educator, and journalist, for his constant creativity, backup and support, readiness for dialogue, and clearing up questions.

Mogens Fich, for having adapted the Bodymap figure to be used on computers, and for patient assistance and support during the preparation of the small cuts of the Bodymap placed by each muscle, as well as the Bodymaps showing the muscles in the Character Structures and in the Ego Functions.

My thanks also go to all the members and teachers at the Bodynamic Institute, whose precise work and insights have supported the development of our system: Merete Holm Brantbjerg, Marianne Bentzen, Erik Jarlnaes, Steen Joergensen, Ditte Marcher, Bente Moerup, Ellen Ollars, Lennart Ollars, Lone Reimert, and Sonja Fich. In fact, we have been working as a team developing this system, and our many different resources have contributed to making the system more complete. Through the years all of our students have also been an important part of this process.

Sonja Fich, Bodynamic analyst, psychotherapist, and relaxation educator, has always been our anatomy specialist, and so when I started this book it was natural that we would be working together. It is a delight to have a wonderful partner like Sonja. As we each have different specialties, we make a very constructive team. That has enabled the two of us to create precise verbal descriptions for the psychological content of practically every muscle in the human body.

So, both Sonja and I would like to thank you all, everyone.

All the books that have served as background material or sources of inspiration in developing the Bodynamic System, and for this publication in particular, are listed in the Bibliography.

The translation from Danish into English would not have been possible without the help of the following people: Bodynamic therapist and English teacher Helle Waehrens, who has translated the descriptions of the muscles, Character Structures, Ego Functions, and the "Use of the Book" and "Anatomical Terms" sections; and physiotherapist, Bodynamic therapist, and trainee Barbara Picton, from Vancouver, Canada, who with her British-Canadian background has given feedback and adjustment to the same parts of the book so that the language has become more precise and in international English.

Bodynamic analyst Erik Jarlnaes has translated the Preface, the Definitions, the Ego Formation through the Coding Elements, and the cases according to the Coding System. Bodynamic therapist and translator Yorgis Toufexis, from Athens, Greece, has edited this part. We have also received supplementary help from Bodynamic therapist and trainee Joel Isacs, from Venice, California, and psychologist Nathalie Albert-Ozga from California.

Thanks to all who have contributed to the translation from Danish into English and to the fine-tuning of the English used. The translation into English has helped us to become more accurate and precise in Danish, and in this process we want to thank especially Helle Waehrens for her invaluable help. We are very grateful for her translation of all the corrections that have occurred in the process of the final editing of this book.

We want to thank printer and graphic designer Jens Peter Jacobsen for his willingness and great help in the original layout of the book. It is due to him that we have been able to complete the book in a way that makes it ready for printing.

I want to extend my thanks for financial support in writing this book to Bodynamic therapist Michael Gad, and to Hildur and Ross Jackson. Their support has made it possible for me to take time off and also to get help typing, which was a necessary condition for me to write this book at all. It has been invaluable help, and I am deeply grateful.

I am also deeply grateful to the Egmont Foundation, which supported the completion of my research and the written account of my results—the background for this book. One reason that the Egmont Foundation funded me is that I am a dyslexic, and the money has been necessary for my work.

Finally, thank you to Ailish Schutz in California for believing in the Bodynamic System and in me personally, for your ongoing generosity, and for making available to me a quiet house where I was able to finish the book.

I am visually, aurally, and motorically dyslexic. It is thanks to my fantastic teacher, Mrs. Freil at the Oester Soegade Gymnasium, that I can write at all in a form that people can read. Because of my father's support and my own stubbornness I am now able to read Danish and also Swedish, Norwegian, English, and German, but my reading is considerably slower than that of nondyslexics. The writing process is also very irritating because my hand is not able to write at the pace of my thinking—and writing on a computer is even slower. My first stage is pen on paper; then I get people to help me make a fair copy on the computer and to develop it from there through the phases that a nondyslexic person would be able to do alone and with considerably more ease. So I want to dedicate this book to all dyslexics and especially to my daughter, Ditte, and one of my grandchildren, Haddi, who are both dyslexics. It is possible if you are persistent enough, able to ask for help and support, and able to receive it when it is offered to you.

So, once again, thank you for all the help and support offered.

Lisbeth Marcher
December 2009

The anatomy, the muscles, and all the elements in the Bodynamic System are always inspiring for me to deal with, and they hold my greatest interest. So of course I wanted to contribute to gathering the essential elements of a book. Lisbeth Marcher and I have worked together in writing other manuals for education. Our professional partnership has always been of great inspiration for me, and we complement each other with our different resources and knowledge in a constructive way. The writing has been an ongoing process through several years, and it has been a challenge to take part in the process of formulating and updating the material. At the same time I have learned a lot both professionally and personally, for which I am very thankful. It is with great pleasure and contentment that we have succeeded in this project.

We have expressed thanks to several people in Lisbeth Marcher's preface. I am very grateful to all these people. Personally I would very much like to thank my close friend and colleague Ellen Ollars, for having been by my side, giving inspiration and support through all the years, and for her willingness to be a sparring partner for me through the whole process—sparring that I appreciate very much. Helle Waehrens, for her perseverance and for good cooperation in the process of translating from Danish to English and vice versa. My family and my circle of friends, for their interest, care, and support. My son, Mogens Fich, for his patient computer assistance, and for being available when I needed it. My husband, Niels Thorball, who died in March 2004, for his natural support of my interest in Bodynamic issues. My close friend and colleague

Lennart Ollars, who died in September 2004, for his engagement and support in the birth of this book. My colleague Erik Jarlnaes, for his interest and support in finishing the book.

Sonja Fich
December 2009

SECTION 1

Introduction to the Bodynamic System

Definitions in the Bodynamic System

We would like to explain why we have chosen specific concepts and how we define them.

Mutual Connection

We define Mutual Connection as the very close relationship that occurs between two or more people; it also requires that each person maintain individuality within that relationship. In a relationship based on Mutual Connection, the partners come forth with their experiences and emotions verbally and/or nonverbally. Their exchanges include their differences of experience and emotion; they grasp and accept those differences; and they rise together to a new level where each person has acquired new knowledge about themselves and about the other. Besides molding new learning for all the individuals involved, Mutual Connection spreads out like concentric waves in water as the people involved pass the new learning on to others in new contacts, etc.

Mutual Connection also exists on a more global level: there is a deep innate knowledge of how all life on earth is in an interaction process with every other, and in spite of differences, like that between a mosquito and an elephant, all forms of life depend on that coexistence, which offers an experience of the global interaction with the all.

The spiritual part of Mutual Connection is close to this description but also involves interaction with the collective unconscious and with what we call individual soul energy—life energy and the Higher Me.

Dignity

We use the term *Dignity* to describe a person's inner sensation and feeling that she is able to own her inner values and deep ethics, respecting them and living according to them. Dignity also involves authentic acceptance of certain commitments, actions, and rights.

In the Danish language dictionary it describes Dignity with a quotation about the thinking of Immanuel Kant (1724-1804): "It is not what we think but what we are within ourselves that gives us true human dignity" (Krarup 1906, 9). Dignity implies that a person is authentic. Dignity usually drives a person toward self-development. Dignity provides the urge for self-acknowledgement and self-development, which arise in our relationships and interactions with others.

The Ego

In spite of our connectedness to the cultural-historical school of psychology's theory of development, founded by the Soviet psychologists, we have chosen to use the word *Ego,* Greek for "I" and therefore not the exclusive province of Freud, Jung, or anyone else. We chose *Ego* over *I* because the latter is very seldom used in English psychology. We didn't choose the word *Self* because in our experience it is often used in a way that is too vague and lacks a clear limit in relation to the Higher Self, and it may be confused with the concept of an inner core of some kind of soul-energy. Teaching in English in the United States, we have experienced that the effect of the word *Ego* is just as powerful in the coding systems as *Jeg* ("I") in Scandinavia.

The Ego consists of a combination of Character Structure and Ego Functions.

The Me

The Me is the part of the person that is activated in survival situations, where actions need to happen quicker than the Ego is capable of in order for the person to survive, for the species to survive, or for the person to be able to manage a high intensity of energy. The actions of the Me are driven by instincts, reflex systems, automatic skills and knowledge, plus genetic knowledge, as well as by combinations of two or more automatic skills that do not involve any thoughts. This means that you can create new skills without thinking (also see M. H. Brantbjerg et al. 2006).

A Definition in Terms of Libet's Half-second Delay

Benjamin Libet was the first to examine and describe the 0.55-second delay that occurs between an impulse to action and the conscious action that results from the impulse. Libet argues that "Consciousness can not start an action, but it can decide that the action shall not be realized," since "awareness of the conscious will to perform the act appears only 0.15-0.2 sec before the act" (Norretranders 1999, 231-250).

James Clark Maxwell examines Libet's theory in the same book (Norretranders 1999, 251-278). Maxwell believes that there is a higher instance, which he calls the Me, that our organism activates when decisions have to be made and executed so fast that there is no time to use the Ego with its delays; and that this Me is beyond the Ego.

In the Bodynamic System we believe in this theory, and we have registered how a person, especially in a situation of shock, stress, or peak experience, acts so rapidly and competently that we often hear our clients say, "I didn't know that I could do this."

We know that in situations of shock, stress, and peak experience the "normal" thinking processes of the Ego are cancelled out by neurological factors and functions, and later by other substances such as excessive production of stress hormones, and possibly by other factors. We also know from our practical work that it is most difficult to make the Ego accept that there is a higher instance beyond the Ego itself.

The Higher Me

The Higher Me is the part of the person that takes over when the Me cannot contain it or act any more. Certain authors have described that process as "dissociation" while others say that the person "goes out of the body." The important part is that this state of being offers new information from the collective unconscious and from other levels of consciousness that are more spiritual.

This state of being can allow the Me a brief rest—an island of calm in the midst of intense stress—and thereby offer new knowledge and new power, making the overall experience what we usually call "spiritual." Spirituality is deeply connected to the body as long as we are alive.

Codes and Coding

In the Bodynamic System we talk of Open Codes, Closed Codes, and Unexplored Codes. These types of codes are formed during childhood. Coding systems are shaped by the interactions and relationships between the child and adults, and between the child and other children.

Open Codes

Open Codes are formed when a child from an age-relevant theme is met by the parents or other significant individuals in a way that offers optimal contact and communication. That way the child can receive and integrate the challenge, support, matching, and guidance that make it possible to learn the theme. As a result the child attains a new level of development from which he or she can continue the experimentation in the same contact or in new ones. Simply put, Open Codes build solid foundations for contact and for higher levels of development.

Closed Codes

Closed Codes are formed when a child from an age-relevant theme is met by the parents (or other significant individuals) in nonoptimal contact. The child shuts down the interest to further explore the potential of the situation and thus arrests any further exploration to a higher level of learning and development. Simply put, Closed Codes build weaker foundations for contact and for higher levels of development.

Unexplored Codes

In a person's life, these are potentials that have remained latent because they were not the focus of any contact situation, and therefore were neither learned optimally (as in the Open Codes) nor arrested (as in the Closed Codes). Any of them could be either learned or arrested in the future, for example fishing, being around animals, having philosophical discussions, and so on.

Imprints

We form a kind of coding system in both the Me and the Higher Me, but the codes formed at those levels involve huge amounts of stress hormones. To access those codes we need to create a setting of similar intense energy. Because those high-energy codes emerge in a different way than developmental codes, and because we have to access them in a different way, we call them Imprints to distinguish them from more ordinary developmental codes.

Hyperresponsive Muscles

When we pull a muscle with our fingers in the direction of its fibers—as we do in Bodymapping—and the muscle responds with involuntary recoil force that is faster and stronger than the initial pull, we say that the muscle is hyperresponsive.

To the palpating hand, a hyperresponsive muscle will feel like a tight elastic band that reacts strongly against being stretched. The force and speed of recoil will be greater than the force and speed applied while stretching the muscle. In regular motor function, hyperresponsive muscles will hold back the psychomotor content, in effect arresting its expression.

Hyporesponsive Muscles

When we pull a muscle with our fingers in the direction of its fibers—as we do in Bodymapping—and the muscle responds with involuntary withdrawal or pullback that is weaker and slower than the pull we exerted, we say that the muscle is hyporesponsive.

To the palpating hand, a hyporesponsive muscle will feel like an elastic band that has gone limp so that when stretched it does not recoil all the way. The force, speed, and distance of recoil will be less than those the hand applied while stretching the muscle. In regular motor function, hyporesponsive muscles resign or withdraw from the psychological impulse, so that in effect its expression fades away and disappears.

Tenseness

We use the word *Tenseness* to describe a muscle that seems to be contracted although the person is not contracting it voluntarily.

Tenseness Systems

The hyperresponse or hyporesponse of the muscles can be observed in a person as Tenseness Systems, comprising arrays of muscles in various parts of the body that remain tense even after a person has voluntarily relaxed her body.*

Character

In the original Greek sense of the word, *Character* is the mark we leave when we scratch or stamp an object like a coin or pottery so that we can distinguish it from other similar objects. It becomes a Coding of a certain structure—and this is exactly what we are dealing with. In more recent times the term *Character* has been employed to describe personal peculiarities, the qualities that characterize a certain person. Likewise, psychomotor material becomes encoded in the brain and takes root in the muscles, so specific psychological behavior patterns develop into specific bodily features and structures and particular life patterns, and vice versa.

Character Structure

We are fully aware that the terms *Character* and *Character Structure* have been used in different psychological systems, which have often implied that character and its structures are fixed and unchangeable. Assuming the risk of being compared with those other systems, we have dared to go back to the original meaning of the word and use it as such.

We define Character Structures as sets of coding experienced by the person at specific age levels and stored in the brain, forming specific behavior patterns, norms, and mind sets. Character Structure coding is embodied in the muscles in a way that allows us to observe if the codes are closed or open.

The Bodynamic System considers that all coding and imprints can be changed through the many different impactful situations that a human being is exposed to. We change involuntarily, often without thinking about it. It happens every day and is connected to the support and challenges we meet through contact with colleagues, friends, partners, children, and so on. Change can also occur through other more structured processes aimed at personal development, such as psychotherapy.

Ego Function

This concept encompasses life themes that run vertically through our age levels. It covers learned functions that the Ego can use, coded in through socialization processes and colored by the different Character Structures.

*Personal communication with the well-known Danish pediatric psychiatrist Axel Arnfred, 1990.

Ego Formation through the Coding Elements

The Bodynamic System is founded on a uniform understanding of human development, psychomotor function, and body sensing or proprioception. This understanding is applied in adult psychotherapy, and also as a means to support development during childhood.

We believe that human beings are characterized by an innate urge for development, and that the Ego is formed by processes arising from that urge, along with a constant subtle movement and balance between two fundamental principles that we call Mutual Connection and Dignity. We believe that it is by means of contact in relationships and interactions with others that we develop our uniqueness. We also believe that this contact has to be of such quality that both individuals and everyone involved are giving something of themselves into the contact and gaining something from the contact. This is illustrated very well in these verses:

> *In a real sense all life is interrelated.*
> *All men are caught in an inescapable network*
> *Of mutuality, tied in a single garment of destiny.*
> *Whatever affects one directly affects all indirectly.*
> *I can never be what I ought to be*
> *Until you are what you ought to be,*
> *And you can never be what you ought to be*
> *Until I am what I ought to be.*
> *This is the interrelated structure of reality.**

We believe that the processes that form the human personality start before birth and continue throughout life. As the child grows to adolescence, each age level represents a window during which the child explores and learns new cognitive, affective, and behavioral codes—Coding Systems—that are particular to that age and often unique to it. Lev Vygotsky (1978) described a similar principle, which he called "nearest proximal zone for development"; he did not describe any connection to the body, however.

The process of motor development take place at the same time. At each age level the child integrates new muscles or parts of muscles into her voluntary motor function, which is how she develops the new patterns of movement that are appropriate

*Martin Luther King Jr., Detroit, 1961.

to that age. This correlation of psychological and motor function implies that, in effect, the Coding Systems that comprise psychological development are actually rooted in the body.

We believe that it is through relationships and interaction with others that we develop our Ego. Every time we try something new, structures are developed in the brain that become Codings after we have tried them many times. In Codings we integrate the whole situation and not just elements of it. Coding happens in contact with other individuals, and it forms within the child a basic knowledge of "who I am," "how I feel," "how I'm going to act," and more knowledge about "the other" and the actions of the other. In this way we can hypothesize that learning about who or how the Ego is happens through experiencing the Ego in interactions. Some Codings are created when the child is by him or herself and in contact with gravity and new movements or in new activities, such as painting or playing.

This understanding compares to a concept proposed by Maja Lisina (1989, 27-28), who wrote that "the development of the Ego-image and imaginings about other people depend to the utmost degree on the character, which the communication with other people had. . . ." This led to new research on "interrelations (friendship, love, popularity), the Ego-image (the social reflection), and the image of other people (the social perception), and thus so to speak was a specific product of the communication."

Bodynamic perceives the Ego-image as our Ego-formation.

Codes and Coding

In the Bodynamic System we talk of Open Codes, Closed Codes, and Unexplored Codes. These types of codes are formed during childhood, their coding patterns shaped by the interactions and relationships between the child and adults, and the child and other children. See the definitions in the previous section.

Coding involves eight elements, which appear in the diagram below. These elements apply equally to Open Codes, Closed Codes, and Unexplored Codes, though they don't necessarily occur in any specific sequence or order. Any given Context may apply more or less of these elements, and the way they are involved in the coding process may be different.

The Coding System exists in an ambience that we call Context. Context may be understood as the basic frame of mind of the person in general and the developing child in particular (the subject); at the same time Context is also the basic frame of mind of the person that the child is communicating with (from the child's point of view, the object). Most likely, Context also includes all elements of the space where the interaction is taking place (a classroom, a living room, etc.) and also factors such as the time of day, the weather, and so on.

Context is central in the coding interaction scheme and impacts all the other elements, as described in the following paragraphs. Context is also an individual's former experience, which together with the actual situation impacts all the elements. These elements are also described in the following paragraphs.

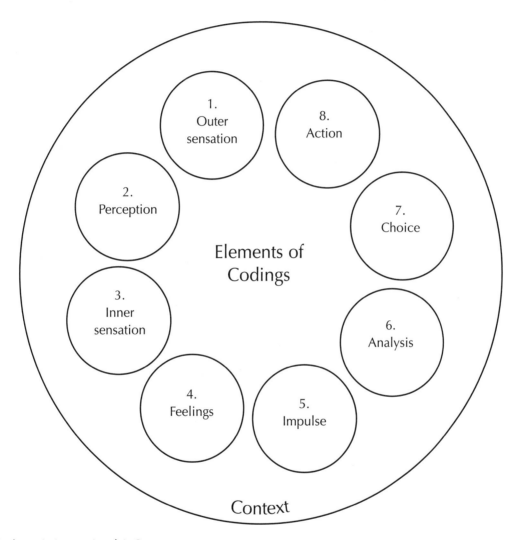

© Bodynamic International ApS

Elements of Coding

1. Outer Sensations and Outer Facts (Exteroception)

This element encompasses all the information we receive from our surroundings by means of our physical senses: *vision, hearing, smell (olfaction), taste,* and *touch* (through the skin: pressure, pain, cold, heat, body hair receptor sensing, tickling, and so on). The outer sensations may also include a sixth sense: receptors that are sensitive to electromagnetic current and can distinguish different grades of frequency, tension (voltage), and intensity.

2. Perception and Interpretation of Facts

After the sensory input is received by our outer senses, its signals are processed in the nervous system in ways that create meaning and structure from the outer events, in our case from being together with another person. The words our culture uses to describe this element are: *experience, interpret, think, believe, understand,* and *meaning,* among others. Sometimes we use words from another element, such as *I see, I hear* (element 1), *I feel* (emotion, element 4), or *inner sensation* (element 3), but such use of other elements dilutes the clarity of the perception and/or interpretation and sets the scene for the beginning of a Closed Code.

3. Inner Sensations and Body Sensing (Interoception and Proprioception)

Our nervous system and muscles carry out our movements without our conscious participation, and they also register sensations unconsciously—although it is possible to do so consciously. Part of the challenge is thus to find words that describe all of these often unconscious modalities of body sensing, and also to have a relatively clear idea where in the body the sensations are located. Some of the words our culture uses to describe this element are: *tension, pressure, hot, cold, movement, vibration,* and *pain,* as well as *stretch, heartbeat, breathing, pulse, streaming, flow, position of the body,* and other words that differentiate the finer aspects of our inner sensing.

There are different inner sensation systems (Gjesing 2004; Jacobsen 2005):

- Limb position and movement, which covers the muscle and joint sensation/proprioception, is a sense that registers and adjusts unconsciously (though it is possible to do it consciously) the interrelated positions of the limbs in relation to gravity and the contraction or extension of muscles and joints.
- Kinesthetic sense—equilibrium and balance—is a kind of movement thinking that consciously registers positions and movements in and with the body.

This is a combination of the touch/feeling sense (outer sensation) and the muscle and joint sense (inner sensation).

- Gravitational and accelerational forces sense gives information about the position of the head in relation to gravity and also gives information about direction and speed.

4. Feelings

The Bodynamic System distinguishes three different layers of affective function, which we call Instincts, Emotions, and Sentiments. These three layers correspond largely to the three brain layers identified by neuroscience. In our scheme:

- Instincts arise in the brain stem (the reptilian brain),
- Emotions arise and are processed in the limbic system of the mesencephalon (the mammalian brain), and
- Sentiments are processed in the part of the brain that is uniquely human, the frontal cortex or telencephalon.

Instincts

Properly speaking, this layer would be called Instinctual Affect, the feelings of reptiles caught in life-or-death situations where survival of the individual or survival of the species becomes an all-consuming compulsion. Instinctual Affect is immediate, very direct, and very powerful, and it is acted out through the Me (see the definitions in the previous section). In our culture we may think that human beings don't really need this layer, but in conditions of great stress such as war, natural disasters, and physical attacks, our organism activates Instinctual Affect to help us survive.

Words that indicate instincts include *rage, mating, lust, angst, calm,* and *dread,* among others.

Emotions (Basic Emotions)

These arise in the limbic system, and we have them in common with mammals that live their lives in groups. The emotions are a layer of affective skill necessary for handling relationships and social structure in the animal group. Research has demonstrated that specific emotions, listed below, are closely correlated to specific levels of various hormones and neurotransmitters in the blood and organs. For that reason, emotions can be detected by special blood tests, and a sensitive nose can detect different emotions.

The Bodynamic System distinguishes seven Basic Emotions, the same that are largely acknowledged by research and psychological theory in general: *anger, fear, sorrow, joy, sensual/sexual desire, disgust,* and *shame.* Basic Emotions present the advantage that they are clearly defined, so a Basic Emotion can't be mistaken for anything else. They are very clear when they appear one at a time, but they may also appear in combinations that we call mixed emotions. Having differentiated and defined the Basic Emotions, we can detect to what extent each one is present in a complex emotional situation.

Sentiments

In Bodynamic we define Sentiments as less direct and more complicated than the Basic Emotions. Sentiments arise from cognitive processing of Basic Emotions; this processing takes the stuff of Basic Emotions and adds cognitive elements such as fantasy, imagination, opinion, belief, symbol, justification, denial, etc. Sentiments can also describe states, for example, feeling unworthy, feeling disillusioned.

Words that indicate Sentiments include *frustrated, nervous, provoked, reluctant, worried, delighted, excited, butterflies in the stomach, weak in the knees, attracted, and shy,* among others. All these expressions have a story to tell that goes beyond the affect itself. Because Sentiments are less direct and less straightforward than Emotions, when we try to describe them it often happens that different people perceive them differently.

5. Impulses

We define Impulses as the start of a behavior of action that spontaneously arises in the interaction with others. The Impulse is a reaction to the stimuli we receive from our inner sensations and emotions, and/or it is an answer from the meaning (perception) that we create from the outer sensation. Phrases that indicate Impulses include *"I want to get closer," "I want to get away," "I need," "I desire," "I wish," "I will have," "I want to be good at,"* and *"I would like to."*

6. Analysis

Here the person analyzes the overall situation in terms of cause and effect. People usually think of analysis as a rational procedure, but that would isolate the cognitive function, which in fact is not the case in real life. A large part of analysis occurs at the gut level because our sensations and our emotions (our kinesthetic and affective intelligence) are able to process information much faster than the mind.

Analysis is necessary when there are competing impulses that might drive the person to inconsistent or contradictory behaviors. What makes the difference in Analysis is that the person takes a step back from the situation to line up and observe different choices and to produce an overview of different consequences. Phrases that indicate analysis are *"When this happens, what then?,"* and *"What would be the consequences?"*

7. Choice

Consciously, preconsciously, or unconsciously we take positions in relation to the possible actions indicated in Analysis, and then we actively choose our preferred option while also excluding other choices in the present. Phrases such as *"I prefer this," "I don't want that one; this one," "OK, I'm ready to choose that one,"* as well as *"Give me that," "It is a good idea to do that,"* and *"I don't want to do that"* are indicative of choices—although some of these do not illustrate clear-cut choices.

8. Action

Action is the result of a long process that has preceded it. The other person (object) did or said something, and the subject is now responding to it. The interaction may be verbal or nonverbal. After a choice has been made, it needs to be followed by action—otherwise nothing happens.

Another possibility of action is inaction. It often happens that in choosing not to act or not to express something, the subject is in fact making a definite decision that can be viewed as the person's choice of an alternative course of action.

Integration

We need to visualize that the brain perceives all these elements as a pattern of wholeness, and that by doing so the brain is creating a structure, the Coding. In situations that involve human interaction, all these elements are active in the interaction with others, and they are more or less active in all individuals involved in the interaction.

Examples of Formation of Coding

Two examples illustrate how to use the Coding Model and the concepts of Open Code and Closed Code.

Example 1: Maria

This is an example from daily life, where Lisbeth Marcher was present.

Lisbeth is visiting friends. Lisbeth and the mother are sitting in the kitchen, which has doors that open both to the living room and to the hall, and between the hall and the living room. This layout allows the daughter, Maria, to run around, her favorite game for now. She is three years old, and she has just learned to run around corners. Her father play-runs after her, and the whole situation is full of energy. Maria laughs; she doesn't want to get caught, and she is very joyful. There is a joyful and light atmosphere in the room. All this is part of the Context for the following.

Suddenly Maria slips on the floor, falls, and hurts herself. The parents comfort her without exaggerating, kiss her leg to make it well, and apply a small bandage on a minor abrasion. Then the father takes her along to find out why she had fallen. They discover that she had actually slipped on water that was spilled on the floor. Holding her father's hand for support, Maria tries out what it is like to slip. Together they mop up the water, Maria senses that the danger of slipping has gone, and they start play-running again.

Many elements of the Coding Model are active in this example. We'll focus on the Coding that took place in the first part of the play-running. Maria is running around. She has done this before, and her running is an Open Coding situation since it allows Maria to explore actively and to move on to a higher level of learning. That way, the Open Coding is actually reinforced. Maria is now running faster, closer to the corners, and she has her father running after her. She has made a lot of progress since a few days ago, when she needed to hold hands with her father in order to feel safe while running. All this means that her cortex keeps receiving and processing new Open Coding: the light, easy, joyful atmosphere among those present, everybody's interest in her, and her mastering the running around corners.

In this context Maria is practicing the Ego Function called Social Balance and the subfunctions (b) degree of pulling oneself together/letting go, (c) degree of "facade" and maintaining one's front (mastering the form and rules of the game), (d) balancing a sense of personal identity against being a group member, and (e) managing stress in exciting situations. The situation enables her to try and to succeed at running closer to the corners, mastering the Ego Function called Social Balance, and in that way developing a new Open Coding.

Using the Coding Elements

What we would like to present next is Lisbeth's interpretation of the same situation—her perception is based on experience—using Coding Elements 1 through 8, which can follow one another at random.

1. Outer sensations: Maria *hears* her father's voice saying "now I'm coming after you" along with his steps, and she notices that we are all smiling.
2. Perception: Maria *perceives* it as a fun game.
3. Inner sensation: Maria *senses* her feet on the floor and the muscles she uses from this age level (2-4 years, the Will Character Structure), muscles used to maintain balance, both physical and psychological—(42) peroneus longus; (44a) sartorius, proximal part; (23) iliotibial tract, 2nd part; and (5) teres major.
4. Feelings: She *feels* delight, joy, and excitement.
5. Impulse: Her *impulse* is to run faster.
6. Analysis: She *analyzes: There are no problems; I can do this and still be safe.*
7. Choice: She *chooses* to run faster and to make sharper turns.
8. Action: She puts her choice into *action.*

All of these Coding Elements constitute a whole that forms the Open Coding. This means that Maria has reached a stage of competence where she can run fast around corners while feeling delighted, joyful, and excited—a stage that enables her to develop even further. At the same time the atmosphere in the group is well-balanced, and she is in contact with everybody in the group. This level of competence gives her an opportunity for further development.

And Then Comes the Fall

Here the experience could have turned into a Closed Code, but we'll describe how an Open Code was developed.

The Fall—Open Code

Maria falls, but she is met at once by her father and the rest of us with the message "Oops; things like this can happen." These are not the precise words we use, but it is the intent in what we say and do. Then Maria and her father go together to explore why she fell. They find the water on the floor. Maria experiments with the water, and she actually slips on purpose to get a good physical sense of what it is like to slip on water—holding on to her father's hand for safety, "so it is not the muscles, me, or the game that is to blame." Maria and her father mop up the water together. Then Maria is able to sense that she can once again have a firm foothold, and the impulse to continue the running game reappears. In this case it is possible to imagine the formation of the following Open Code: "It is OK to fail, to be comforted, to get help to find out what the problem was, to solve it, and to go on with further experiments—while the contact is still intact, intense, and alive."

The Situation Described through the Coding Elements

1. Outer sensation: *seeing* her father running after her and *hearing* his steps
3. Inner sensation of the *sense of balance* and that the muscles cannot "hold" her, *sensing* herself slipping
3. Inner sensation: *sensing* the pain
2. Perception: *It may be dangerous to run so fast that I slip.*
4. Feelings: *feeling* sad and afraid,
5. Impulse: and *wanting* to make it go away.
5. Impulse: *I could stop playing the game.*
6. Analysis: *I could get help.*
1. Outer sensation: *seeing*
3. Inner sensation: and *sensing* her Dad helping her up
4. Feelings: *experiencing* joy,
7. Choice, and 8. Action: *receiving* and taking in help,
8. Action: and then going out together with Dad to explore the problem,
8. Action: find the water,
3. Inner sensation: e.g., the *sensation* of balance and the muscles
8. Perception: *perceive* what it is like to slip,
8. Action: and to mop up the water,
1. Outer sensation: and *see* how it disappears,
3. Inner sensation: e.g., the involved muscles: *sense* that she has a firm foothold,
2. Perception and 7. Choice: so the game may continue.

All these elements make up a whole that forms an Open Coding: "She can run, fall, and get help in figuring out why she fell, so that she can continue the game of running fast around corners feeling delighted"—in effect leading Maria to a new stage of competence that allows her to develop even further. The Open Code immediately gave Maria the desire to continue the game, and her father got the message and participates in the game.

Often more Ego Functions are involved in such a situation, but we have chosen to describe only Social Balance for the sake of clarity.

The Fall—Closed Code

Here we will see how the fall could have produced a Closed Code. Let's go back to the situation when Maria falls and imagine this course of events: Maria's mother gets very scared, hurries over, picks up Maria, makes a grand display of pity, tells her how dangerous it is to run around corners, and then scolds the father for playing such irresponsible games. Then they go to the kitchen, where the mother starts reading a book to Maria while the father disappears with the dog. By doing so, the mother has focused on the pain. She tells Maria that running around corners is dangerous, and the message becomes even more serious because mother's voice and manner show great fear (in voice and manner). She blames the father rather than the water on the floor.

This scenario will make Maria form a Closed Code: "Play-running around corners is dangerous, and the joy disappears; dad causes pain (the pain from the fall), so dad is a fool; mom is afraid, and Maria is afraid. Sitting still and listening to a story is safe, so mom saved me."

1. Inner sensation: the muscles cannot "hold" her–(42a) peroneus longus, (44a) sartorius, proximal part, (23) iliotibial tract, 2nd part, (5) teres major; she falls (sense of balance) and feels the pain at the fall on the floor
3. Outer sensation: the mother's voice is shrill, and Maria also sees other body signals from her mother
2. Perception: *Mom is afraid.*
4. Feelings: Maria is scared and becomes afraid
1. Outer sensation: *Mom says running around corners is dangerous.*
2. Perception: *To run fast and play-running is dangerous.*
1. Outer sensation: *Mom says that Dad is to blame.*
2. Perception: *Dad is a fool; he hurt me* (here the perception is mixed with the inner sensation of the pain from the fall).
5. Impulse: to get away from the play-run with Dad
6. Analysis: *It is better to be quiet and still (it does not hurt).*
7. Choice: to do something quiet
8. Action: to sit still and quiet in the kitchen and listen to a story with Mom.

All these elements form a whole, and in this case a Closed Code, which prevents Maria from reaching a new level of competence in running around corners while she is in contact with the group and in balance with her own joy and the good atmosphere in the group. Maria has stopped the game, Mom is angry with Dad, Dad has left with the dog, so the good balance in the family (group) has disappeared.

If a similar situation is repeated several times, it may have the effect that Maria later will not enjoy running fast and especially not around corners. At the same time she'll probably experience that if she is too fast, she loses contact, or she'll give up what is good for her in order to maintain contact.

Here is an interesting twist: Maria has indirectly learned by the fall that sitting quietly and reading a book is safe and it provides safe contact with her mother, so Maria may turn into one of those children who prefers to sit at home instead of using her body in a powerful way. This may continue into her adulthood. Reading, sitting quietly, and being in contact with her mother is an Open Code that involves other muscles, and it is a resource even though it is based on a Closed Code.

Example 2: Susan

This is an example from Lisbeth Marcher's therapy practice with an adult client.

Susan came to me when she was in her thirties. Her complaints were that she was afraid and she had pain in one leg. She had just rented a new "dream apartment," but she could not bring herself to move there, which she further described by saying "It's like I can't get out the door." I asked her if her leg had hurt before, but she could not remember anything of that sort. Then I encouraged her to describe the pain in her leg, where it was localized, and how painful it was—on a scale from one to ten. With this research she experienced that the pain was on the back side of her right thigh and got worse when she activated biceps femoris and semitendinosus (the back of the right thigh). I now had her walk through the door to the therapy room and at the same time activate the muscles of the back of her thigh. When she did so, she suddenly recalled a fall she had had when she was three years old.

Susan's childhood experience as she narrated it—the facts: Susan was playing by herself, running back and forth in the rooms of the new apartment that the family had just moved into. While running through the door leading to the hall, she stumbled, fell down, and hurt herself. She experienced a lot of pain in her leg, was carried to the kitchen, sat down at the table, and started drawing—it was safe, and she experienced nearly no pain. Her parents were busy in the new apartment, and to them it looked as if Susan was "cozy and OK" in the kitchen, so they let go of the contact. Susan remained silent, the parents forgot about the fall, and only on the third day did they realize that something was really wrong. They took Susan to the hospital and found out that one of the bones in her leg had been fractured.

So the process was: Susan ran through the door, the surroundings were new, she fell and broke her leg, she didn't get enough contact, and the fracture was not noticed. Susan's words for her experience: to move and walk through a door will produce pain in the leg as well as no contact, keeping silent, and losing self-worth. This description is a conclusion of the perceptual or the analyzed part of the Coding.

In the therapy session I stayed in contact with Susan and said, "Somebody should have been there—somebody that had enough time to look at you and understand that your leg was broken." Then I helped Susan through all the elements in the Coding System that had formed a Closed Code at that time:

0. Context: the sensation of excitement of something new, new rooms, new apartment
1. Outer sensation: focus on the door and the corridor on the other side
2. Perception: *Going through the door means falling, pain, and danger.*
3. Inner sensation: sensation of moving forward from the back side of the leg—(24b) biceps femoris, long head, proximal part, deep; (25) semitendinosus, proximal part; (28a) gastrocnemius, lateral head, proximal part; (31) flexor hallucis longus. These muscles come into play in the Will Character Structure. At the same time they are involved in the Ego Function called Self-assertion

with the subfunctions (a) manifesting one's own power and (c) forward momentum and sense of direction.

4. Feelings: joy changing to sadness and becoming afraid
5. Impulse: to move away from new doors
2. Perception: *It is dangerous to move.*
5. Impulse: *It is better to stop moving.*
2. Perception: *I am not good at moving.*
6. Analysis: don't go through new doors
7. Choice: be quiet and paint

In therapy we try to form new Open Codes. This means that I stayed in contact with Susan in the therapy session and questioned her about the different Coding Elements. The first thing we did was to work with the first three elements:

1. Outer sensation: Susan *hears* my voice and *sees* my body position.
2. Perception: she *perceives* that I am open.
3. Inner sensation: at the same time she *senses* and uses the muscles of the back side of the leg that have to do with moving forward through the door.

We did this together several times, had fun, and stayed in contact, and then Susan said:

2. Perception: *It is not dangerous to go through a door.*
4. Feelings: *It is almost amusing.*

In this way a new Coding was formed and new resources were created.

At that point another issue emerged: "When you move house, you are left alone." We talked about it a little, and I suggested that she could invite a friend or friends to be there with her on the day she moved, and we discussed who those friends might be. Back in the therapy setting, I arranged with one of my colleagues for him to stay outside in the corridor, and that he would make contact with Susan when she walked out through the door. Again I asked her to leave the therapy room and at the same time sense and use the muscles on the back side of her leg, then close the door, stay outside for a minute, and come back. When she closed the door she realized that she was not alone and got contact from my colleague. In this way a new Open Coding was created: "Susan can leave the room, close the door, and she will not be left alone." The session ended with her phoning and arranging that two of her friends would be there for her during the actual move.

Susan came to see me twice after her successful move. Her friends had been there, so she was not alone. She came to finish the therapy and also to find out what was still missing. The pain in her leg had gone after the first therapy session. The last part of therapy was for her to learn to reach out for help and to be able to sense and understand the importance of contact in new situations.

To create new resources, or more to the point, to form new Open Codes, is the way we prefer to work in the Bodynamic System. We decipher and melt away the Closed Codes in order to make space for new resources. We saw one example in Susan's therapy when she walked through the door, sensing and activating the back side of her leg, having fun, and making contact. At the start of therapy the old Closed Code was buried deep in the preconscious, its facts totally forgotten except for their disturbing effect on Susan's life. Then the precise questioning with much focus on bodily sensations and movements charged the old Code with so much energy that it gradually emerged into consciousness. Once the old Code was remembered, it could also be changed.

Healing happens by means of contact, empathy, and understanding or insight; by creating new resources, in this case going out through the door and experiencing that she was not alone; and by means of doing the movements and experiencing the contact that changes the perception, all the while remembering to focus on all Coding Elements at a pace that suits the process.

Susan relaxed, and she experienced that it was not dangerous to go through the door. She was not afraid, and her leg stopped hurting. Later in her therapy:

6. Analysis: "To move to a new apartment is the same as being alone."

This changed to: "To go through a door (in the therapy room) to a new hall, you make contact, and it is amusing (you are not left alone)." And later, "To have friends in her new apartment when she moved gave her contact and safety."

The consequence was that Susan could suddenly visit new customers and new restaurants without her heart pounding, which she had accepted as a natural experience in these situations. Susan also learned to ask for contact when she needed it, and she could feel and sense that it was possible, not every time and not always right away, but it was a basic possibility. It is possible for her to ask for contact and to get the contact without losing her dignity in moving forward with full power in the direction of her choice.

When we do therapy this way, we allow the client to experience both Mutual Connection and Dignity—the two core principles in the Bodynamic System. Part of the incredible experience of doing such therapy is that the quality of contact that changes the client also changes the therapist, the therapist's colleague, and Susan's family and friends, because Susan brings something new into their relationships. This makes me think of a quote by Maja Lisina, psychologist and psychiatrist, who in my mind has expanded our understanding of relationships in the direction of wholeness:

> Communication processes (also meaning processes of being together) are social processes, and therefore they can not be reduced just to being contact between two or more individuals. Expressed figuratively, people in communication situations do not act like Adam and Eve, which means not as if they were the only people in the universe.
>
> When two human beings establish contact, they are both linked to the rest of humanity with thousands of invisible threads. (Lisina 1989)

Using This Book

Initially it was thought that *Body Encyclopedia* would be a scholarly book for body-psychotherapists training in the Bodynamic System and for other kinds of body-psychotherapists, but it is also useful for all psychotherapists interested in including the signals of the body in the therapeutic process.

It may also be useful as a manual for physiotherapists, chiropractors, sports coaches, rolfers, masseurs, and others who are interested in understanding the psychological patterns connected to the physical body. In fact, it may be used by anyone who is interested in knowing more about the connection between body and mind.

In using this book, you will gain knowledge of many of the muscles in the body and find suggestions for working with issues that are connected to the muscle in question—suggestions that may be used in psychotherapeutic work, self-development, and for those who are simply personally curious.

An example: after jogging, the muscles close to your shinbone hurt. One of the muscles in this area is (39) tibialis anterior. Curiosity about your discomfort could be a reason for looking up this muscle in the book. Under "Child's Developmental Stage/Age" it says that this muscle takes part in the bouncing movements in the ankle and foot. Discovering this, you may decide to change your training by including exercises to improve elasticity in your foot and ankle joints, or you may decide that better running shoes are necessary.

You might follow your curiosity into another direction and enjoy reading about the three Character Structures that include (39) tibialis anterior—Autonomy, Will, and Opinions. Or you may be interested in discovering the psychological functions of its Ego Function. For instance with the Ego Function Grounding and Reality Testing and the subfunction (b) relationship between reality and fantasy/imagination, associated with the Character Structure Opinions, you will read, "testing one's imagination and thoughts." You might be led to consider whether to test or check out your own imaginings and thoughts when interacting with others, or whether you just "know" that your imaginings/fantasies are correct. As you continue to read about the Character Structure Opinions, you recognize how some of the issues from this Character Structure show up in your daily life. By choosing to look at them, you could reflect on ways to make changes, if you want to.

Let's look at another example. The text states that people holding the Late position of Opinions are "very persistent in one's opinions." Two muscles in the hand that become active at this stage/age, (83) opponens digiti minimi and (80) opponens pollicis, are muscles the child uses to grip the pen when writing. On the pages where these muscles are described, three Ego Functions are mentioned. One of them is the Ego Function Self-Assertion with the subfunction (a) self-assertion (manifesting one's power). Besides (83) opponens digiti minimi and (80) opponens pollicis, a third muscle, found under the nose, is listed, (*) depressor septi. The two muscles in the hand bring the thumb and the little finger together forming a hand gesture we often use in discussion. The muscle found under the nose is part of the facial expression we commonly use when snorting to emphasize our opinions.

When you read this description of the muscles, do you recognize anything? Is there something you'd like to examine further? The next time you are in a discussion, notice the muscles of your hand. Do they hold on/tighten up, or are they active in another way? On the other hand, if it is difficult to hold onto your opinions, try activating these muscles, making the movements while you are in a discussion, and notice whether it makes a difference. Find the muscles on your hand—feel them, use them— and discover what you sense and feel when doing so.

Exploring an Ego Function or subfunction may be to become aware from within yourself of the different muscles/areas of muscles in the body and at the same time "taste" how the resource of the Ego Function presents itself—is it recognizable, inactive, etc.?

In a similar way you can explore a Character Structure, and here it's possible to experience sensations and a feeling for the age in question. Sometimes it can be a powerful tool, and you may even find that you start to remember periods from your life story. With this in mind, we suggest that you be careful working with the muscles connected with shock because you might contact memories of traumatic episodes, become confused, or experience unpleasant body sensations.

As you see from these examples, it is possible to start your exploration from the muscles, the Character Structures, or the Ego Functions, and freely move back and forth between them. The numbers of the muscles may also be used to find your way in this book. There is an alphabetical list with numbers and pages at the end of the book.

The contents of this book—among other things, the issues indicated under "Psychological Function"—are not meant as a key nor a direction of action but as a source of inspiration that therapists may use for ideas to support their interaction with clients. Reading this book may provide an opportunity to sense and experience more about yourself, especially if you "play" with the child's movements that arise from the actions of the muscles you take an interest in, at the same time focusing on the psychological issues connected to those muscles.

It is our wish that *Body Encyclopedia* give the reader an understanding of the Bodynamic System and that it become as fruitful and inspiring a tool to professionals and interested others as it has been and still is to those of us who have contributed to creating the system and giving it the form in which it is now published.

Anatomical Terms

We use the internationally recognized *nomina anatomica* nomenclature used in *Gray's Anatomy, 39th Edition* (2005), as well as Erik Andreasen and F. Bojsen-Møller's *Bevægeapparatet, Anatomi I (The Anatomy of the Motion Apparatus/System), 8th Edition* (1988).

In the Bodynamic System we divide the muscles even further; we use the word *part* with a descriptive specification of direction, for example "superior part." The specifications of direction are according to the above texts.

Terms Used for Direction

Head, Neck, and Torso

cranial–caudal or superior–inferior = toward the cranium–toward the coccyx

ventral–dorsal or anterior–posterior = front side, toward the stomach–back side, toward the back

Arms and Legs

proximal–distal = toward the root of the arm or leg–away from the root toward the hand or foot

anterior–posterior = in front–behind

palmar–dorsal = toward the palm–toward the back of the hand

plantar–dorsal = toward the sole of the foot–toward the top of the foot

medial–lateral = toward the midline of the body–away from the midline of the body

Forearm and Hand

ulnar–radial = toward the little finger–toward the thumb

Lower Part of the Leg and Foot

tibial–fibular = toward the shin bone (tibia)–toward outside of the leg (fibula)

The Body as a Whole

superficial–profound = near the surface–deep

medial–lateral = toward the midline of the body–away from the midline of the body

Terms Used for Different Movements

flexion = bending
extension = stretching

rotation = turning, rotating
medial rotation = rotating toward the midline of the body
lateral rotation = rotating away from the midline of the body

abduction = moving away from the body
adduction = moving toward the body

pronation = turning the forearm/ankle so the palm/sole of foot turns toward
  the floor
supination = turning the forearm/ankle so the palm/the sole of the foot
  turns away from the floor

opposition = little finger and thumb are moved toward each other

Section 2

The Bodynamic Psycho-Motor Anatomy

Descriptions of Muscles and Connective Tissue

This section of the book begins with two images of the body, the front (anterior) and the back (posterior). In these drawings you can see how the different muscles are marked on the Bodymap. These marks are placed as close as possible to where the muscle is located in the body while allowing for ease of understanding the drawing.

The superficial muscles are indicated as lines. The deep muscles are indicated as dots. Where the lines cross each other, the diagonal lines indicate the superficial muscles and the straight lines are the deeper muscles. The muscles to be tested and marked on the Bodymap are numbered. This numbering is for identification only and has no relevance to understanding the content of this book. The muscles are described in the order that is most often used when testing for a Bodymap.

Some anatomical structures are not tested, in part because they are difficult or impossible to palpate; they have been included in the Bodynamic System, however, because they do impact both motion and psychology. They are placed on the diagram as close as possible to where they are found in the body. They do not have a number, and instead are indicated with an asterisk (*).

In the Bodynamic System, all of the muscles and anatomical structures, both tested and not tested, are included and described on the appropriate "Character Structures" and "Ego Functions" pages.

Contents of the Right-hand Pages

Every muscle and anatomical structure has its own page. At the top are the "Name," "Origin," and "Insertion." Latin names are used, and only the main attachments have been given. Then follows "Anatomical Function," where anatomical nomenclature is used to describe the movement (for example, *flexion* means "bend").

"Map" is a description of where the muscle is placed according to whether it is superficial or deep in relation to other muscles.

"Is contracted by" is a description of the movement that occurs when the muscle is activated. With movement the muscle is often easier to locate and feel.

"Map" and "Is contracted by" are described as simply as possible to make the book more readable and understandable. It may be a good idea also to consult an anatomical atlas and other material mentioned in the Bibliography, especially if the reader has little experience in anatomical studies.

The muscle is then included in the Bodynamic System's "Character Structure" and "Ego Function" (usually one or two). The Character Structure indicates when the muscle first becomes active. The Ego Function indicates the aspects of the ego that develop throughout life. More detailed information about the Character Structure System and the Ego Function System can be found in Sections 3 and 4. We have also described empirically tested hypotheses relating to psychological themes that are connected to the specific muscle—called "Psychological Function." The psychological ability starts developing at the same time as the child starts using the specific muscle voluntarily, and these abilities/potentials are available throughout our lives.

"Child's developmental stage/age" describes how the muscle takes part in the motor development at a particular stage or age, and for some muscles where it comes naturally we also mention some of the social and psychological issues connected to the stage of development.

"Bodymapping" describes how the muscle is tested and marked on a Bodymap.

The description of the client's and the tester's position is similar to the way our students are instructed. Of course the muscles may be tested otherwise. What is important is that the client's position is such that the muscles are relaxed and inactive. For example, it is not appropriate to test the legs and the torso in a standing position, but it is possible to test the client's arms and shoulders, and neck and face when he or she is sitting on a chair.

The client must wear loose-fitting clothes—sweat pants, T-shirt, or the like.

The test takes place by identifying and locating each muscle in turn, palpating and registering its elasticity—the "muscle-response." These results are marked on the test figure, and in this way the final Bodymap is built up, using specific colors, into a well-defined map of the person's muscle response. This map shows a pattern, a constellation, which is unique for each person in his or her stage of life.

When marking the muscle response, four shades of red are used for the hyperresponsive muscles, and four shades of blue are used for the hyporesponsive muscles; green is used for the neutral responsive muscles. In this book, a black line is used to show which line corresponds to the particular muscle.

The test is a nonverbal, nonprojective test, as it shows the different degrees of elasticity in the client's muscles due to the tester's direct palpation of the muscles. The client need do nothing but relax.

Further validation and evaluation of the Bodymap is not found in this book. For more information, refer to the article by Jørgensen and Marcher (1997). It is possible to download a test figure for making a Bodymap and to see which Stabilo pencils are used for Bodymapping at www.bodymap.dk.

Contents of the Left-hand Pages

One or more anatomical drawings of the specific muscle are presented for the muscles that are tested. When the number of the muscle is in a circle, it indicates where the muscle with this particular number is found and tested—in one or more places. The same is the case if there is a line from the number with a black dot to a place on the body. Opposite, if there is an arrow, it means that a muscle has to be found deeply from the muscles/bones that are shown on the drawing.

An extract of a Bodymap, with an indication of where the test response is marked, is shown in black. There is more information in the descriptions under "Bodymapping."

Bodymap of the Front of the Body

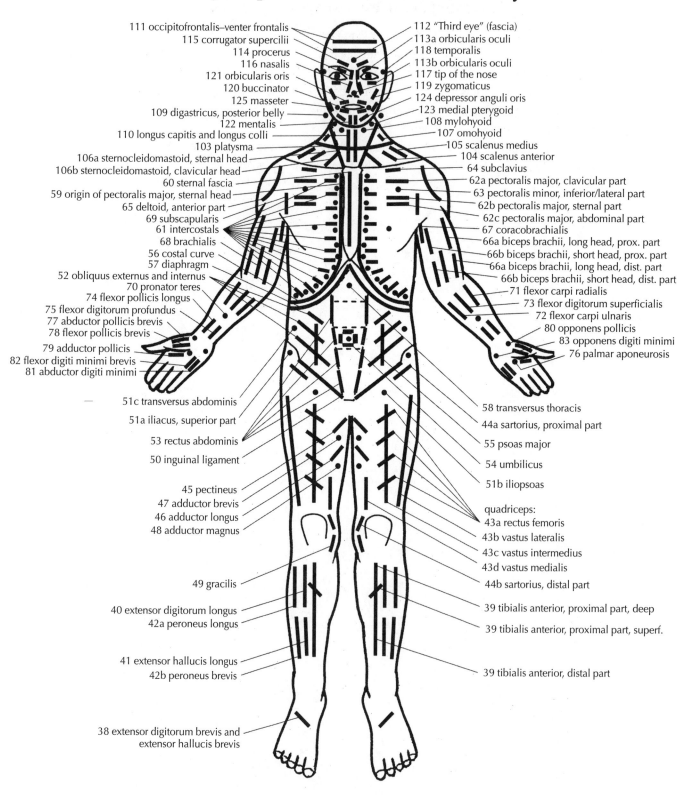

111 occipitofrontalis–venter frontalis
115 corrugator supercilii
114 procerus
116 nasalis
121 orbicularis oris
120 buccinator
125 masseter
109 digastricus, posterior belly
122 mentalis
110 longus capitis and longus colli
103 platysma
106a sternocleidomastoid, sternal head
106b sternocleidomastoid, clavicular head
60 sternal fascia
59 origin of pectoralis major, sternal head
65 deltoid, anterior part
69 subscapularis
61 intercostals
68 brachialis
56 costal curve
57 diaphragm
52 obliquus externus and internus
70 pronator teres
74 flexor pollicis longus
75 flexor digitorum profundus
77 abductor pollicis brevis
78 flexor pollicis brevis
79 adductor pollicis
82 flexor digiti minimi brevis
81 abductor digiti minimi

112 "Third eye" (fascia)
113a orbicularis oculi
118 temporalis
113b orbicularis oculi
117 tip of the nose
119 zygomaticus
124 depressor anguli oris
123 medial pterygoid
108 mylohyoid
107 omohyoid
105 scalenus medius
104 scalenus anterior
64 subclavius
62a pectoralis major, clavicular part
63 pectoralis minor, inferior/lateral part
62b pectoralis major, sternal part
62c pectoralis major, abdominal part
67 coracobrachialis
66a biceps brachii, long head, prox. part
66b biceps brachii, short head, prox. part
66a biceps brachii, long head, dist. part
66b biceps brachii, short head, dist. part
71 flexor carpi radialis
73 flexor digitorum superficialis
72 flexor carpi ulnaris
80 opponens pollicis
83 opponens digiti minimi
76 palmar aponeurosis

— 51c transversus abdominis
51a iliacus, superior part
53 rectus abdominis
50 inguinal ligament
45 pectineus
47 adductor brevis
46 adductor longus
48 adductor magnus
49 gracilis
40 extensor digitorum longus
42a peroneus longus
41 extensor hallucis longus
42b peroneus brevis
38 extensor digitorum brevis and
extensor hallucis brevis

58 transversus thoracis
44a sartorius, proximal part
55 psoas major
54 umbilicus
51b iliopsoas
quadriceps:
43a rectus femoris
43b vastus lateralis
43c vastus intermedius
43d vastus medialis
44b sartorius, distal part
39 tibialis anterior, proximal part, deep
39 tibialis anterior, proximal part, superf.
39 tibialis anterior, distal part

Bodymap of the Back of the Body

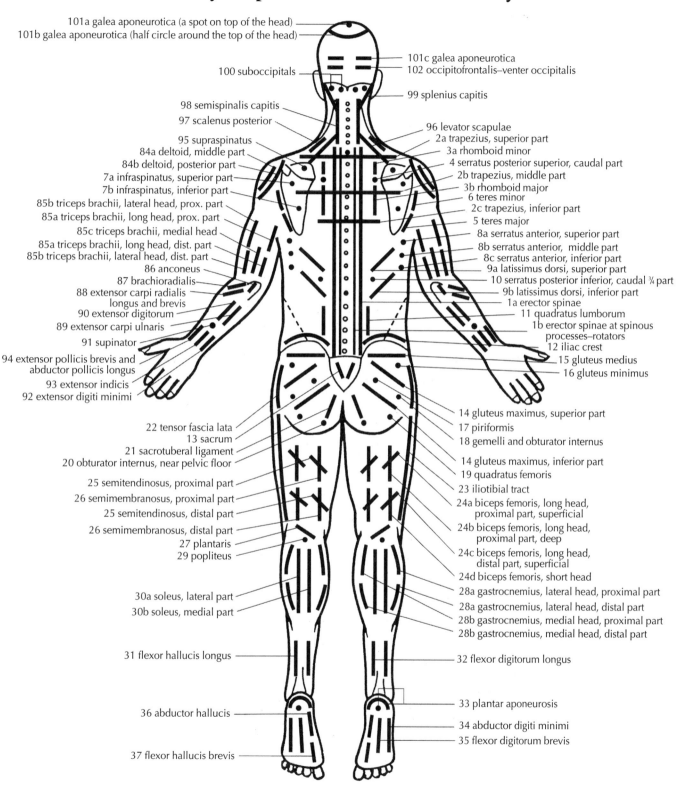

101a galea aponeurotica (a spot on top of the head)
101b galea aponeurotica (half circle around the top of the head)

100 suboccipitals

101c galea aponeurotica
102 occipitofrontalis–venter occipitalis

99 splenius capitis

98 semispinalis capitis
97 scalenus posterior

96 levator scapulae
2a trapezius, superior part
3a rhomboid minor
4 serratus posterior superior, caudal part
2b trapezius, middle part
3b rhomboid major
6 teres minor
2c trapezius, inferior part
5 teres major
8a serratus anterior, superior part
8b serratus anterior, middle part
8c serratus anterior, inferior part
9a latissimus dorsi, superior part
10 serratus posterior inferior, caudal ¾ part
9b latissimus dorsi, inferior part
1a erector spinae
11 quadratus lumborum
1b erector spinae at spinous
   processes–rotators
12 iliac crest
15 gluteus medius
16 gluteus minimus

95 supraspinatus
84a deltoid, middle part
84b deltoid, posterior part
7a infraspinatus, superior part
7b infraspinatus, inferior part
85b triceps brachii, lateral head, prox. part
85a triceps brachii, long head, prox. part
85c triceps brachii, medial head
85a triceps brachii, long head, dist. part
85b triceps brachii, lateral head, dist. part
86 anconeus
87 brachioradialis
88 extensor carpi radialis
   longus and brevis
90 extensor digitorum
89 extensor carpi ulnaris
91 supinator
94 extensor pollicis brevis and
   abductor pollicis longus
93 extensor indicis
92 extensor digiti minimi

22 tensor fascia lata
13 sacrum
21 sacrotuberal ligament
20 obturator internus, near pelvic floor

14 gluteus maximus, superior part
17 piriformis
18 gemelli and obturator internus

14 gluteus maximus, inferior part
19 quadratus femoris
23 iliotibial tract
24a biceps femoris, long head,
   proximal part, superficial
24b biceps femoris, long head,
   proximal part, deep
24c biceps femoris, long head,
   distal part, superficial
24d biceps femoris, short head
28a gastrocnemius, lateral head, proximal part
28a gastrocnemius, lateral head, distal part
28b gastrocnemius, medial head, proximal part
28b gastrocnemius, medial head, distal part

25 semitendinosus, proximal part
26 semimembranosus, proximal part
25 semitendinosus, distal part
26 semimembranosus, distal part
27 plantaris
29 popliteus

30a soleus, lateral part
30b soleus, medial part

31 flexor hallucis longus

32 flexor digitorum longus

33 plantar aponeurosis

36 abductor hallucis

34 abductor digiti minimi
35 flexor digitorum brevis

37 flexor hallucis brevis

35

Muscles and Connective Tissue

Name:	**Connective tissue of the back level with thoracic vertebrae 3–5**

Number: *

Origin:

Insertion:

Anatomical function:

Map: Connective tissue between erector spinae and rhomboids level with thoracic vertebrae 3-5.

Is contracted by:

Character structure(s):   EXISTENCE

Ego function: CONNECTEDNESS, (a) bonding.

Psychological function: Give in/allow oneself to bond through physical contact.

Ego function: CONNECTEDNESS, (c) feeling support and self-support.

Psychological function: Receive support for being in the world.

Ego function: MANAGEMENT OF ENERGY, (d) self-containment, feeling "backed."

Psychological function: Through integration of support, the experience of self-support is achieved, which leads to the possibility of containment of high-level energy.

Child's developmental stage/age: The place on the fetus or child's back where it has contact with the uterus most frequently.

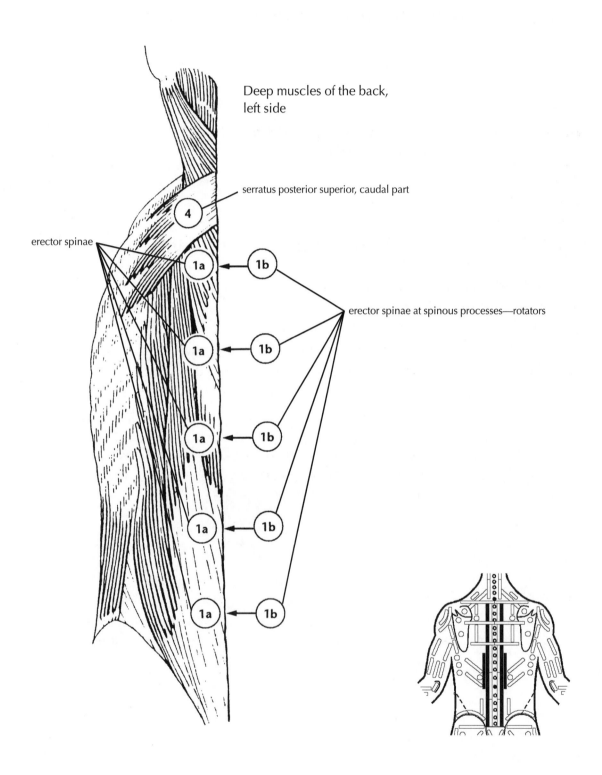

Deep muscles of the back, left side

serratus posterior superior, caudal part

erector spinae

erector spinae at spinous processes—rotators

Name:	Erector spinae	Number: 1a

	A complex muscle system that consists of three subgroups, each made up of overlapping slips of muscle.
Origin:	Sacrum; ilium; lumbar spinous processes.
Insertion:	(1) iliocostalis: on all the ribs. (2) longissimus: on lumbar and thoracic transverse processes of all vertebrae. (3) spinalis: on all thoracic spinous processes.
Anatomical function:	(1) + (2) extension and side flexion of the spinal column. (3) extension of the spinal column.
Map:	Is found as muscle bodies on each side of the spinal column from sacrum to neck. Lies deep to latissimus dorsi, trapezius, rhomboids, serratus posterior superior, and serratus posterior inferior.
Is contracted by:	Lying on the stomach: tuck chin toward the chest and lift the head and upper part of the body from the floor. Sitting position: press head backward with the chin tucked toward the chest; or curl the spine forward and roll up into a sitting position.
Character structure(s):	Deepest fibers: NEED 1a* Lateral fibers level with thoracic vertebrae 8-12: SOLIDARITY/PERFORMANCE–PUBERTY Most likely the superficial fibers are activated at different ages/stages.
Ego function:	POSITIONING, (a) stance toward life.
Psychological function:	NEED: holding on to life. Extension of the erector spinae integrates the sense of locality and grounding. SOL/PERF-PUB: preserve dignity in stressful situations (also conflicts), e.g., if humiliated by a teacher (hold one's head high no matter what). To be able to relate to life using the observing ego and hold on to reality at the same time.
Ego function:	GROUNDING AND REALITY TESTING, (c) experience and grounding of extrasensory perceptions.
Psychological function:	NEED: centering of the spiritual extrasensory energy system grounded in reality from an energetic sense/perception. SOL/PERF-PUB: centering of the spiritual extrasensory energy system grounded in reality from an abstract, philosophical, and cognitive process/way of thinking.
Child's developmental stage/age:	NEED: The child lies on her stomach and uses the muscles to pull herself up, orienting herself in the room. Preserving contact with the ground while integrating orientation and grounding, thus integrating attitude to life. Preserve oneself in an upright position, sitting and standing, reflexive (reflex from the ischial tuberosity). SOL/PERF-PUB: Adjusting and balancing the upright position of the spinal column.

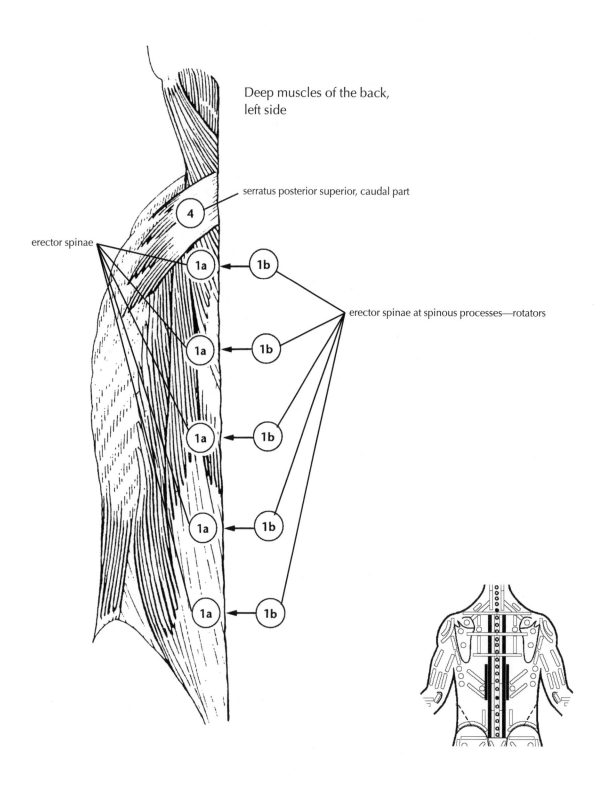

Deep muscles of the back,
left side

serratus posterior superior, caudal part

erector spinae

erector spinae at spinous processes—rotators

| **Name:** | **Erector spinae** | **Number: 1a** |

Bodymapping:

Client's position:	On the stomach.
Tester's position:	Opposite the side that is tested.
Activation in test position:	Lift head with the chin tucked toward the chest, and raise the upper part of the body from the floor as well.
Test location:	In the middle where the muscle is full. Start testing erector spinae in the lumbar part and then continue testing up to vertebra prominens (on C7) in five different locations along the muscle. Test the lateral fibers of erector spinae level with thoracic vertebrae 8-12.
Test direction:	Inferiorly (caudally).

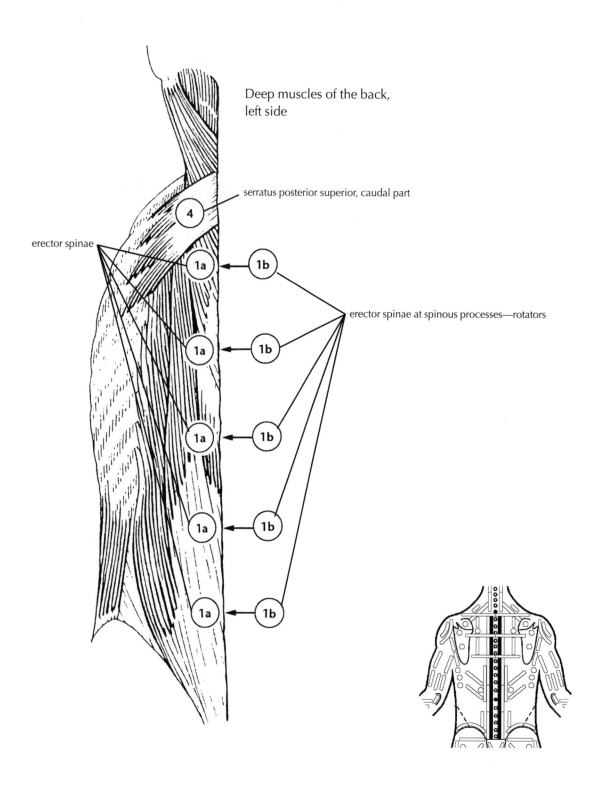

Deep muscles of the back, left side

serratus posterior superior, caudal part

4

erector spinae

1a ← **1b**

erector spinae at spinous processes—rotators

1a ← **1b**

1a ← **1b**

1a ← **1b**

1a ← **1b**

	Deepest layer in the transversospinal system. The fibers run almost horizontally, never passing more than one thoracic vertebra.
Origin:	Transverse processes of each vertebra.
Insertion:	Base of the spinous process of next higher vertebra.
Anatomical function:	Rotates the spinal column.
Map:	Are found deep in erector spinae, latissimus dorsi, trapezius, and rhomboids close to the spinous processes.
Is contracted by:	Rotating the spinal column; however, there is very little movement activated by the small rotators at the spinous processes.
Character structure(s):	OPINIONS SOLIDARITY/PERFORMANCE
Ego function:	POSITIONING, (d) stance toward values and norms.
Psychological function:	Integration of norms and values.
Ego function:	CENTERING, (c) being oneself in one's different roles.
Psychological function:	Integration of one's roles.
Child's developmental stage/age:	Fine adjustment of rotation, adjusting to balance. Stabilizes the back so the child is able to use arms and legs with more strength/power.

Bodymapping:

Client's position:	On the stomach.
Tester's position:	Opposite the side that is tested.
Activation in test position:	As a rule, it is not necessary.
Test location:	By the medial fibers of erector spinae. Test deeply and close to the spinous processes.
Test direction:	Slightly laterally and caudally.

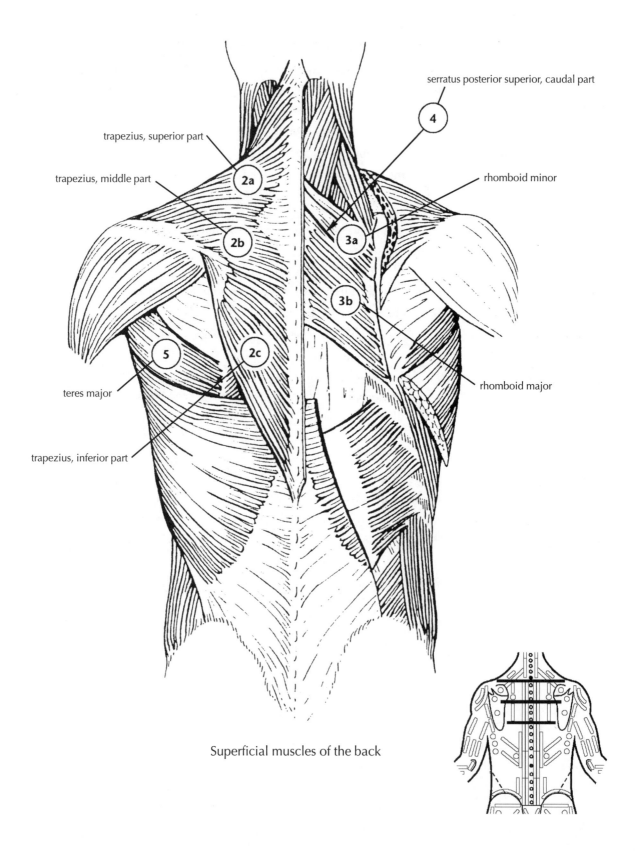

serratus posterior superior, caudal part

(4)

trapezius, superior part

(2a)

rhomboid minor

trapezius, middle part

(2b)

(3a)

(3b)

(5)

(2c)

teres major

rhomboid major

trapezius, inferior part

Superficial muscles of the back

Name:	**Trapezius**	**Number: 2a, b, c**

Origin:	(a) Superior part: occiput, ligamentum nuchae, and spinous process C7. (b) Middle part: spinous processes T1-5. (c) Inferior part: spinous processes T6-12.
Insertion:	(a) Superior part: lateral third of clavicle, acromion process of scapula. (b) Middle part: spine of scapula. (c) Inferior part: root of spine of scapula.
Anatomical function:	Different parts of the muscle lift, lower, and rotate the scapula. Extends the neck and bends sideways, and rotates the neck so the face turns to the opposite side.
Map:	Is found from the cranium out to the scapulas and down the back of the chest forming a point at T12. The paired muscles form a diamond shape.
Is contracted by:	(a) Superior part: lift your shoulders toward the ears. Note: first pull shoulder blades together slightly, and then lift from that position to exclude levator scapulae. (b) Middle part: pull scapulas toward each other. (c) Inferior part: pull scapulas down the back and then toward each other.
Character structure(s):	Superior part: AUTONOMY Middle part: NEED Inferior part: LOVE/SEXUALITY
Ego function:	CONNECTEDNESS, (c) feeling support and self-support.
Psychological function:	AUT: ask for help, and get the help needed to do it on one's own. NEED: get support to fulfill one's needs. LOVE/SEX: get support to become a sensual/sexual person, and get support in constructive alliances.
Ego function:	MANAGEMENT OF ENERGY, (d) self-containment, feeling "backed."
Psychological function:	AUT–NEED–LOVE/SEX: through integration of support from others, the experience of self-support is achieved, which allows the possibility of containing high energy.
Ego function:	2 (c) Inferior part: GENDER SKILLS. (c) experience of gender role. (e) manifestation of sensuality and sexuality.
Psychological function:	(c) LOVE/SEX: conscious knowledge of own gender and the matching feminine or masculine energy. (e) LOVE/SEX: through support, the right to assert oneself as a sensual and sexual person is achieved.
Child's developmental stage/age:	(a) Superior: takes part in crawling to stabilize the scapulas. (b) Middle: stabilizes the scapulas when the child lifts his head and shoulder up while supporting himself with his arms, and when creeping. (c) Inferior: takes part in the movement when the child throws a small ball with an underhand motion. Getting up from a lying position to a standing position by pushing up from one arm behind. Takes part in flirting with the shoulder together with pectoralis major, clavicular head.

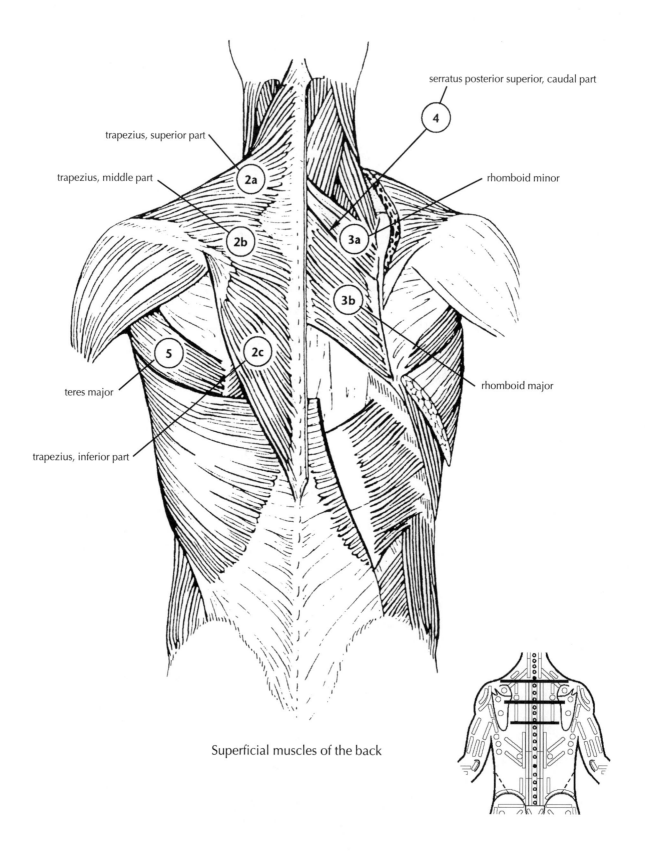

serratus posterior superior, caudal part

rhomboid minor

trapezius, superior part

trapezius, middle part

rhomboid major

teres major

trapezius, inferior part

Superficial muscles of the back

Name: **Trapezius** **Number: 2a, b, c**

Bodymapping:

Client's position: On the stomach.

Tester's position: Opposite the side that is tested.

Activation in test position:
(a) Superior part: lift the head or move the shoulder and head toward each other (give resistance if necessary).
(b) Middle part: pull the scapulas together or stretch arm along floor/mat into abduction so hand is level with shoulder and palm is toward the floor/mat. Lift arm off the floor/mat.
(c) Inferior part: first stretch arm out above the shoulder diagonally away, then lift the arm off the floor/mat.

Test location: On the upper, middle, and lower part of the muscle.

Test direction: Pull medially in the direction of the fibers.

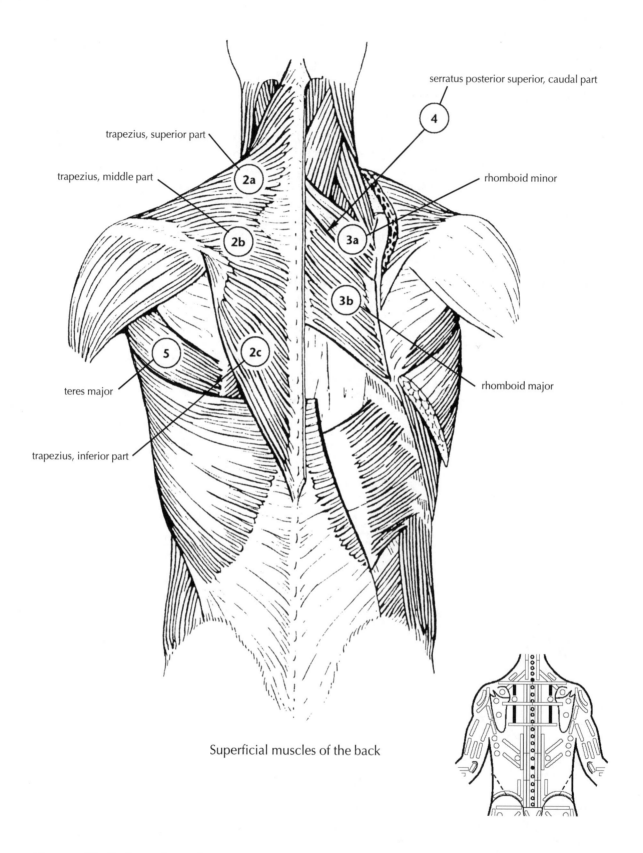

trapezius, superior part

trapezius, middle part

serratus posterior superior, caudal part

4

2a

rhomboid minor

2b

3a

3b

5

2c

teres major

rhomboid major

trapezius, inferior part

Superficial muscles of the back

Name:	**Rhomboids minor and major**	Number: 3a, b

Origin:	(a) Minor: C7 and T1 spinous processes. (b) Major: T2–T5 spinous processes.
Insertion:	(a) Minor: medial border of the scapula at the root of the spine. (b) Major: medial border of the scapula below the spine.
Anatomical function:	Pull scapula diagonally medially and upward (medial rotation of scapula).
Map:	Minor is found between C7–T1 and the root of spine of scapula. Major is found more caudally along the vertebral border of the scapula. Both muscles lie superficially.
Is contracted by:	Moving the arm across the back with a slightly bent elbow or by moving the edges of the scapulas toward each other.
Character structure(s):	Minor: WILL Major: LOVE/SEXUALITY
Ego function:	CENTERING, (c) being oneself in one's different roles.
Psychological function:	WILL: being in your role from your center. LOVE/SEX: living your role with integrity from your center.
Ego function:	SELF-ASSERTION, (b) asserting oneself in one's roles.
Psychological function:	WILL: to manifest different roles (experience the difference between doing wrong and being wrong). LOVE/SEX: have self-confidence in manifesting roles (the observing ego has developed/is manifesting itself).
Ego function:	GENDER SKILLS, (c) experience of gender role.
Psychological function:	WILL: experience of "mother is like this, and father is like that." LOVE/SEX: integration of the gender role; "women do this, and men do that."
Child's developmental stage/age:	WILL: stabilizes scapula when the child throws a ball overhand. LOVE/SEX: the child adds power and accuracy in its overhand throw.
Bodymapping:	
Client's position:	On the stomach.
Tester's position:	Opposite the side that is tested.
Activation in test position:	Pull the same side's arm across the back with a slightly bent elbow.
Test location:	(a) Minor: between T1 spinous process and spine of scapula. (b) Major: more caudally.
Test direction:	Pull medially in the direction of muscle fibers.

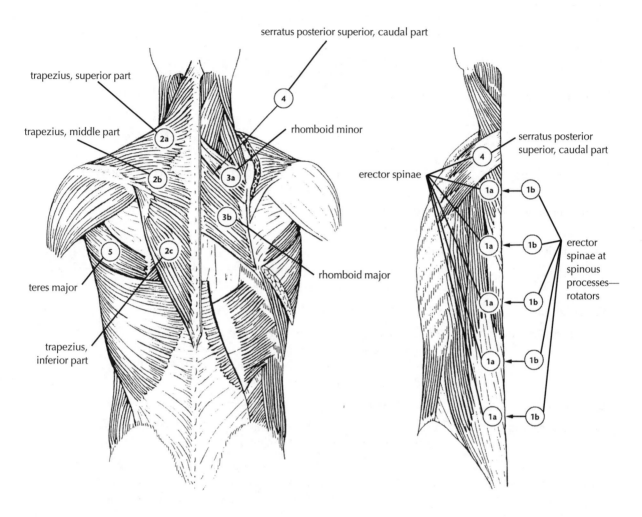

serratus posterior superior, caudal part

trapezius, superior part

trapezius, middle part

rhomboid minor

erector spinae

trapezius, inferior part

teres major

rhomboid major

serratus posterior superior, caudal part

erector spinae at spinous processes—rotators

Superficial muscles of the back

Deep muscles of the back, left side

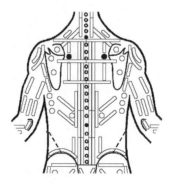

Name:	**Serratus posterior superior**	Number: 4

Origin:	Spinous processes C7–T2.
Insertion:	Cranial borders of ribs 2–5.
Anatomical function:	Raises the ribs to increase thoracic cavity; assists in inhalation.
Map:	Is found deep between C7 and the border of scapula, deep to trapezius and rhomboid minor.
Is contracted by:	Taking a deep breath into the upper back.
Character structure(s):	Cranial part: WILL (is not tested separately) Caudal part: LOVE/SEXUALITY
Ego function:	CONNECTEDNESS, (b) heart contact/opening.
Psychological function:	WILL: have an open heart to do something for the world/others; altruism. LOVE/SEX: have an open heart to give and receive; you cannot give the heart away, but you can give from the heart and receive with the heart.
Ego function:	Caudal part: GENDER SKILLS, (c) experience of gender role.
Psychological function:	LOVE/SEX: have an open heart in filling yourself out and accept/integrate the social gender role; "women do this, and men do that."
Child's developmental stage/age:	The child fills lungs fully into the upper part of the chest at the back. The child copies gender roles, e.g., playing house.

Bodymapping:	
Client's position:	On the stomach.
Tester's position:	Opposite the side that is tested.
Activation in test position:	A deep inhalation all the way up in the upper back part of the chest confirms the position of the muscle (gasp for breath if necessary); "take a deep breath, push against my finger with your breath"; when the client is breathing normally again, test the muscle.
Test location:	Between C7 and level with the spine of the scapula—test the muscle between the two locations.
Test direction:	Pull laterally in the direction of the muscle fibers.

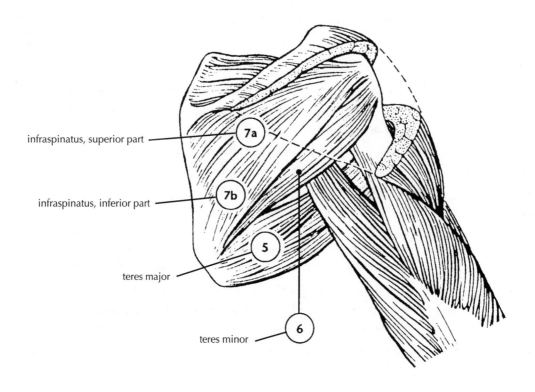

infraspinatus, superior part — **7a**

infraspinatus, inferior part — **7b**

teres major — **5**

teres minor — **6**

Right shoulder blade, dorsal view

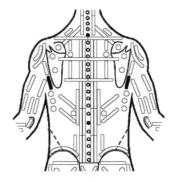

The Bodynamic Psycho-Motor Anatomy

Name:	**Teres major**	**Number: 5**
Origin:	Inferior angle of scapula.	
Insertion:	Medial lip of bicipital groove of humerus.	
Anatomical function:	Medially rotates, adducts, and extends the arm.	
Map:	Is found superficially, laterally to the scapula, superior to latissimus dorsi.	
Is contracted by:	Turning the arm medially in the shoulder joint with the palm backward and extending the arm.	
Character structure(s):	WILL	
Ego function:	SOCIAL BALANCE, (c) degree of "facade" and maintaining one's front.	
Psychological function:	Ability to master appearances in relation to the world; e.g., to keep a secret/not to show emotions (hold the arm in a position as if ready to "draw a gun."	
Child's developmental stage/age:	The child is able to catch a big ball with her arms; the muscle stabilizes the shoulder joint when lifting heavy things, gives power to an underhand throw, and provides the ability to throw with an overhand motion.	

Bodymapping:

Client's position:	On the stomach.
Tester's position:	Opposite the side that is tested.
Activation in test position:	The arm lies by the side with palm upward; extend, medially rotate, and adduct the upper arm.
Test location:	Where the muscle is full.
Test direction:	Medially in the direction of muscle fibers.

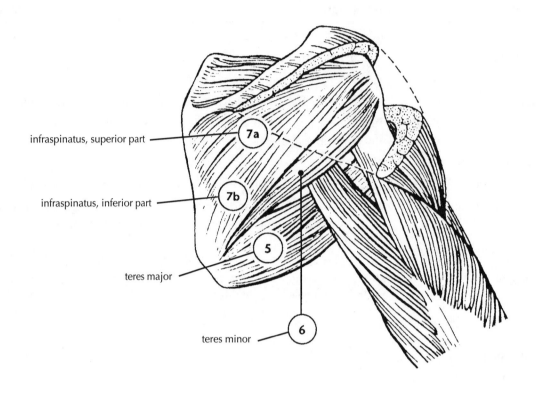

infraspinatus, superior part — 7a

infraspinatus, inferior part — 7b

5

teres major

teres minor — 6

Right shoulder blade, dorsal view

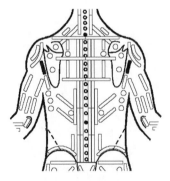

The Bodynamic Psycho-Motor Anatomy

Name:	Teres minor	Number: 6

Origin:	Upper axillary border of scapula.
Insertion:	Greater tubercle of humerus.
Anatomical function:	Laterally rotates and adducts the arm; is part of the rotator cuff.
Map:	Is found between the lateral border of the scapula and posterior deltoid, superior to teres major and inferior to infraspinatus.
Is contracted by:	Rotating the arm laterally in the shoulder joint, and then moving it slightly backward and toward the body.
Character structure(s):	LOVE/SEXUALITY
Ego function:	SOCIAL BALANCE, (c) degree of "facade" and maintaining one's front.
Psychological function:	To show or not show your love or attraction to another person; among other things in establishing alliances ("we are sweethearts, and we won't tell anybody").
Ego function:	GENDER SKILLS, (e) manifestation of sensuality and sexuality.
Psychological function:	Flirting.
Child's developmental stage/age:	The child is able to coordinate throwing a ball against a wall and catching it again with an underhand motion. This muscle also takes part in flirting with movements of the shoulder and arm.

Bodymapping:	
Client's position:	On the stomach.
Tester's position:	Opposite the side that is tested.
Activation in test position:	Lie with arm along the side and palm upward, then turn the arm so palm is downward (lateral rotation); if necessary lift the arm off the mat into extension.
Test location:	At the lateral edge of scapula, in the fullness of the muscle.
Test direction:	Along the edge of scapula in the direction of muscle fibers; i.e., caudally and medially.

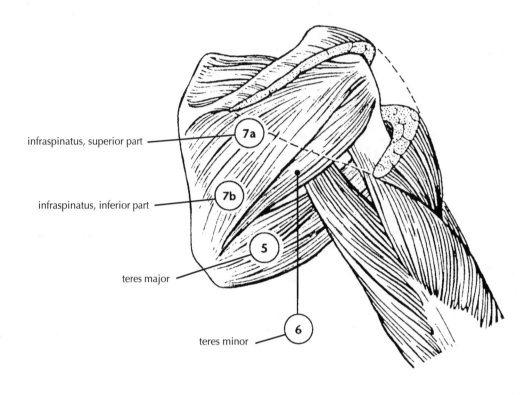

infraspinatus, superior part — **7a**

infraspinatus, inferior part — **7b**

teres major — **5**

teres minor — **6**

Right shoulder blade, dorsal view

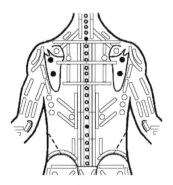

The Bodynamic Psycho-Motor Anatomy

Name:	Infraspinatus	Number: 7a, b

Origin:	Infraspinous fossa of the scapula.
Insertion:	Greater tubercle of humerus.
Anatomical function:	Lateral rotation and abduction of the arm; is part of the rotator cuff.
Map:	On scapula below the spine of the scapula.
Is contracted by:	Moving the arm upward in a cheering/waving position.
Character structure(s):	(a) Superior part: SOLIDARITY/PERFORMANCE (b) Inferior part: OPINIONS
Ego function:	SOCIAL BALANCE, (c) degree of "facade" and maintaining one's front.
Psychological function:	SOL/PERF: loyalty in a group; there are matters you don't talk about; ability to separate private affairs from group affairs. OPINIONS: ability to keep a straight face while telling jokes.
Child's developmental stage/age:	The child is able to throw a rather heavy ball with an overhand motion and plays games where one has to throw a ball and hit others.

Bodymapping:

Client's position:	On the stomach.
Tester's position:	Opposite the side that is tested.
Activation in test position:	Laterally rotate upper part of arm as it lies by the side, or abduct the arm in a cheering/waving position.
Test location:	In two locations: cranially test on the muscle below the spine of the scapula, where the muscle fibers are thick. Caudally test near the inferior angle of the scapula, where the muscle fibers are thinner.
Test direction:	Medially, inferiorly (caudally).

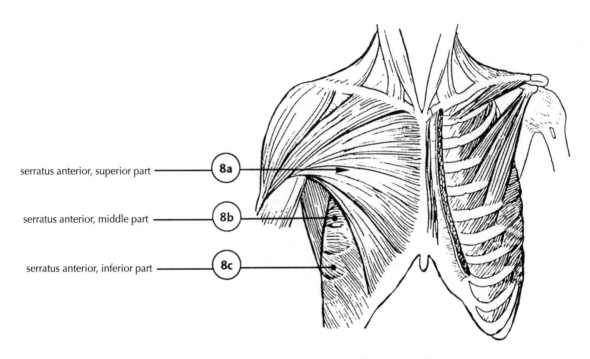

serratus anterior, superior part — **8a**

serratus anterior, middle part — **8b**

serratus anterior, inferior part — **8c**

Chest, ventral view

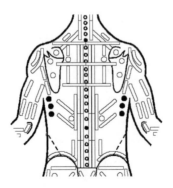

Name:	Serratus anterior	Number: 8a, b, c

Origin:	Outer surface of nine upper ribs.
Insertion:	Medial border of the scapula.
Anatomical function:	Stabilizes, lowers, or rotates scapula; pulls scapula forward and assists in abduction and flexion of arm.
Map:	Is found laterally on the chest wall under the armpit on the ribs.
Is contracted by:	Widening the back or moving the scapulas apart.
Character structure(s):	(a) Superior part: EXISTENCE (b) Middle part: NEED (c) Inferior part: AUTONOMY
Ego function:	CONNECTEDNESS, (b) heart contact/opening
Psychological function:	EX: you are wanted and loved for who you are. NEED: you are loved no matter what needs you have. AUT: you are loved for your curiosity and impulses.
Ego function:	PATTERNS OF INTERPERSONAL SKILLS, (a) reaching out.
Psychological function:	EX: reaching out with your breath and receiving the contact all the way to the heart through the eyes and by the breath. NEED: ability to stabilize the body to contain sensations and emotions, and at the same time satisfy one's needs. AUT: space to enjoy oneself and freedom to explore the world and to own one's emotions without losing contact.
Child's developmental stage/age:	EX: the child is able to have an influence on those he comes into contact with. NEED: the child pushes himself up lying on his stomach. AUT: the child stands on all fours. The muscle is integrated in activities of creeping, crawling, and pulling oneself up into a standing position, and it is active in the stabilization of these actions.

Bodymapping:

Client's position:	(1) On the stomach. (2) On the back.
Tester's position:	(1) Stomach: opposite the side that is tested. (2) Back: on the side that is tested.
Activation in test position:	(1) Stomach: press hands and elbows to floor while lying prone. (2) Back: lift the arm vertically with the fingers stretched toward the ceiling, or widen the back (only a small movement).
Test location:	1st under pectoralis major on the ribs. 2nd and 3rd in different locations on the muscle.
Test direction:	(1) Stomach: pull medially toward yourself in the direction of the fibers. (2) Back: pull medially on the client in the direction of the fibers.

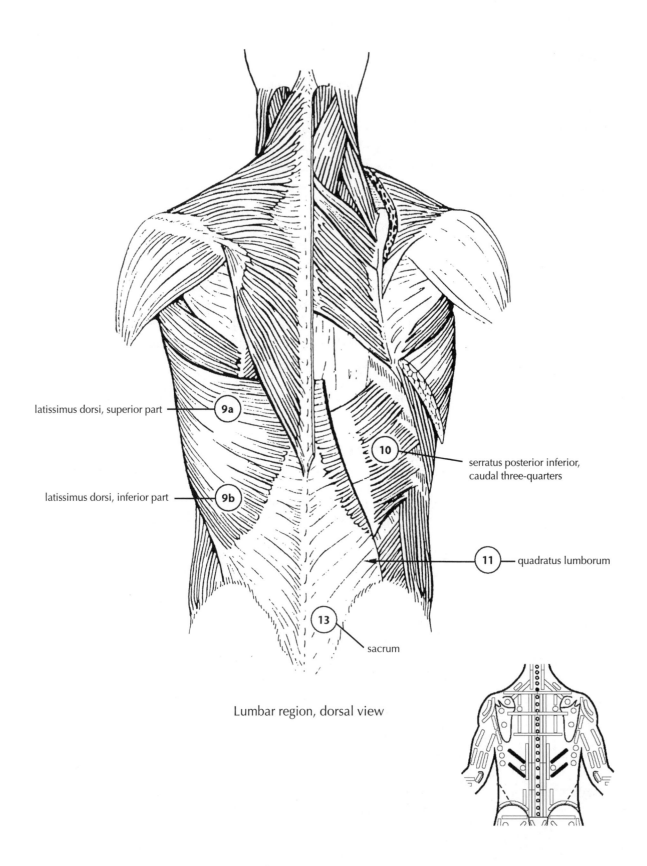

latissimus dorsi, superior part — **9a**

latissimus dorsi, inferior part — **9b**

10 — serratus posterior inferior, caudal three-quarters

11 — quadratus lumborum

13

sacrum

Lumbar region, dorsal view

The Bodynamic Psycho-Motor Anatomy

Name:	**Latissimus dorsi**	Number: 9a, b

Origin:	Thoracolumbar aponeurosis from T7 to iliac crest; lower three or four ribs; inferior angle of scapula.
Insertion:	Bicipital groove of the humerus.
Anatomical function:	The only muscle that connects the pelvis (legs) and shoulders (arms); extends, adducts, and medially rotates the arm (humerus).
Map:	Is found superficially on the lower part of the back; covered by trapezius on the upper part of the muscle.
Is contracted by:	Turning the palms of the hands toward each other behind you; imagine holding a large ball on your back and pressing on it.
Character structure(s):	(a) Superior part: WILL (b) Inferior part: OPINIONS-SOLIDARITY/PERFORMANCE
Ego function:	CONNECTEDNESS, (c) feeling support and self-support.
Psychological function:	WILL: the experience of being able to get support from others while doing activities in the world. OPINIONS-SOL/PERF: to be able to receive support while expressing one's own ideas/opinions and remaining true to oneself in a group.
Ego function:	MANAGEMENT OF ENERGY, (d) self-containment, feeling "backed."
Psychological function:	WILL: maintaining and containing emotions (sometimes opposing); staying in contact with awareness of both oneself and the surroundings. OPINIONS-SOL/PERF: Feeling supported and able to think and communicate from a balanced position.
Child's developmental stage/age:	WILL: throw a small ball with both an underhand and overhand motion. OPINIONS-SOL/PERF: throw a large ball with precision both with an underhand and overhand motion. Latissimus dorsi is involved in straightening the back and widening it simultaneously.

Bodymapping:	
Client's position:	On the stomach.
Tester's position:	Opposite the side that is tested.
Activation in test position:	Lift the arm slightly off the floor with the palm upward; pull/stretch it toward the feet slightly medially.
Test location:	(a) Superior part: test below inferior angle of scapula. (b) Inferior part: test in thoracolumbar area at level of lower ribs.
Test direction:	Medially, inferiorly (caudally) in the direction of the fibers.

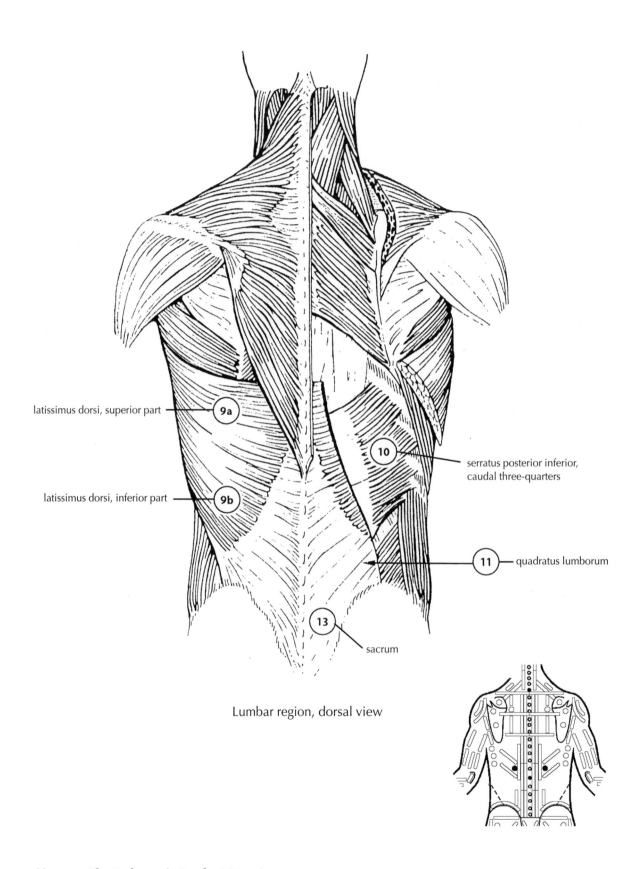

latissimus dorsi, superior part   **9a**

latissimus dorsi, inferior part   **9b**

10   serratus posterior inferior, caudal three-quarters

11   quadratus lumborum

13   sacrum

Lumbar region, dorsal view

Name:	**Serratus posterior inferior**	**Number: 10**

Origin:	Spinous processes T11–T12 and L1–L3.
Insertion:	Inferior borders of last four ribs (9-12).
Anatomical function:	Helps in exhalation.
Map:	Is found over the lower ribs deep to latissimus dorsi.
Is contracted by:	Coughing or puffing out the last bit of air on exhalation.
Character structure(s):	Cranial one-quarter: OPINIONS (is not tested separately) Caudal three-quarters: SOLIDARITY/PERFORMANCE
Ego function:	CONNECTEDNESS, (b) heart contact/opening.
Psychological function:	OPINIONS: having bosom friends, best friends, and buddies, and at the same time being able to have one's own opinions. SOL/PERF: maintaining one's individuality in gatherings.
Child's developmental stage/age:	The child has strength in throwing, e.g., shot put. Strength in exhalation: the child is able to puff out air in physical training, e.g., karate.

Bodymapping:

Client's position:	On the stomach.
Tester's position:	Opposite the side that is tested.
Activation in test position:	Cough and/or puff out the last air from an exhalation.
Test location:	Over the lower ribs, deep to latissimus dorsi and laterally to erector spinae. Contract latissimus dorsi to distinguish serratus posterior inferior.
Test direction:	Medially, slightly caudally in the direction of the muscle fibers.

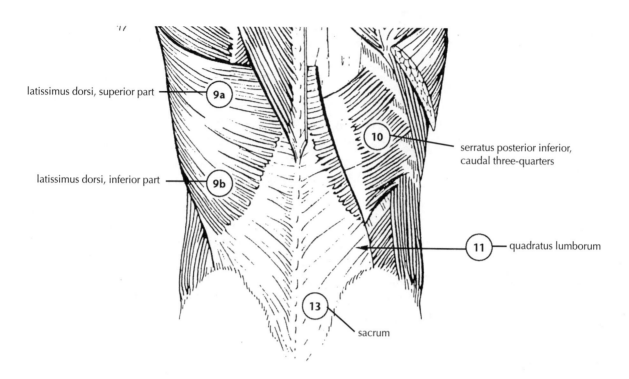

latissimus dorsi, superior part — **9a**

latissimus dorsi, inferior part — **9b**

10 — serratus posterior inferior, caudal three-quarters

11 — quadratus lumborum

13 — sacrum

Lumbar region, dorsal view

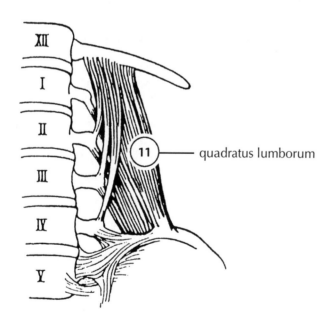

XII

I

II

III

IV

V

11 — quadratus lumborum

Quadratus lumborum, ventral view

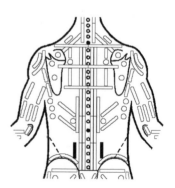

The Bodynamic Psycho-Motor Anatomy

Name:	**Quadratus lumborum**	Number: 11

Origin:	Posterior iliac crest.
Insertion:	Rib 12, transverse processes of lumbar vertebrae.
Anatomical function:	Lowers the ribs and laterally flexes the spinal column; raises the hip.
Map:	Is found deep to erector spinae, between the lower ribs and the edge of the "hip bone." Connects upper and lower parts of the body.
Is contracted by:	In a standing position move (pull) one hip up toward the ribs with a stretched leg.
Character structure(s):	AUTONOMY
Ego function:	SOCIAL BALANCE, (a) balancing own needs/feelings/desires against others' expectations.
Psychological function:	Maintaining the awareness of oneself and one's own impulses while mirroring others.
Child's developmental stage/age:	Is involved in the movements of creeping and crawling, and when the child has all the weight on one leg or stands on one leg.

Bodymapping:

Client's position:	On the stomach.
Tester's position:	Opposite the side that is tested.
Activation in test position:	Stretch the leg along the floor/mat on the opposite side of the side that is tested.
Test location:	Laterally to erector spinae, test deeply into the muscle between the hip bone and the lower ribs.
Test direction:	Medially and inferiorly (caudally).

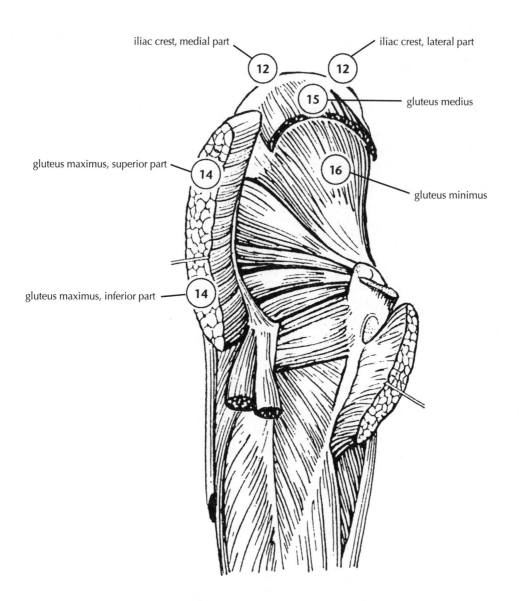

iliac crest, medial part — 12

iliac crest, lateral part — 12

15 — gluteus medius

gluteus maximus, superior part — 14

16 — gluteus minimus

gluteus maximus, inferior part — 14

Deep muscles of the hip, right side,
dorsal view

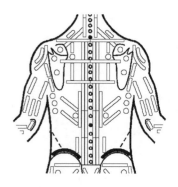

The Bodynamic Psycho-Motor Anatomy

Name:	**Iliac crest**	Number: 12

Origin:	
Insertion:	
Anatomical function:	Muscles (e.g., quadratus lumborum and obliquus externus and internus) and connective tissue originate and insert on the iliac crest.
Map:	Iliac crest is found in the area of the waistline.
Is contracted by:	
Character structure(s):	Medial part: PERINATAL Lateral part: PUBERTY
Ego function:	MANAGEMENT OF ENERGY, (b) containment of high-level energy.
Psychological function:	PERINATAL: medial part relates to birth–the power in the stretching reflexes/coming forward with your own power (erection of the torso). PUB: lateral part–making one's way out in the world and preserving one's dignity, and also having a good sense of strategies and tactics.
Child's developmental stage/age:	PERINATAL: reflex contraction in erector spinae begins from the hip bone so the back gains its first curve. PUB: full rotation in rapid movements–ability to contract diagonally, e.g., in football/soccer tackling.
Shock:	Commonly the lateral part of muscle and connective tissue is impacted by shock.

Bodymapping:	
Client's position:	On the stomach.
Tester's position:	Opposite the side that is tested.
Activation in test position:	
Test location:	Find the iliac crest. Push up the skin slightly and test in two locations, medially and laterally, on the edge of the iliac crest. Test a general impression of muscle and connective tissue. The tissue may be very tight.
Test direction:	Laterally and inferiorly (caudally).

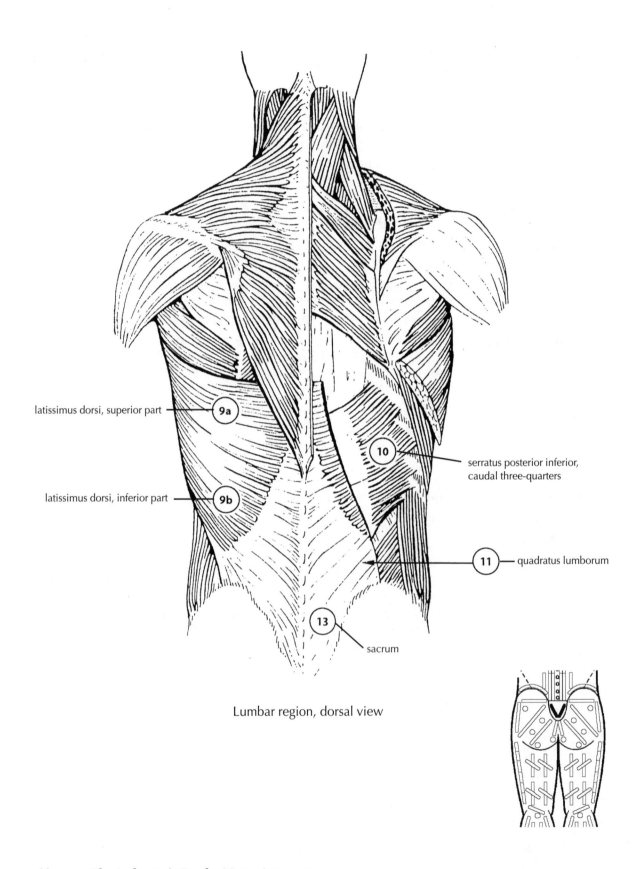

latissimus dorsi, superior part — **9a**

latissimus dorsi, inferior part — **9b**

10 — serratus posterior inferior, caudal three-quarters

11 — quadratus lumborum

13 — sacrum

Lumbar region, dorsal view

The Bodynamic Psycho-Motor Anatomy

Name: Sacrum   **Number: 13**

Origin:	
Insertion:	
Anatomical function:	Erector spinae and fascia thoracolumbalis originate from the sacrum.
Map:	Sacrum is found wedged between the hip bones. Together the bones form the pelvis.
Is contracted by:	Sitting or standing: make the movement of a "hollow back." Lying on the stomach, the fibers are activated by lifting the upper part of the torso. They work as stabilizers when the stretched legs are lifted.
Character structure(s):	PERINATAL
Ego function:	CENTERING, (d) feelings of self-esteem.
Psychological function:	Ability to feel that one's power comes from one's center.
Ego function:	SELF-ASSERTION, (c) forward momentum and sense of direction.
Psychological function:	Ability to have a focused life-energy/life direction; a fundamental code of knowledge for navigating through stress.
Child's developmental stage/age:	Part of the stretch reflex required for pushing oneself through the birth canal during birth.

Bodymapping:

Client's position:	On the stomach.
Tester's position:	On the side, testing both left and right sides.
Activation in test position:	Lift the extended legs, or lift the upper part of the body.
Test location:	Where the sacrum is broadest.
Test direction:	Inferiorly (caudally).

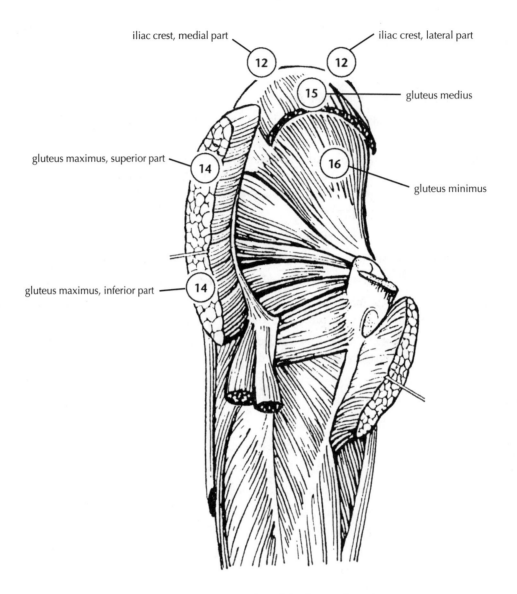

iliac crest, medial part — **12**

iliac crest, lateral part — **12**

15 — gluteus medius

gluteus maximus, superior part — **14**

16 — gluteus minimus

gluteus maximus, inferior part — **14**

Deep muscles of the hip, right side,
dorsal view

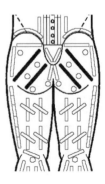

Name:	**Gluteus maximus**	Number: 14

Origin:	Posterior sacrum; superior gluteal line of ilium; coccyx; and sacrotuberous ligament.
Insertion:	Gluteal tuberosity of femur and iliotibial tract (which attaches to lateral condyle of tibia).
Anatomical function:	Extension of the hip joint; lateral rotation of the extended hip; assists in adduction and abduction of hip joint–stabilizes sacroiliac joint. The iliotibial tract permits both gluteus maximus and tensor fascia lata to stabilize the extended knee.
Map:	Is found superficially in the buttocks.
Is contracted by:	Tightening gluteus maximus/tightening buttocks. Moving the leg backward at the hip joint.
Character structure(s):	Superior part: OPINIONS Inferior part: SOLIDARITY/PERFORMANCE
Ego function:	CENTERING, (b) filling out from the inside.
Psychological function:	OPINIONS: Putting one's energy behind one's own opinions SOL/PERF: Putting one's energy into one's own performances.
Ego function:	PATTERNS OF INTERPERSONAL SKILLS, (g) taking on chores (assignments).
Psychological function:	OPINIONS: expressing one's attitude and thus staying in contact with the task. SOL/PERF: ability to keep one's energy purposely on the task.
Ego function:	GENDER SKILLS, (e) manifestation of sensuality and sexuality.
Psychological function:	OPINIONS: playing with your sensuality and sexuality verbally, for instance in jokes or secret messages. SOL/PERF: ability to keep your manifestation of sensuality/sexuality, regardless of the situation.
Child's developmental stage/age:	The child is able to stand on one leg and extend the other leg. Long jumps/triple jumps. Walking with a push-off movement and with strength in running and jumping. It is also used when moving from a sitting position to a standing position.

Bodymapping:

Client's position:	On the stomach.
Tester's position:	On the side that is tested.
Activation in test position:	Tighten the buttocks, or straighten the leg and lift backward at the hip.
Test location:	Superior and inferior on the fullness of the muscle. Remember that the fat layer may be thick, and the muscle layer is about 2-4 inches.
Test direction:	From sacrum and diagonally laterally across the buttock.

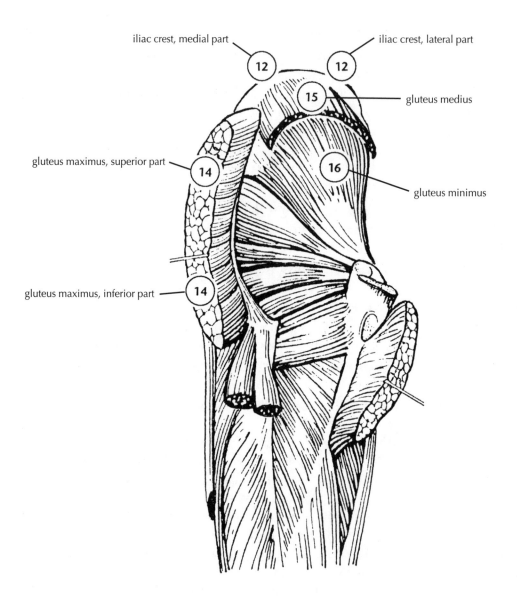

iliac crest, medial part — **12**

iliac crest, lateral part — **12**

15 — gluteus medius

gluteus maximus, superior part — **14**

16 — gluteus minimus

gluteus maximus, inferior part — **14**

Deep muscles of the hip, right side,
dorsal view

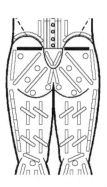

Name:	**Gluteus medius**	Number: 15

Origin:	Iliac crest; ilium between superior and middle gluteal lines.
Insertion:	Greater trochanter of femur.
Anatomical function:	Abducts, rotates thigh medially and laterally, assists in flexion and extension of the hip joint.
Map:	Is found on the edge of the hip bone and one inch below the lateral aspect of the iliac crest, laterally to gluteus maximus.
Is contracted by:	Moving the leg to the side (abducting).
Character structure(s):	LOVE/SEXUALITY
Ego function:	CENTERING, (b) filling out from the inside.
Psychological function:	Letting sensuality/sexuality fill while staying centered.
Ego function:	PATTERNS OF INTERPERSONAL SKILLS, (g) taking on chores (assignments).
Psychological function:	Ability to join/engage in tasks related to gender role.
Ego function:	GENDER SKILLS, (b) experience of gender. (c) experience of gender role. (e) manifestation of sensuality and sexuality.
Psychological function:	(b) to be conscious of one's gender. (c) to be conscious of one's gender role. (e) ability to manifest one's gender identity.
Child's developmental stage/age:	The child is able to stand on one leg, move the other in all directions, and rotate more with pelvis while walking. At the end of this stage the child is able to use a hula hoop.

Bodymapping:

Client's position:	On the stomach.
Tester's position:	Opposite the side that is tested.
Activation in test position:	Move the leg to the side along the mat/floor (abduction). Lift the leg slightly from the mat/floor. Give resistance to the movement if necessary.
Test location:	Find the iliac crest and move fingers caudally and laterally, separated from gluteus maximus.
Test direction:	Inferiorly (caudally)/laterally.

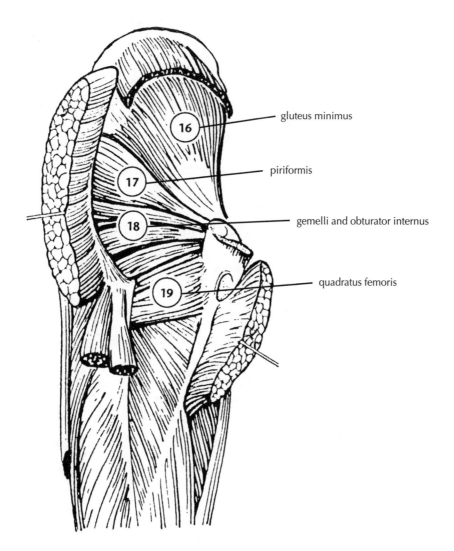

gluteus minimus

piriformis

gemelli and obturator internus

quadratus femoris

Deep muscles of the hip, right side,
dorsal view

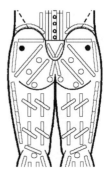

Name:	**Gluteus minimus**	Number: 16

Origin:	Posterior ilium between middle and inferior gluteal lines.
Insertion:	Anterior surface of greater trochanter of femur.
Anatomical function:	Abducts, rotates thigh medially and laterally, assists in flexion and extension of the hip joint.
Map:	Is found caudally to gluteus medius and deep to gluteus maximus and to gluteus medius.
Is contracted by:	Medially rotate the leg in the hip joint so the big toe turns toward the other leg.
Character structure(s):	WILL
Ego function:	CENTERING, (b) filling out from the inside.
Psychological function:	Using the emotions and the action-energy from one's center.
Ego function:	PATTERNS OF INTERPERSONAL SKILLS, (g) taking on chores (assignments).
Psychological function:	Ability to do things with delayed gratification of one's own needs.
Ego function:	GENDER SKILLS, (b) experience of gender.
Psychological function:	Physical sensation of one's gender and containment of being a boy or a girl.
Child's developmental stage/age:	The child brings foot position to parallel from being turned out during the autonomy stage. The ability to push off through the foot begins at this age. Takes part in rotation of the hip joint while walking, while standing on one leg and lifting the other leg out laterally, while walking on a broad tree trunk, and when changing direction.

Bodymapping:

Client's position:	On the stomach.
Tester's position:	Opposite the side that is tested.
Activation in test position:	Medially rotate the leg in the hip joint.
Test location:	Locate inferiorly to gluteus medius, and test deeply to find the muscle fibers that medially rotate.
Test direction:	Inferiorly (caudally).

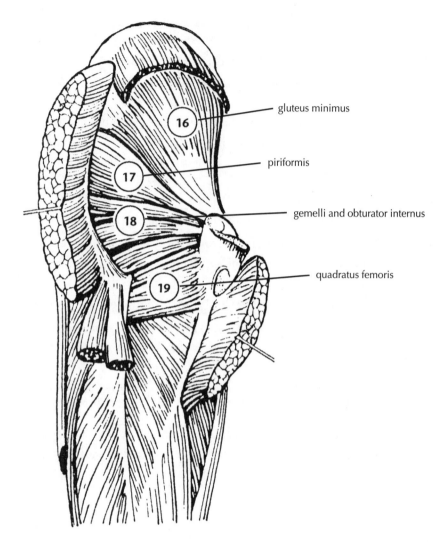

gluteus minimus

piriformis

gemelli and obturator internus

quadratus femoris

Deep muscles of the hip, right side,
dorsal view

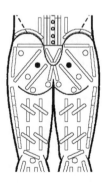

Name:	**Piriformis**	Number: 17

Origin:	Anterior surface of sacrum.
Insertion:	Greater trochanter of femur.
Anatomical function:	Abducts, extends, and laterally rotates thigh at the hip joint. Is able to pull the sacrum forward.
Map:	Is found in the third layer deep to gluteus maximus and gluteus medius, and caudally to gluteus minimus.
Is contracted by:	Standing or sitting position: bend slightly in the knee, place the big toe on the floor, turn the knee laterally from the hip joint.
Character structure(s):	AUTONOMY
Ego function:	CENTERING, (b) filling out from the inside.
Psychological function:	Filling oneself with lust/desire and impulses.
Ego function:	GENDER SKILLS, (b) experience of gender.
Psychological function:	Consciousness of oneself and one's gender.
Child's developmental stage/age:	The muscle takes part in creeping and crawling when the child pulls the leg up and forward and also slightly laterally, allowing the "tail" to wag slightly in the movement. Crawling with a lifted "tail" makes it possible to follow impulses of delight and curiosity.

Bodymapping:	
Client's position:	On the stomach.
Tester's position:	Opposite the side that is tested.
Activation in test position:	Bend slightly in the knee and pull the leg up, or rotate laterally in the hip joint (creeping movement).
Test location:	Between greater trochanter and the middle part of the edge of the sacrum.
Test direction:	Inferiorly (caudally), laterally.

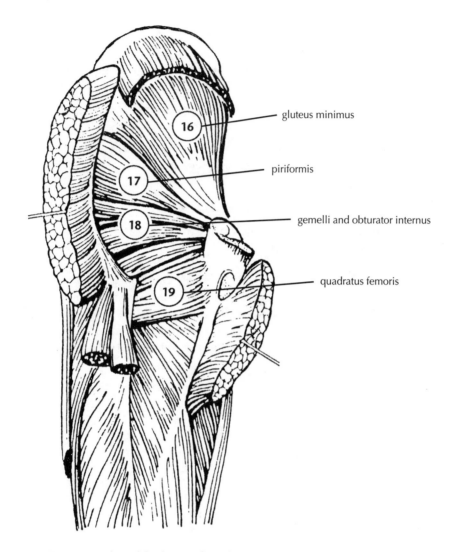

gluteus minimus — 16

piriformis — 17

gemelli and obturator internus — 18

quadratus femoris — 19

Deep muscles of the hip, right side,
dorsal view

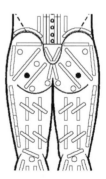

Name:	**Gemelli and obturator internus**	**Number: 18**

Origin:	Ischium; internal surface of obturator foramen.
Insertion:	Greater trochanter of femur–medial surface.
Anatomical function:	Laterally rotates thigh at the hip joint; assists in adduction and abduction of the hip joint.
Map:	Are found one inch caudally to piriformis and deep to gluteus maximus halfway along the horizontal line between coccyx and the greater trochanter.
Is contracted by:	Turning the leg laterally at the hip joint. Sitting and standing position: Place heel on the floor, push off slightly so the body rolls over on the opposite ischial tuberosity, or turn the leg laterally. Focus close to the ischial tuberosity.
Character structure(s):	NEED
Ego function:	CENTERING, (b) filling out from the inside.
Psychological function:	Allow yourself to fill up with your needs.
Ego function:	MANAGEMENT OF ENERGY, (e) containment of sensuality.
Psychological function:	Contain sensuality and sexuality/passion.
Ego function:	GENDER SKILLS, (d) containment of sensuality and sexuality.
Psychological function:	Contain sensuality and sexuality/passion.
Child's developmental stage/age:	The muscles take part in the first attempts at crawling (creeping); when the child rolls with delight or moves closer toward something that she needs.

Bodymapping:

Client's position:	On the stomach.
Tester's position:	Opposite the side that is tested.
Activation in test position:	Rotate leg laterally in the hip joint.
Test location:	Move the fingers distally from the test location for piriformis, between the ischial tuberosity and the greater trochanter, horizontally with the coccyx.
Test direction:	Inferiorly (caudally), laterally.

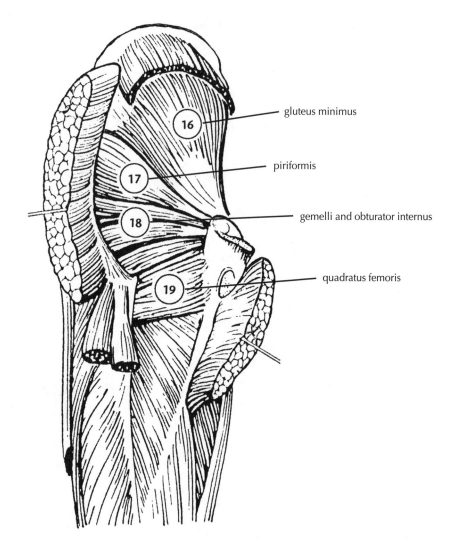

gluteus minimus — 16

piriformis — 17

gemelli and obturator internus — 18

quadratus femoris — 19

Deep muscles of the hip, right side,
dorsal view

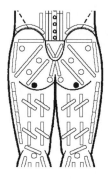

Name:	**Quadratus femoris**	Number: 19

Origin:	Ischial tuberosity.
Insertion:	Tubercle of femur, posterior aspect of greater trochanter.
Anatomical function:	Laterally rotates and adducts thigh in the hip joint.
Map:	Is found between greater trochanter and ischial tuberosity and deep to the distal gluteal fold.
Is contracted by:	Rotating the stretched leg laterally in the hip joint; tucking the tailbone in between the legs.
Character structure(s):	WILL
Ego function:	CENTERING, (b) filling out from the inside.
Psychological function:	Holding onto or keeping the sensation of oneself as being OK, even if one has acted in a wrong way.
Ego function:	MANAGEMENT OF ENERGY, (b) containment of high-level energy.
Psychological function:	Ability to build up high energy (containment of all emotions, including shame and anger).
Child's developmental stage/age:	The muscle enables the child to change direction while walking. Pelvis is free, "tail" is lifted (instead of stuck/locked).

Bodymapping:

Client's position:	On the stomach.
Tester's position:	Opposite the side that is tested.
Activation in test position:	Rotate laterally in the hip joint.
Test location:	Between greater trochanter and ischial tuberosity and superiorly and deep to the distal gluteal fold.
Test direction:	Laterally and inferiorly (caudally).

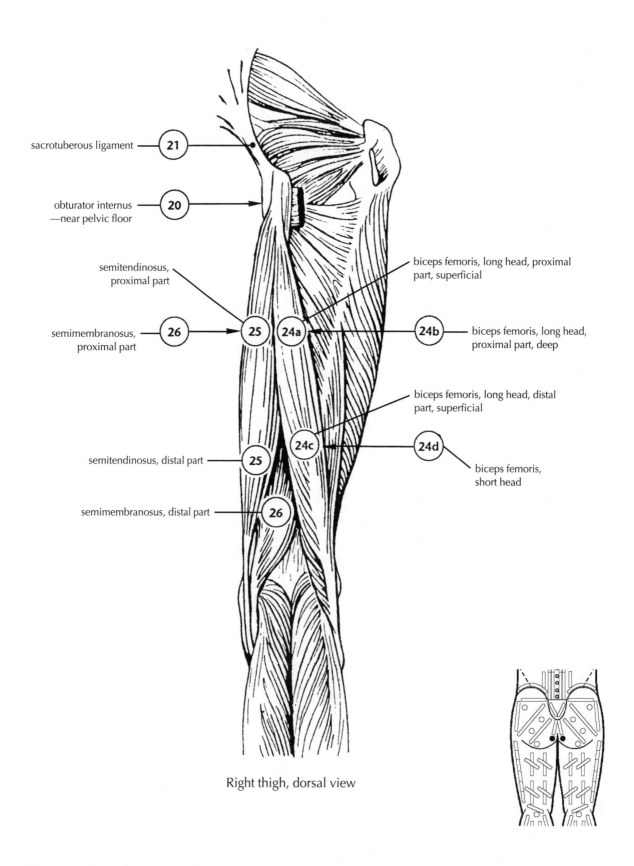

sacrotuberous ligament — ㉑ →

obturator internus —near pelvic floor — ⑳ →

semitendinosus, proximal part

semimembranosus, proximal part — ㉖ → ㉕ ㉔ₐ ← ㉔ᵦ — biceps femoris, long head, proximal part, superficial

biceps femoris, long head, proximal part, deep

biceps femoris, long head, distal part, superficial

semitendinosus, distal part — ㉕

㉔c ㉔d — biceps femoris, short head

semimembranosus, distal part — ㉖

Right thigh, dorsal view

	The part of the muscle medially to ischial tuberosity, near pelvic floor.
Origin:	Internal pelvic surface of obturator membrane and surrounding bones.
Insertion:	Trochanteric fossa.
Anatomical function:	Laterally rotates the leg at the hip joint.
Map:	Is found medial to the ischial tuberosity; continues through obturator foramen into the pelvis.
Is contracted by:	Turning the leg laterally at the hip joint with a focus on the ischial tuberosity.
Character structure(s):	AUTONOMY
Ego function:	CENTERING, (b) filling out from the inside.
Psychological function:	Experience ownership of one's own impulses.
Ego function:	MANAGEMENT OF ENERGY, (b) containment of high-level energy. (e) containment of sensuality.
Psychological function:	Contain impulses of desire and sensuality, and be conscious of giving and holding back.
Child's developmental stage/age:	The muscle takes part in conscious learning of the functions of moving the bowels and urinating.

Bodymapping:

Client's position:	On the stomach.
Tester's position:	Opposite the side that is tested.
Activation in test position:	Rotate the leg laterally.
Test location:	Find the ischial tuberosity, move fingers medially to it, pull the skin along and around the ischial tuberosity, and test the muscle underneath the skin.
Test direction:	Around laterally in circles, inferiorly (caudally).

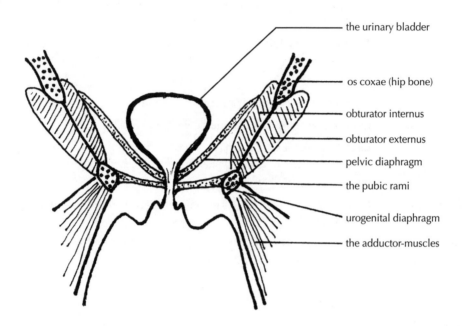

the urinary bladder

os coxae (hip bone)

obturator internus

obturator externus

pelvic diaphragm

the pubic rami

urogenital diaphragm

the adductor-muscles

	Pelvic diaphragm: coccygeus, sphincter ani externus, levator ani, urogenital diaphragm.
Origin:	Pelvic diaphragm is bowl-shaped, formed by coccygeus and levator ani. The edges of the bowl are inserted to the internal surface of the true pelvis, to the lower edge of pubic symphysis in front and posteriorly to the point of the coccyx.
Insertion:	Sphincter ani externus: ring-shaped muscle fibers around the anus below the pelvic diaphragm. Urogenital diaphragm: a triangular fibrous-muscular sheet stretched between the ischiopubic rami and symphysis pubis; the posterior edge lies just in front of the anus.
Anatomical function:	Coccygeus: strengthens pelvic floor together with sacrotuberous ligament. Levator ani: supports and lifts pelvic floor. Sphincter ani externus: closes anus. Urogenital diaphragm: closes and supports the urogenital opening and maintains the openings to urethra and vagina.
Map:	These muscles are found in the "saddle area" of the body between the coccyx, pubis, and the ischial tuberosities.
Is contracted by:	Tightening the openings in the "saddle area," the anus and urethra.
Character structure(s):	Coccygeus: NEED Sphincter ani externus: WILL Levator ani: AUTONOMY Urogenital diaphragm: LOVE/SEXUALITY
Ego function:	MANAGEMENT OF ENERGY, (b) containment of high-level energy.
Psychological function:	Contain high levels of energies–trying to preserve the floor or release the floor of the pelvis. NEED: creates the bottom of the pelvis, raises the energy–ability to administer energy of desire or energy of fear (wag the tail or turn the tail between the legs). AUT: master emotions. WILL: let go of and hold back what comes from oneself. LOVE/SEX: master the energy around sensuality and sexuality.
Ego function:	GENDER SKILLS, (b) experience of gender.
Psychological function:	Sensation of pleasure/lust (goes for all four character structures).
Shock:	In shock, the sphincter muscles release or collapse if one goes "dead"/is paralyzed–the muscles hold back/retain as long as one acts (reflex system).
Child's developmental stage/age:	NEED: the child's legs, which have been flexed, now start extending/stretching out and rotating in the hip joint, beginning to have an awareness of sensation in the muscles. AUT: the pelvic diaphragm is a floor to contain the emotions/feelings; the child is able to sense when the diaper is full, sense peeing and bowel movements, and he starts sensing the private parts. WILL: control of sphincters begins. LOVE/SEX: sensation of lust energy around the private parts (and when peeing) and by looking at others' private parts and playing "doctor."

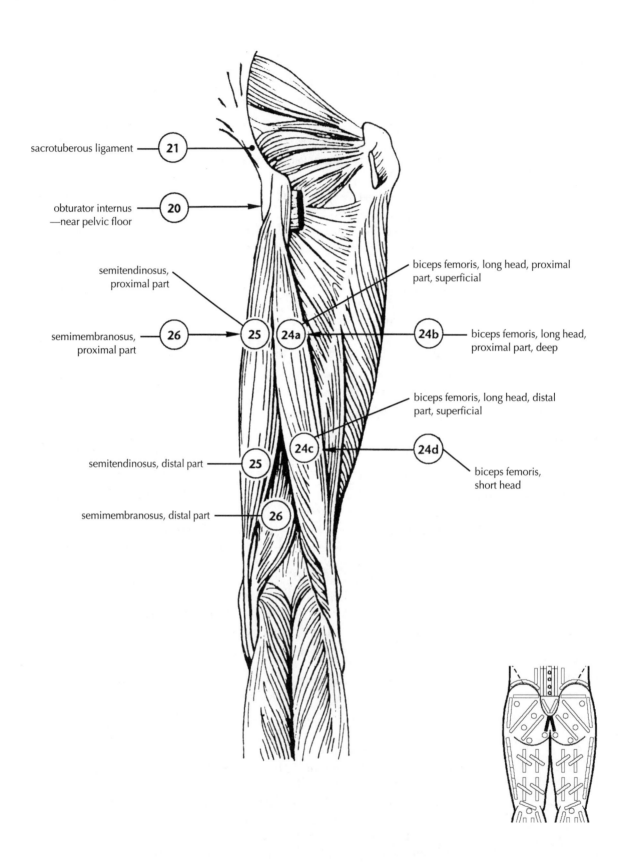

sacrotuberous ligament — **21**

obturator internus
—near pelvic floor — **20**

semitendinosus,
proximal part

semimembranosus, — **26** → **25** **24a**
proximal part

biceps femoris, long head, proximal
part, superficial

24b — biceps femoris, long head,
proximal part, deep

biceps femoris, long head, distal
part, superficial

semitendinosus, distal part — **25**

24c **24d**

biceps femoris,
short head

semimembranosus, distal part — **26**

Name:	Sacrotuberous ligament	Number: 21

Origin:	Middle of ischium.
Insertion:	Sacrum and ilium.
Anatomical function:	The ligament is connected to the origins of erector spinae, is part of the origins of gluteus maximus, and is connected to the hamstring muscles. It is part of the reflex-system that keeps the body upright both in standing and sitting position.
Map:	Is found between ischial tuberosity and the edge of sacrum.
Is contracted by:	
Character structure(s):	PERINATAL–EXISTENCE
Ego function:	CENTERING, (b) filling out from the inside.
Psychological function:	PERINATAL: fundamental experience of right to be filled by using one's total power/energy. EX: the right to exist and the right to mutual connection is taken for granted/with complete naturalness.
Ego function:	SOCIAL BALANCE, (e) balance of managing stress and resolving it.
Psychological function:	PERINATAL: ability to tolerate stress and to maneuver oneself out of stress (birth). EX: ability of combining spiritual and physical energy.
Child's developmental stage/age:	During birth, the sacrotuberous ligament is part of the stretching reflex during second-stage labor, when the child pushes from the heels.
Bodymapping:	
Client's position:	On the stomach.
Tester's position:	Opposite the side that is tested.
Activation in test position:	
Test location:	Test between sacrum and ischial tuberosity; test for the overall impression of the ligament and the fibers of the origins of gluteus maximus.
Test direction:	Laterally and inferiorly (caudally).

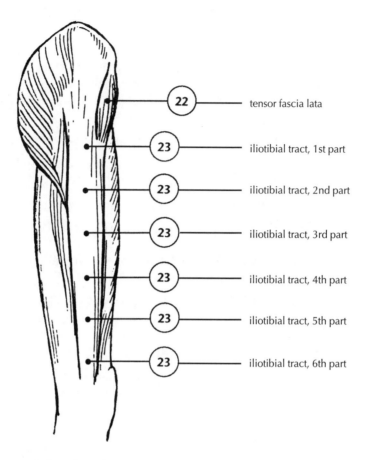

22 — tensor fascia lata

23 — iliotibial tract, 1st part

23 — iliotibial tract, 2nd part

23 — iliotibial tract, 3rd part

23 — iliotibial tract, 4th part

23 — iliotibial tract, 5th part

23 — iliotibial tract, 6th part

Right hip, lateral view

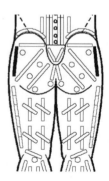

Name:	**Tensor fascia lata**	Number: 22

Origin:	Iliac crest, just posterior to anterior superior iliac spine.
Insertion:	Iliotibial tract, which attaches to lateral condyle of tibia.
Anatomical function:	Medial rotation and flexion of hip joint The iliotibial tract permits both gluteus maximus and tensor fascia lata to stabilize the extended knee.
Map:	Is found just posterior and inferior to the anterior superior iliac spine.
Is contracted by:	Rotating the leg medially in the hip joint.
Character structure(s):	NEED
Ego function:	SOCIAL BALANCE, (b) degree of pulling oneself together/letting go.
Psychological function:	Self-regulating of one's own needs.
Ego function:	MANAGEMENT OF ENERGY, (c) self-containment.
Psychological function:	Mastering the building up of needs.
Child's developmental stage/age:	The muscle is active when the child is rolling and creeping; also when getting up into a sitting position from a lying position.

Bodymapping:

Client's position:	On the back or on the stomach.
Tester's position:	On the side that is tested.
Activation in test position:	On the back: rotate the leg medially in the hip joint. On the stomach: press the knee in the floor/mat, or move the leg laterally with the heel laterally.
Test location:	Find the edge of the hip bone and anterior superior iliac spine, move the hand inferiorly, laterally, and test where the belly of the muscle is full.
Test direction:	Inferiorly (caudally).

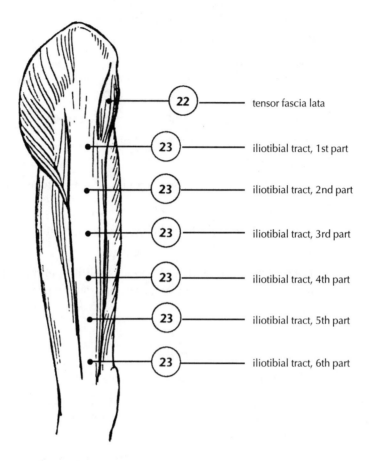

22	tensor fascia lata
23	iliotibial tract, 1st part
23	iliotibial tract, 2nd part
23	iliotibial tract, 3rd part
23	iliotibial tract, 4th part
23	iliotibial tract, 5th part
23	iliotibial tract, 6th part

Right hip, lateral view

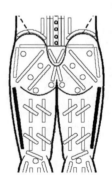

Name:	Iliotibial tract	Number: 23

Origin:	Iliac crest.
Insertion:	Lateral condyle of tibia.
Anatomical function:	The tract is the area for insertion of tensor fascia lata and parts of gluteus maximus. Helps keep the muscles of the leg together; assists in tightening the large fascia system around the leg as a "stocking"; works together with these muscles and affects the mobility in the hip joint and the knee joint, among others, by stabilizing the extended knee.
Map:	Is found from the iliac crest of the femur to the knee joint; along the outside of the thigh as a strengthening in fascia lata (the fasciae of the thigh).
Is contracted by:	Turning the leg laterally and backward in the hip joint; activate tensor fascia lata or gluteus maximus.
Character structure(s):	1st part: AUTONOMY 2nd part: WILL 3rd part: LOVE/SEXUALITY 4th part: OPINIONS 5th part: SOLIDARITY/PERFORMANCE 6th part: PUBERTY
Ego function:	SOCIAL BALANCE, (b) degree of pulling oneself together/letting go. MANAGEMENT OF ENERGY, (c) self-containment.
Psychological function:	AUT: containing oneself in proportion to desire impulses, ideas, and emotions. WILL: containing oneself in proportion to emotions, action impulses, and extrasensory perception. LOVE/SEX: in proportion to the rising of sexual and sensual energy. OPINIONS: in proportion to thoughts, feelings, and opinion formations. SOL/PERF: in proportion to solidarity and performance (release the contact to be able to perform/release oneself to be able to show solidarity). PUB: in proportion to goal in life, group, individuality, philosophical and spiritual thoughts.
Child's developmental stage/age:	The movements of the leg/knee get stronger and more precise as the child gets older/along in age.

Bodymapping:

Client's position:	On the back, or on the stomach.
Tester's position:	On the side that is tested.
Activation in test position:	Activate either tensor fascia lata or gluteus maximus.
Test location:	From the greater trochanter to the knee joint, place the hand in the middle. Test three locations superior to the hand and three locations inferior to the hand.
Test direction:	Inferiorly (caudally).

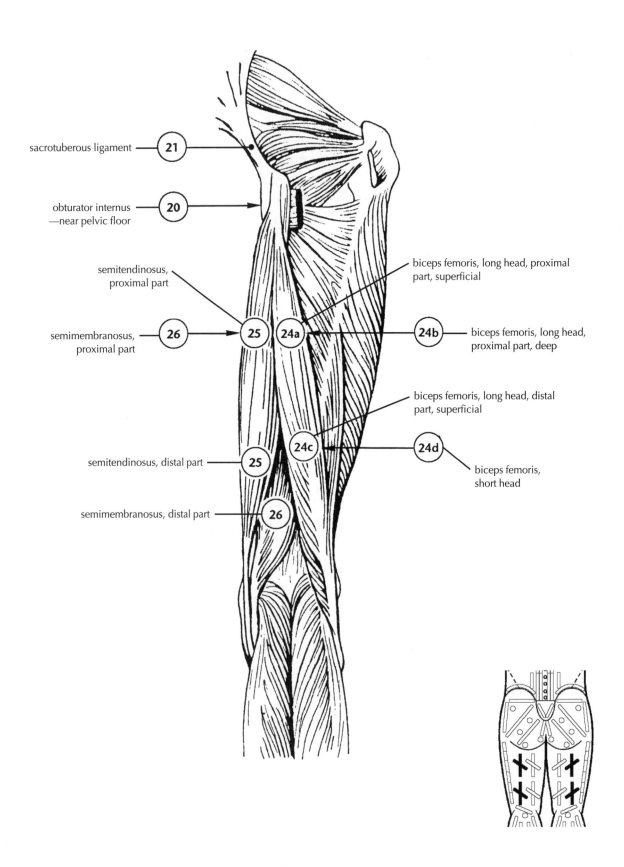

sacrotuberous ligament — (21)

obturator internus
—near pelvic floor — (20)

semitendinosus,
proximal part — (25)

semimembranosus, — (26) → (25) (24a)
proximal part

biceps femoris, long head, proximal
part, superficial

(24b) — biceps femoris, long head,
proximal part, deep

biceps femoris, long head, distal
part, superficial

semitendinosus, distal part — (25) (24c) (24d)

biceps femoris,
short head

semimembranosus, distal part — (26)

Name:	Biceps femoris (lateral hamstring)	Number: 24a, b, c, d

Origin:	Long head: ischial tuberosity. Short head: linea aspera on posterior shaft of femur.
Insertion:	Head of fibula, lateral condyle of tibia.
Anatomical function:	Long head and short head: laterally rotate and flex the knee joint. Long head also extends and assists in lateral rotation of the hip joint.
Map:	Is found posterior-laterally on the back of the thigh running from the ischial tuberosity to the lateral side of the knee. The tendon forms the lateral border of the hollow of the knee.
Is contracted by:	Extending the hip joint (proximal part), and flexing the knee joint (distal part).
Character structure(s):	(a) Long head, proximal part, superficial: OPINIONS (b) Long head, proximal part, deep: WILL (c) Long head, distal part, superficial: SOLIDARITY/PERFORMANCE (d) Short head: LOVE/SEXUALITY
Ego function:	POSITIONING, (b) staying power.
Psychological function:	OPINIONS: combining feelings and thoughts while forming opinions. WILL: using one's emotions and will to stay in power. SOL/PERF: making one's performance and solidarity become visible. LOVE/SEX: making one's sensual and sexual attractions become visible.
Ego function:	SELF-ASSERTION, (c) forward momentum and sense of direction.
Psychological function:	OPINIONS: being able to state one's opinions and then change them if new information is introduced. WILL: able to change direction while keeping the goal in mind. SOL/PERF: step out with one's performance and solidarity. LOVE/SEX: act on one's sensual and sexual attractions.
Ego function:	24 (d): Short head. GENDER SKILLS, (e) manifestation of sensuality and sexuality.
Psychological function:	LOVE/SEX: Ability to manifest and act on one's sensuality and sexuality.
Child's developmental stage/age:	This muscle takes part in the push-off in walking, running, bouncing, and jumping. OPINIONS: long jumps and push-off with the big toe. WILL: bouncing forward and push-off in the ankle joint. SOL/PERF: triple jump/skipping, push-off from big toe and breadth of foot. LOVE/SEX: hop on one foot and push off with the four lateral toes.

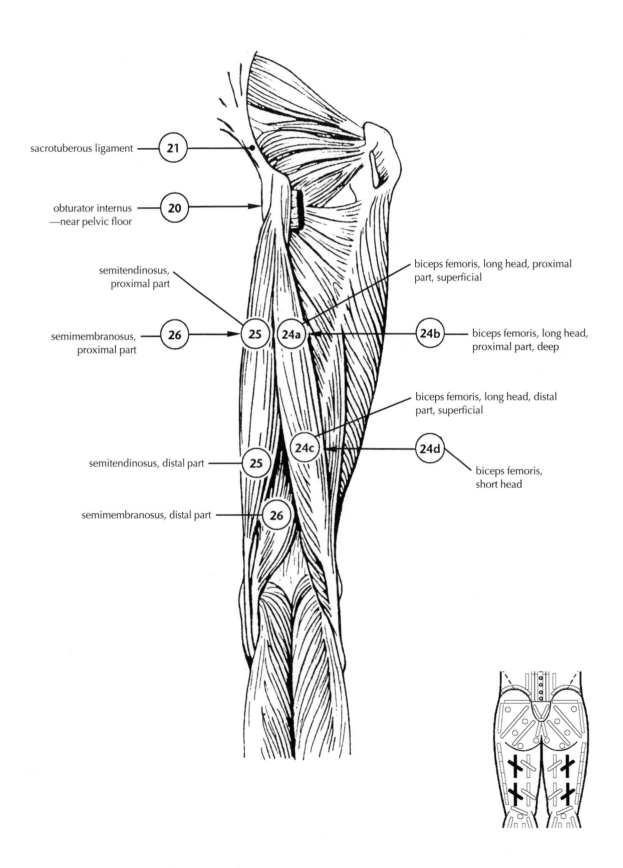

sacrotuberous ligament — **21**

obturator internus
—near pelvic floor — **20**

semitendinosus,
proximal part

semimembranosus,
proximal part — **26** → **25** **24a**

biceps femoris, long head, proximal
part, superficial

24b — biceps femoris, long head,
proximal part, deep

biceps femoris, long head, distal
part, superficial

semitendinosus, distal part — **25**

24c **24d**

biceps femoris,
short head

semimembranosus, distal part — **26**

Name:	Biceps femoris (lateral hamstring)	Number: 24a, b, c, d

Bodymapping:

Client's position:	On the stomach.
Tester's position:	By the leg that is tested.
Activation in test position:	Bend the knee and lift the leg simultaneously, toes turned out.
Test location:	Find the separation of vastus lateralis by stretching the knee.
	Find ischial tuberosity, and bend the knee to find the tendon at the hollow of the knee.
	Follow the muscle proximally.
	(a) + (b) Long head, proximal part is tested superficially and deeply.
	(c) Long head, distal part is tested superficially.
	(d) Short head is tested by pressing/going in laterally and deeply (bend the knee passively if necessary).
Test direction:	Distally.

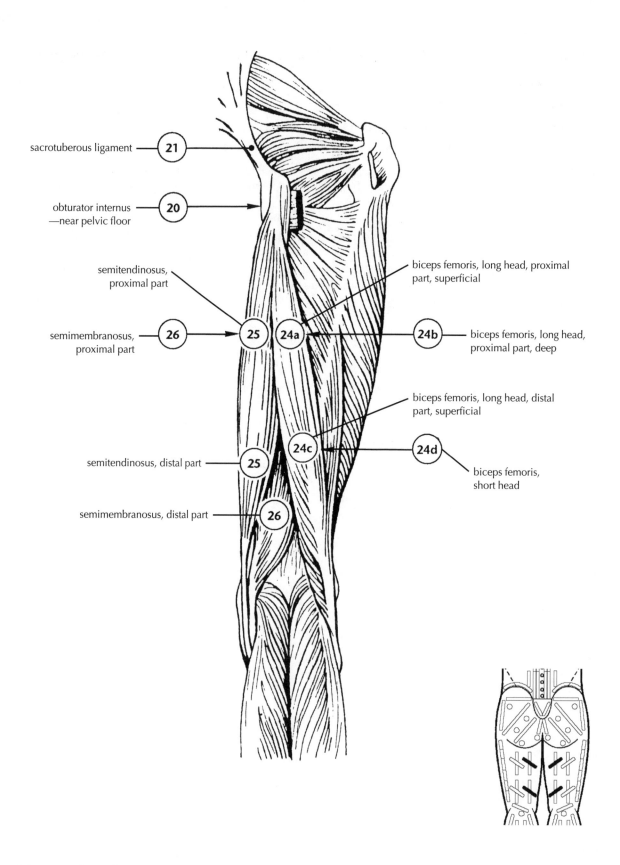

sacrotuberous ligament — **21**

obturator internus — **20**
—near pelvic floor

semitendinosus, — **25**
proximal part

semimembranosus, — **26** — **25** — **24a**
proximal part

biceps femoris, long head, proximal part, superficial

24b — biceps femoris, long head, proximal part, deep

biceps femoris, long head, distal part, superficial

semitendinosus, distal part — **25**

24c — **24d**

biceps femoris, short head

semimembranosus, distal part — **26**

Name:	**Semitendinosus (medial hamstring)**	**Number: 25**
Origin:	Ischial tuberosity.	
Insertion:	Proximal part of the medial (anterior) tibial shaft.	
Anatomical function:	Hip joint: extends and assists in medial rotation. Knee joint: flexes and medially rotates the flexed knee (toes in).	
Map:	Is found posterior-medially on the back of the thigh, running from the ischial tuberosity to the medial side of the knee; its tendon forms the medial border of the hollow of the knee.	
Is contracted by:	Extending the hip joint (proximal part); flexing the knee joint (distal part).	
Character structure(s):	Proximal part: WILL Distal part: OPINIONS	
Ego function:	POSITIONING, (b) staying power.	
Psychological function:	WILL: add power and will to one's choice. OPINIONS: form opinions.	
Ego function:	SELF-ASSERTION, (c) forward momentum and sense of direction.	
Psychological function:	WILL: go for one's choice. OPINIONS: coming forward and stating one's opinions and one's points of view.	
Child's developmental stage/age:	WILL: push-off in walking and jumping (up). OPINIONS: push-off in jumping over a rope; game called "the grass grows."	

Bodymapping:	
Client's position:	On the stomach.
Tester's position:	By the leg that is tested.
Activation in test position:	Bend the knee joint with the toes in.
Test location:	Find the ischial tuberosity and the tendon at the hollow of the knee. Test proximally and distally in different locations along the muscle.
Test direction:	Distally.

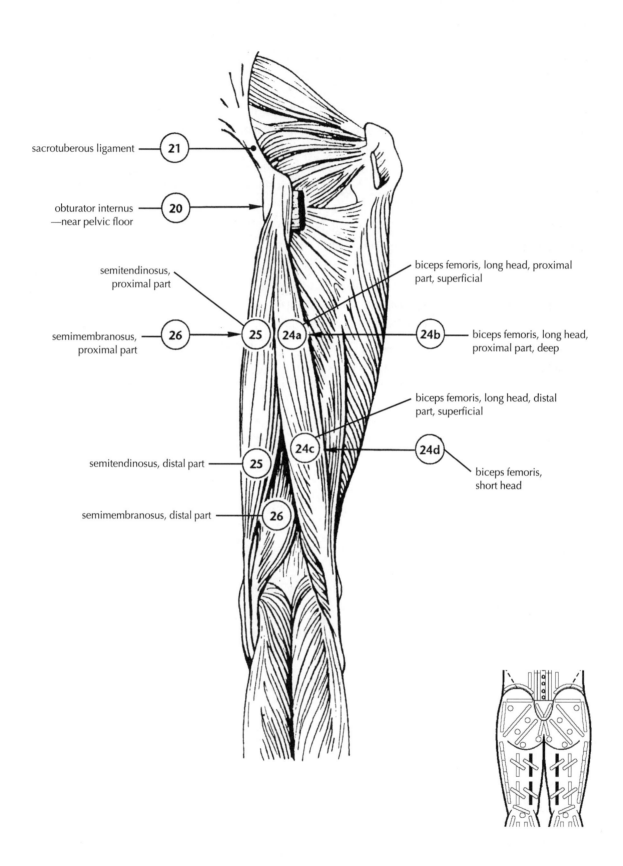

sacrotuberous ligament — 21

obturator internus
—near pelvic floor — 20

semitendinosus,
proximal part

semimembranosus,
proximal part — 26 → 25 24a

biceps femoris, long head, proximal
part, superficial

24b — biceps femoris, long head,
proximal part, deep

biceps femoris, long head, distal
part, superficial

24c

24d — biceps femoris,
short head

semitendinosus, distal part — 25

semimembranosus, distal part — 26

Name:	**Semimembranosus (medial hamstring)**	Number: 26

Origin:	Ischial tuberosity.
Insertion:	Posterior medial tibial condyle.
Anatomical function:	Hip joint: extends and assists in medial rotation. Knee joint: flexes and medially rotates the flexed knee.
Map:	Is found posterior-medially on the back of the thigh running from ischial tuberosity to the medial side of the knee. Superiorly it lies deep to semitendinosus, and inferiorly it lies superficially.
Is contracted by:	Extending the hip joint (proximal part); flexing the knee (distal part).
Character structure(s):	Proximal part: NEED Distal part: AUTONOMY
Ego function:	POSITIONING, (b) staying power.
Psychological function:	NEED: want to have what one needs. AUT: keep (maintain) one's curiosity and stay activated.
Ego function:	SELF-ASSERTION, (c) forward momentum and sense of direction.
Psychological function:	NEED: move toward what one needs. AUT: move forward, driven by curiosity.
Child's developmental stage/age:	Stand and walk/go forward, stay activated no matter what happens.

Bodymapping:

Client's position:	On the stomach.
Tester's position:	By the leg that is tested.
Activation in test position:	Bend knee joint with the heel turned out (toes in).
Test location:	Find ischial tuberosity and the tendons at the back of the knee. Test proximally, deep to semitendinosus; and test distally, laterally to semitendinosus, where semimembranosus is placed superficially.
Test direction:	Distally.

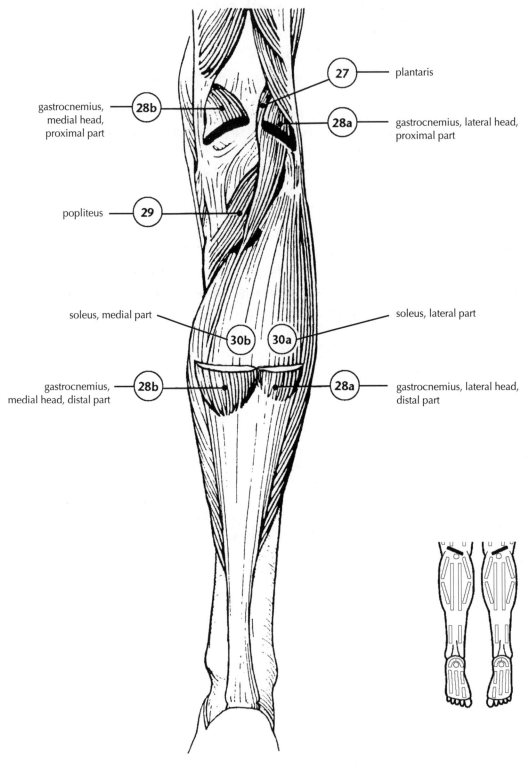

27 — plantaris

28b — gastrocnemius, medial head, proximal part

28a — gastrocnemius, lateral head, proximal part

29 — popliteus

soleus, medial part — 30b

30a — soleus, lateral part

28b — gastrocnemius, medial head, distal part

28a — gastrocnemius, lateral head, distal part

Right calf, dorsal view

Name:	**Plantaris**	Number: 27

Origin:	Lateral condyle and posterior aspect of femur.
Insertion:	Calcaneous via Achilles tendon.
Anatomical function:	With gastrocnemius, this muscle plantar flexes the ankle joint (points the foot) and assists in flexion of the knee joint. (A connection is made with the plantar fascia under the foot.)
Map:	Is found between the two heads of gastrocnemius (just above the joint line at the back of the knee). Plantaris lies medially to the lateral head of gastrocnemius, and the tendon continues all the way down to calcaneus.
Is contracted by:	Stretching fully in ankle joint as if jumping; or, resisting a push from the ball of the foot while curling the toes.
Character structure(s):	SOLIDARITY/PERFORMANCE
Ego function:	SOCIAL BALANCE, (e) balance of managing stress and resolving it.
Psychological function:	Contains stressful situations; experiences that it is possible to get through stressful situations.
Ego function:	MANAGEMENT OF ENERGY, (b) containment of high-level energy.
Psychological function:	Being flexible in staying or running away from threatening situations.
Child's developmental stage/age:	Running and jumping. Landing firmly (then you have tightened the arch of the foot) Fine tuning of different jumping techniques.
Shock:	Is related to jumping and running reflex, which is activated in shock.

Bodymapping:	
Client's position:	On the stomach.
Tester's position:	By the leg that is tested.
Activation in test position:	Support the client's knee so the ankle joint is free; stretch the foot out thoroughly while the knee remains passively flexed. Sometimes one only feels this muscle when it releases.
Test location:	Locate the lateral head of gastrocnemius, and test at the medial part of the origin (just above the joint line in the knee).
Test direction:	Distally in the direction of the fibers.

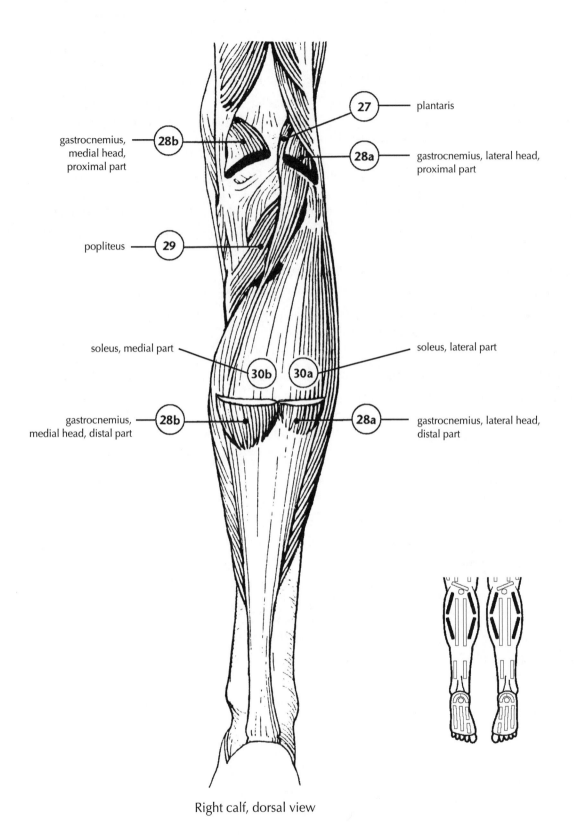

gastrocnemius, medial head, proximal part — **28b**

27 — plantaris

28a — gastrocnemius, lateral head, proximal part

popliteus — **29**

soleus, medial part — **30b**   **30a** — soleus, lateral part

gastrocnemius, medial head, distal part — **28b**   **28a** — gastrocnemius, lateral head, distal part

Right calf, dorsal view

Name:	Gastrocnemius	Number: 28a, b

Origin:	(a) Lateral head: lateral epicondyle of femur. (b) Medial head: medial epicondyle of femur.
Insertion:	Calcaneus via Achilles tendon.
Anatomical function:	Knee joint: flexes knee joint. Foot: plantar flexes the foot; medial head supinates the foot.
Map:	Is found superficially on the back of the leg from just above the knee joint line down to the Achilles tendon.
Is contracted by:	Standing on the toes, i.e., stretching the ankle joint while bending the knee slightly.
Character structure(s):	(a) Lateral head, proximal part: WILL distal part: OPINIONS (b) Medial head, proximal part: NEED distal part: AUTONOMY
Ego function:	SELF-ASSERTION, (a) self-assertion (manifesting one's power).
Psychological function:	(a) WILL: power behind action and choice. OPINIONS: strength behind opinions. (b) NEED: demand one's need to be fulfilled. AUT: assert one's independence.
Child's developmental stage/age:	(a) WILL: stamp. OPINIONS: karate kick with precision. (b) NEED: used in rolling when pushing off through the foot and ankle. AUT: push-off with the foot in creeping (together with flexor hallucis brevis) and in walking movements.

Bodymapping:

Client's position:	On the stomach.
Tester's position:	By the leg that is tested; support the client's leg so the ankle joint is free.
Activation in test position:	Palpate the whole muscle, differentiating it from the other muscles in the calf. Contract by pointing the foot; if necessary, give resistance on the sole of the foot.
Test location:	Test in two different locations on both heads of the muscle.
Test direction:	Distally.

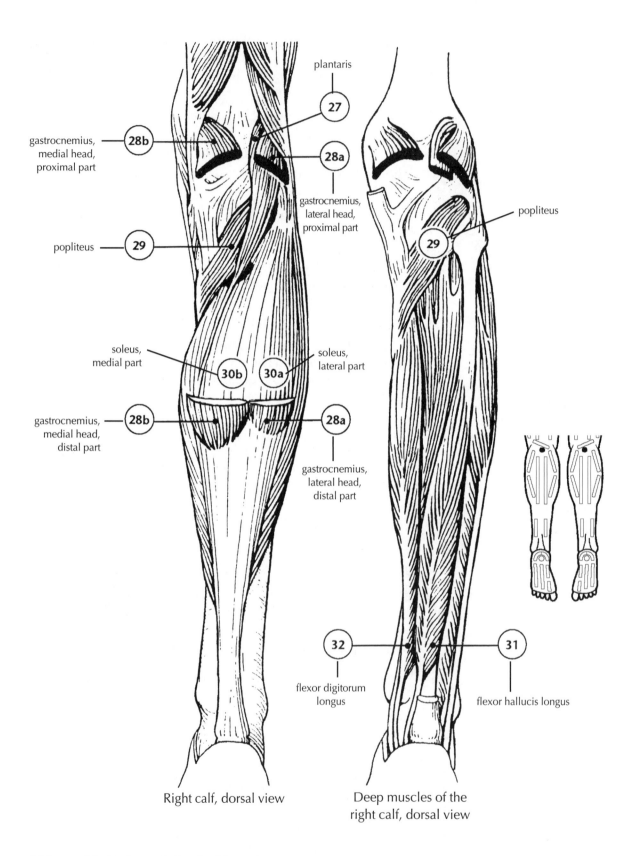

plantaris

27

gastrocnemius,
medial head,
proximal part

28b

28a

gastrocnemius,
lateral head,
proximal part

popliteus

29

popliteus

29

soleus,
medial part

30b

30a

soleus,
lateral part

gastrocnemius,
medial head,
distal part

28b

28a

gastrocnemius,
lateral head,
distal part

32

31

flexor digitorum
longus

flexor hallucis longus

Right calf, dorsal view

Deep muscles of the
right calf, dorsal view

Name:	**Popliteus**	Number: 29

Origin:	Lateral condyle of femur.
Insertion:	Posterior proximal tibial shaft.
Anatomical function:	Initiates knee flexion through medial rotation of the tibia to "unlock" the extended knee; the only muscle that "unlocks" the extended knee.
Map:	Is found proximally at the back of the knee between the heads of gastrocnemius, proximally to soleus.
Is contracted by:	The first bend in the knee joint from a locked knee. When the knee joint is bent, rotate the lower leg so the toes turn in.
Character structure(s):	OPINIONS
Ego function:	GROUNDING AND REALITY TESTING, (a) ability to stand one's ground, feel rooted and supported by it.
Psychological function:	Stand on the ground and sense its support; stick to one's opinions.
Ego function:	SOCIAL BALANCE, (e) balance of managing stress and resolving it.
Psychological function:	Ability to be realistic in stressful situations.
Ego function:	MANAGEMENT OF ENERGY, (b) containment of high-level energy.
Psychological function:	Preserve one's own ethics in high-level energy situations.
Child's developmental stage/age:	Stability and flexibility in the knee.
Shock:	In shock the muscle suddenly tightens up (hyper) and you collapse—or the muscle collapses (hypo) and you cannot move; the knees are not able to unlock.

Bodymapping:	
Client's position:	On the stomach.
Tester's position:	By the leg that is tested.
Activation in test position:	Bend knee 90 degrees; go deep and press firmly into the hollow of the knee between the two heads of gastrocnemius. Client medially rotates lower leg (big toe in).
Test location:	Proximally on the lower leg, between the two heads of gastrocnemius and proximally to soleus.
Test direction:	Distally, medially.

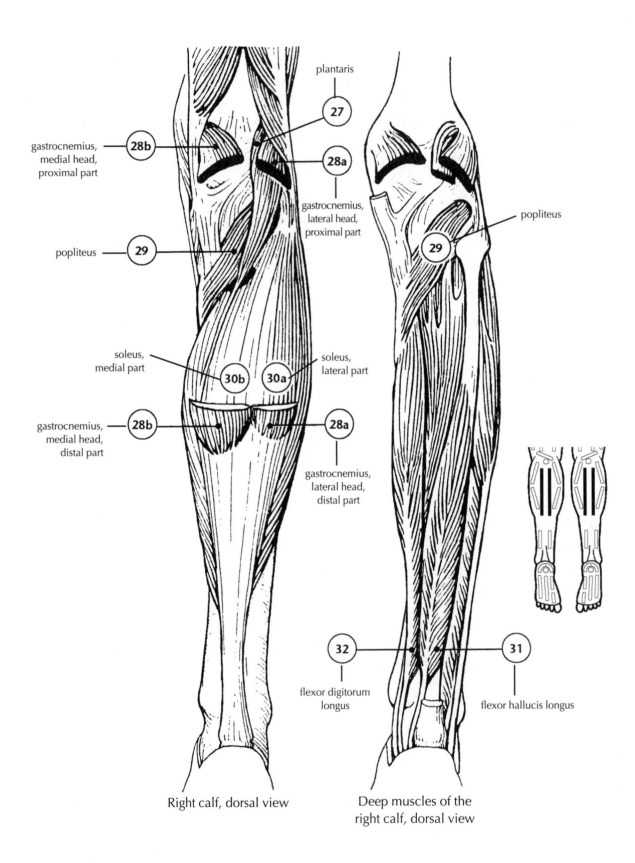

plantaris **27**

gastrocnemius, medial head, proximal part **28b**

28a gastrocnemius, lateral head, proximal part

popliteus **29**

popliteus

29

soleus, medial part **30b**   **30a** soleus, lateral part

gastrocnemius, medial head, distal part **28b**   **28a**

gastrocnemius, lateral head, distal part

32   **31**

flexor digitorum longus   flexor hallucis longus

Right calf, dorsal view

Deep muscles of the right calf, dorsal view

Name:	Soleus	Number: 30a, b

Origin:	Soleal line of tibia; posterior head and upper shaft of fibula.
Insertion:	Calcaneus via Achilles tendon.
Anatomical function:	Ankle joint: plantar flexion of the foot.
Map:	Is found deep to gastrocnemius; it is big and broad and superficial on either side of gastrocnemius.
Is contracted by:	Pointing the foot and ankle. Bending the knees and then standing on the toes (i.e., stretching the ankle joint).
Character structure(s):	a) Lateral part: AUTONOMY b) Medial part: NEED
Ego function:	POSITIONING, (c) standing on one's own.
Psychological function:	Maintain one's life energy (antigravity reflex). AUT: stand up for one's emotions and impulses. NEED: stand up for what one needs.
Child's developmental stage/age:	AUT: standing and walking. NEED: getting up into a standing position.

Bodymapping:

Client's position:	On the stomach.
Tester's position:	By the leg that is tested.
Activation in test position:	Is contracted by pointing the foot and ankle joint; if necessary bend knee slightly and give resistance under the foot.
Test location:	Locate soleus between the heads of gastrocnemius; move fingers laterally and test lateral part; go back to the middle and move medially to test medial part.
Test direction:	Distally, respectively laterally and medially.

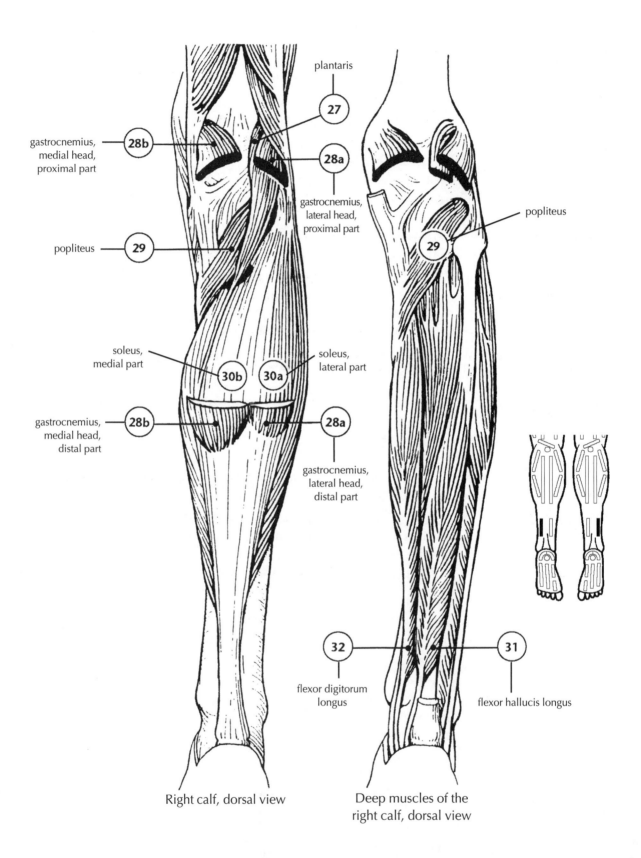

plantaris

27

gastrocnemius,
medial head,
proximal part

28b

28a

gastrocnemius,
lateral head,
proximal part

popliteus

29

popliteus

29

soleus,
medial part

30b

30a

soleus,
lateral part

gastrocnemius,
medial head,
distal part

28b

28a

gastrocnemius,
lateral head,
distal part

32

31

flexor digitorum
longus

flexor hallucis longus

Right calf, dorsal view

Deep muscles of the
right calf, dorsal view

Name:	**Flexor hallucis longus**	Number: 31

Origin:	Posterior fibula.
Insertion:	Distal phalanx of big toe (plantar surface).
Anatomical function:	Big toe: flexion. Ankle joint: assists with plantar flexion and supination (inversion) of the foot.
Map:	Is found in the calf deep to soleus and the Achilles tendon.
Is contracted by:	Press the big toe against the floor. Bend the big toe; lift the inner part of the sole of the foot if necessary so the weight of the foot leans on the outer edge of the foot (supinate).
Character structure(s):	WILL SOLIDARITY/PERFORMANCE
Ego function:	GROUNDING AND REALITY TESTING, (a) ability to stand one's ground, feel rooted and supported by it.
Psychological function:	To feel rooted and supported by the ground. WILL: ability to distinguish reality, fantasy, and extrasensory sensations. SOL/PERF: ability to preserve the sense of reality.
Ego function:	COGNITIVE SKILLS, (c) understanding (getting something well enough to go forward with it).
Psychological function:	WILL: make a choice once you have seen all the consequences. SOL/PERF: understand something well enough to stand up for it and come forward with it.
Ego function: Psychological function:	SELF-ASSERTION, (a) self-assertion (manifesting one's power). WILL: hold on to one's power. SOL/PERF: come forward with one's attitudes to life.
Child's developmental stage/age:	WILL: curl one's toes (hold on to the ground), pick up/collect things with the toes. The child jumps (starts to jump downward); starts to push off from the big toe. The muscle stabilizes in activities that require changing direction. SOL/PERF: the muscle is active in the final push off in walking.

Bodymapping:	
Client's position:	On the stomach.
Tester's position:	By the leg that is tested.
Activation in test position:	Support the ankle joint so it is relaxed and slightly bent; give resistance to the big toe in flexion—little movement, little resistance.
Test location:	Go deep from the lateral side of the Achilles tendon.
Test direction:	Distally.

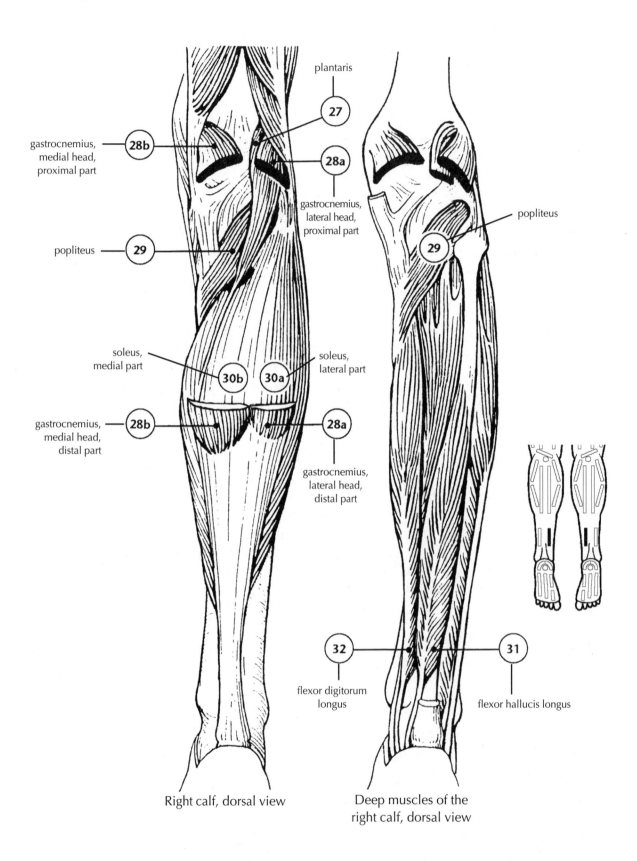

plantaris

27

gastrocnemius,
medial head,
proximal part

28b

28a

gastrocnemius,
lateral head,
proximal part

popliteus

29

popliteus

29

soleus,
medial part

30b

30a

soleus,
lateral part

gastrocnemius,
medial head,
distal part

28b

28a

gastrocnemius,
lateral head,
distal part

32

31

flexor digitorum
longus

flexor hallucis
longus

Right calf, dorsal view

Deep muscles of the
right calf, dorsal view

Name:	**Flexor digitorum longus**	Number: 32

Origin:	Posterior tibia.
Insertion:	Distal phalanges of the four lateral toes (plantar surface).
Anatomical function:	Toe joints: flexion of the four lateral toes. Ankle joint: assists with plantar flexion and supination of the foot.
Map:	Is found in the lower leg deep to soleus and the Achilles tendon.
Is contracted by:	Curling the toes; gripping the mat/floor.
Character structure(s):	NEED LOVE/SEXUALITY
Ego function:	GROUNDING AND REALITY TESTING, (a) ability to stand one's ground, feel rooted and supported by it.
Psychological function:	NEED: preserve the sensation of grounding and at the same time sense one's needs. LOVE/SEX: relate realistically to one's love fantasies.
Ego function:	COGNITIVE SKILLS, (c) understanding (getting something well enough to go forward with it).
Psychological function:	NEED: to feel and express one's needs. LOVE/SEX: to know, because of norms and values, that there are things you don't do (feeling embarrassed enough "to make your toes curl").
Ego function:	SELF-ASSERTION, (a) self-assertion (manifesting one's power).
Psychological function:	NEED: stand up for one's needs, make demands (claim one's rights). LOVE/SEX: have the courage to be vulnerable and show one's vulnerability.
Child's developmental stage/age:	NEED: both fingers and toes reflexively grasp when baby is feeding—originally a pumping reflex. LOVE/SEX: ability to curl the toes; be shy. Push off with the toes while walking. The child is fascinated by her toes and feet.

Bodymapping:

Client's position:	On the stomach.
Tester's position:	By the leg that is tested.
Activation in test position:	Rest foot and ankle on a pillow. Give resistance to flexion of the toes—little movement, little resistance.
Test location:	Go deep from the medial side of the Achilles tendon.
Test direction:	Distally.

Name:	Lumbricals	Number: *

Origin:	From the tendons of flexor digitorum longus.
Insertion:	Medial side of proximal phalanx of 2nd–5th toes.
Anatomical Function:	Flexion of the metatarsophalangeal joints.
Map:	Are found in second layer in the foot attached to the long flexor tendons of the four lateral toes.
Is contracted by:	Bending the four little toes; these muscles provide springiness/elasticity to the action of the foot.
Character structure(s):	SOLIDARITY/PERFORMANCE
Ego function:	SOCIAL BALANCE, (d) balancing sense of personal identity against being a group member.
Psychological function:	Balancing performing and being on equal terms at the same time.
Child's developmental stage/age:	Now the child has gained springiness in the foot and is able to bounce and spring with a push-off from the foot.

Name:	**Quadratus plantae**	**Number: ***

Origin:	Calcaneus.
Insertion:	Lateral side of the flexor digitorum longus tendon.
Anatomic function:	Flexes toes and supports the convexity of the sole of the foot.
Map:	Is found in the second layer in the convexity of the sole of the foot.
Is contracted by:	Flexing (curling) the four smaller toes toward the floor/mat.
Character structure(s):	LOVE/SEXUALITY
Ego function:	GROUNDING AND REALITY TESTING, (a) ability to stand one's ground, feel rooted and supported by it.
Psychological function:	Relate realistically to fantasy and dreams.
Child's developmental stage/age:	Stabilizes the convexity of the sole of the foot, providing the spring/elasticity required for jumping. When the child is playing fantasy games, he/she is still able to maintain a sense of his/her own reality, e.g., games like Batman, princess, and playing "house."

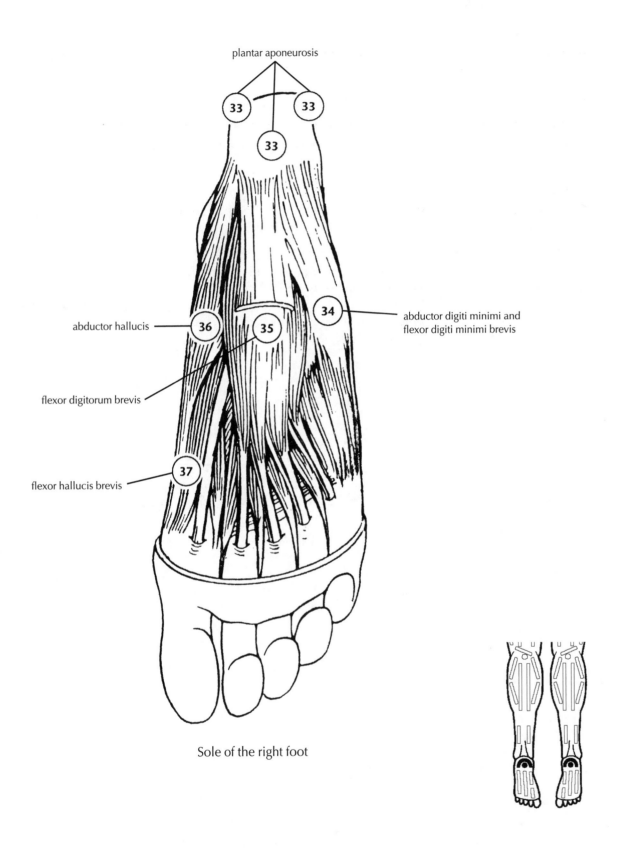

plantar aponeurosis

abductor digiti minimi and
flexor digiti minimi brevis

abductor hallucis

flexor digitorum brevis

flexor hallucis brevis

Sole of the right foot

The Bodynamic Psycho-Motor Anatomy

Name:	**Plantar aponeurosis**	Number: 33

Origin:	Calcaneus, plantar surface.
Insertion:	The bases of the five toes.
Anatomical function:	Supports the long arches under the foot. Holds the concavity in the sole of the foot. The arch may be tight or loose or flexible.
Map:	Is found as a tendon sheet in the sole of the foot connecting the calcaneus to the metatarsophalangeal joints.
Is contracted by:	Lift the heel or the toes from the floor/mat. Is contracted constantly during walking, being tightened through the action of the muscles and the mechanics in the walking movement.
Character structure(s):	PERINATAL
Ego function:	GROUNDING AND REALITY TESTING, (a) ability to stand one's ground, feel rooted and supported by it.
Psychological function:	A clear sensation of oneself as a physical person.
Ego function:	COGNITIVE SKILLS, (c) understanding (getting something well enough to go forward with it).
Psychological function:	Integration of intuitive sensations.
Ego function:	SELF-ASSERTION, (c) forward momentum and sense of direction.
Psychological function:	A deep sense of the right to come vigorously forward with oneself.
Child's developmental stage/age:	Extension reflex during birth. The child contacts with the heels of the mother's uterus and then starts extension of the legs. The beginning of the walking reflex.

Bodymapping:

Client's position:	On the stomach.
Tester's position:	By the foot that is tested; support and stabilize the foot.
Activation in test position:	
Test location:	First examine the hard skin, and note where and how much. Push the hard skin away and test the tissue on the side or under the heel in three different locations along the curve of the heel.
Test direction:	Toward the middle of the heel.

Name:	**Insertions of abductor, flexors, and extensors on proximal phalanx of the little toe** **Number:** *

Origin:

Insertion:

Anatomical function:

Map: Is found on the proximal phalanx of the little toe.

Is contracted by:

Character structure(s):   EXISTENCE
NEED

Ego function: GROUNDING AND REALITY TESTING, (a) ability to stand one's ground, feel rooted and supported by it.

Psychological function: Sense one's right to existence and connection; being.

Ego function: COGNITIVE SKILLS, (c) understanding (getting something well enough to go forward with it).

Psychological function: An integration of physical and energetic sensation.

Child's developmental stage/age: A catch/grasp reflex.
The child grasps with the little toe reflexively ("pumps") during breast- and bottle-feeding.

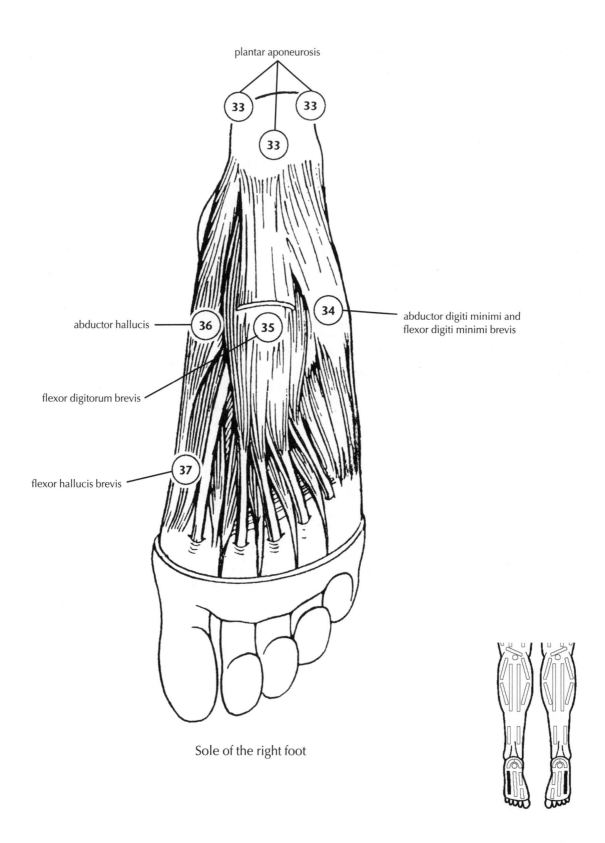

plantar aponeurosis

33
33
33

abductor hallucis

36
35

abductor digiti minimi and
flexor digiti minimi brevis

34

flexor digitorum brevis

flexor hallucis brevis

37

Sole of the right foot

Name:	**Abductor digiti minimi and flexor digiti minimi brevis Number: 34**
Origin:	Abductor: calcaneus. Flexor: base of 5th metatarsal bone.
Insertion:	Base of proximal phalanx of little toe.
Anatomical function:	Both muscles flex and abduct the little toe.
Map:	Are found on the little-toe side of the sole of the foot; the abductor lies in the first layer of muscle deep to plantar aponeurosis, and the flexor in the third layer.
Is contracted by:	Spreading the toes; move the little toe away from the other toes (abductor). Curl the little toe down under the sole of the foot or down into the mat/floor (flexor).
Character structure(s):	Flexor digiti minimi brevis: NEED Abductor digiti minimi: OPINIONS
Ego function:	GROUNDING AND REALITY TESTING, (a) ability to stand one's ground, feel rooted and supported by it.
Psychological function:	NEED: sensing one's needs through contact (grounding through contact), or by contacting others. OPINIONS: providing (or forming) a platform for one's opinions.
Ego function:	COGNITIVE SKILLS, (c) understanding (getting something well enough to go forward with it).
Psychological function:	NEED: determining one's needs through sensations. OPINIONS: the right to test your ideas/imaginings and in this way gain a relaxed sense of grounding (the right to ask for explanation).
Child's developmental stage/age:	Provides balance and support because it provides lateral stability to the foot. Push off through the little toe in walking.

Bodymapping:

Client's position:	On the stomach.
Tester's position:	By the foot that is tested.
Activation in test position:	Is contracted by spreading the toes.
Test location:	Where the belly of the muscle is full; slightly laterally and/or plantar (the two muscles are tested together).
Test direction:	Toward the heel.

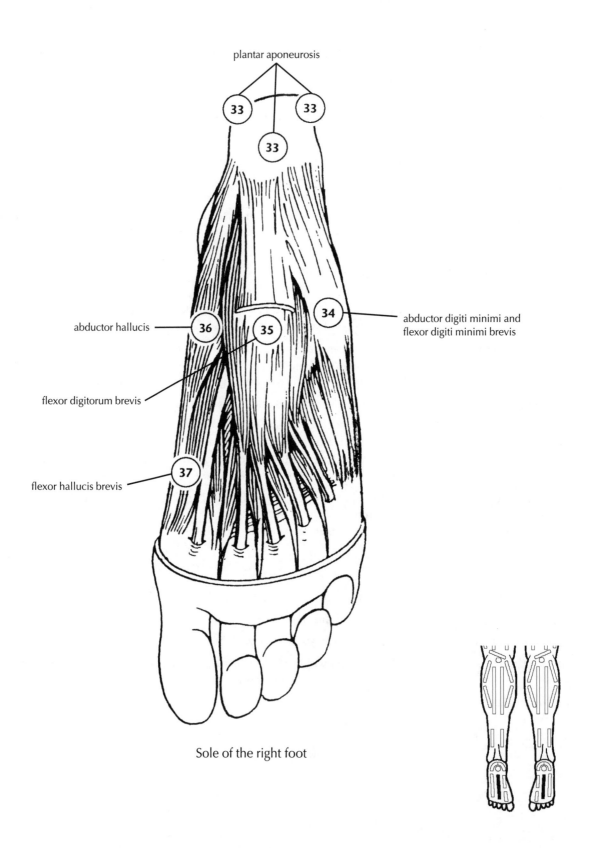

plantar aponeurosis

33 **33**

33

abductor digiti minimi and
flexor digiti minimi brevis **34**

abductor hallucis **36** **35**

flexor digitorum brevis

flexor hallucis brevis **37**

Sole of the right foot

Name:	**Flexor digitorum brevis**	**Number: 35**

Origin:	Calcaneus.
Insertion:	Middle phalanges of the four lateral toes.
Anatomical function:	Flexes the toes and supports the convexity of the foot.
Map:	Is found between the heel and the proximal phalanx of the four lateral toes; lies in the first layer of muscles deep to the plantar aponeurosis.
Is contracted by:	Flexing (curling) the four little toes toward the mat/floor.
Character structure(s):	NEED
Ego function:	GROUNDING AND REALITY TESTING, (a) ability to stand one's ground, feel rooted and supported by it.
Psychological function:	To feel grounded/well-rooted in acceptance of one's needs.
Ego function:	COGNITIVE SKILLS, (c) understanding (getting something well enough to go forward with it).
Psychological function:	Awareness of how one can satisfy one's needs.
Child's developmental stage/age:	When the child is sucking, this muscle takes part in the reflex movement patterns. This reflex movement is a remnant from animals' pumping action.

Bodymapping:

Client's position:	On the stomach.
Tester's position:	By the foot that is tested.
Activation in test position:	Is tightened by curling the toes down under the sole of the foot.
Test location:	Deep to plantar aponeurosis; between the heel and the proximal phalanx of the four lateral toes.
Test direction:	Toward the heel.

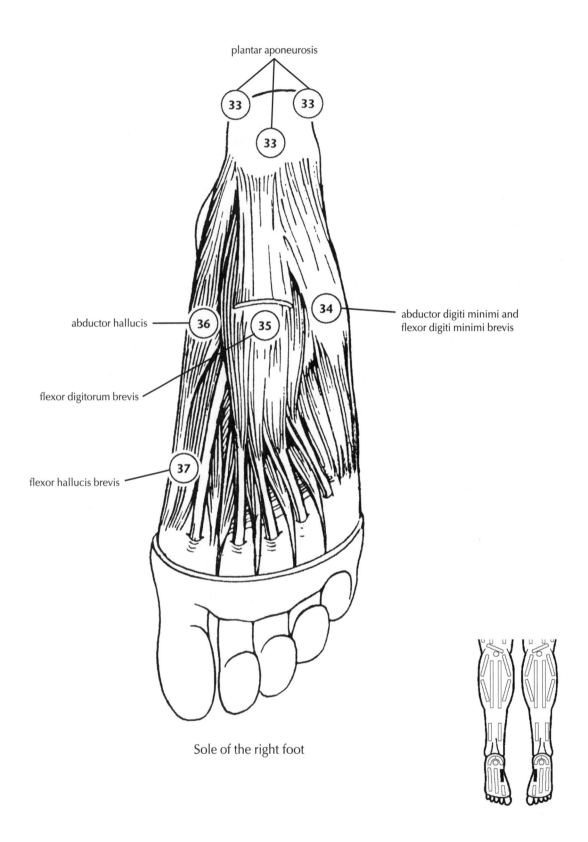

plantar aponeurosis

33

33

33

abductor hallucis — 36

35

34 — abductor digiti minimi and
flexor digiti minimi brevis

flexor digitorum brevis

flexor hallucis brevis — 37

Sole of the right foot

Name:	**Abductor hallucis**	Number: 36

Origin:	Calcaneus.
Insertion:	Base of proximal phalanx of big toe.
Anatomical function:	Abducts the big toe and supports the convexity of the foot.
Map:	Is found superficially on the medial (big toe) side of foot toward the heel.
Is contracted by:	Moving the big toe away from the other toes. If this is difficult, move it passively, hold it there, and activate the muscle.
Character structure(s):	SOLIDARITY/PERFORMANCE
Ego function:	GROUNDING AND REALITY TESTING, (a) ability to stand one's ground, feel rooted and supported by it.
Psychological function:	Following a direction and/or changing it, while at the same time preserving the sense of grounding.
Ego function:	COGNITIVE SKILLS, (c) understanding (getting something well enough to go forward with it).
Psychological function:	Preserving one's vision (inner direction) even though altering the course now and then.
Ego function:	SELF-ASSERTION, (c) forward momentum and sense of direction.
Psychological function:	Ability to express one's sense of self-direction and be flexible at the same time.
Child's developmental stage/age:	The final push off with the big toe in walking; stabilizing the big toe when changing direction.

Bodymapping:

Client's position:	On the stomach.
Tester's position:	By the foot that is tested.
Activation in test position:	Is tightened by abducting the big toe (spreading the toes).
Test location:	In the muscle belly in the arch of the foot.
Test direction:	Toward the heel.

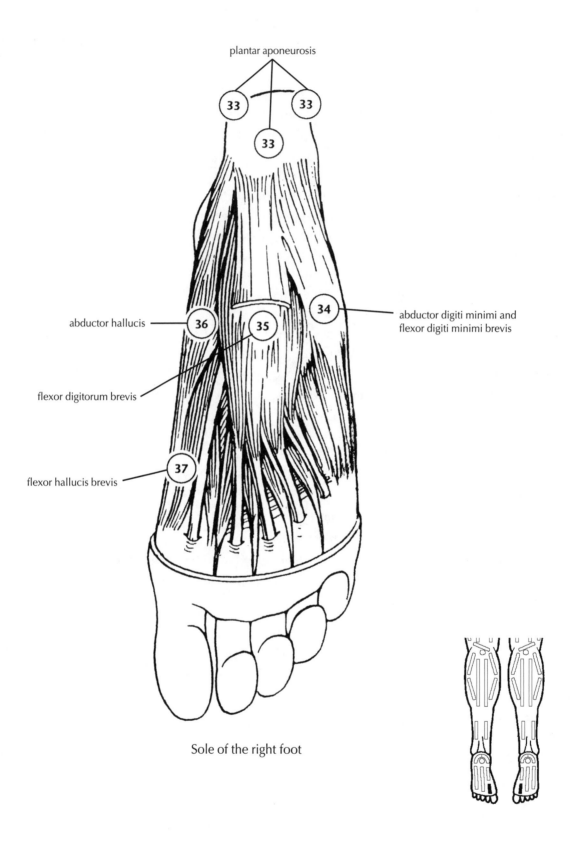

plantar aponeurosis

33   33

33

abductor hallucis — 36

35

34 — abductor digiti minimi and flexor digiti minimi brevis

flexor digitorum brevis

flexor hallucis brevis — 37

Sole of the right foot

Name:	**Flexor hallucis brevis**	**Number: 37**

Origin:	Cuboid bone.
Insertion:	Base of proximal phalanx of big toe.
Anatomical function:	Flexes the big toe and supports the concavity (arch) of the foot.
Map:	Is found behind the pad of the big toe, in the third layer deep to the plantar aponeurosis.
Is contracted by:	Flexing (curling) the big toe toward the floor/mat.
Character structure(s):	AUTONOMY
Ego function:	GROUNDING AND REALITY TESTING, (a) ability to stand one's ground, feel rooted and supported by it.
Psychological function:	Maintaining the sense of grounding while moving forward with curiosity.
Ego function:	COGNITIVE SKILLS, (c) understanding (getting something well enough to go forward with it).
Psychological function:	The ability to understand cognitive coherence through motor sensation ("motor memory").
Child's developmental stage/age:	Used in walking, especially when the child begins to walk quickly and "run," and when walking on the toes.

Bodymapping:

Client's position:	On the stomach.
Tester's position:	By the foot that is tested.
Activation in test position:	Flex or curl the big toe.
Test location:	Proximal to the big toe pad on the sole of the foot.
Test direction:	Toward the heel.

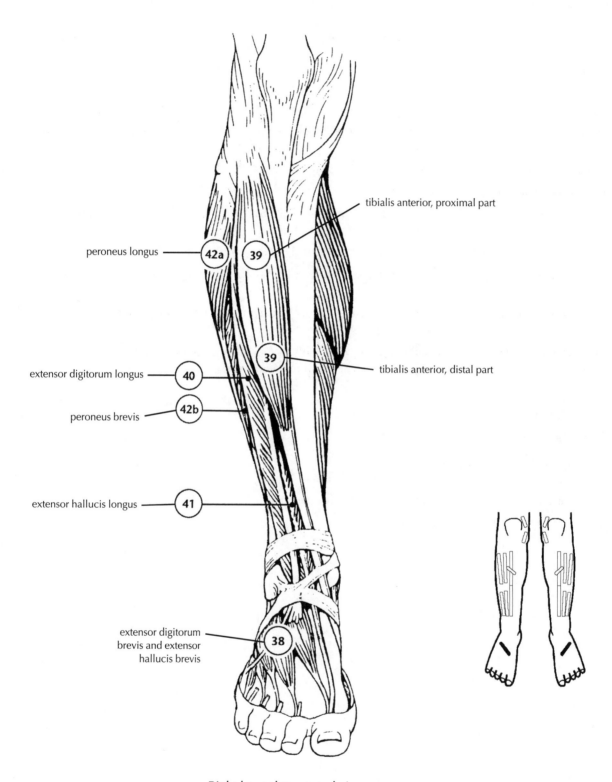

tibialis anterior, proximal part

peroneus longus — **42a** **39**

extensor digitorum longus — **40**

39 tibialis anterior, distal part

peroneus brevis — **42b**

extensor hallucis longus — **41**

extensor digitorum brevis and extensor hallucis brevis — **38**

Right lower leg, ventral view

Name:	**Extensor digitorum brevis and extensor hallucis brevis Number: 38**
Origin:	Anterior calcaneus on dorsal surface.
Insertion:	Digitorum: extensor expansion of 2nd, 3rd, and 4th toes. Hallucis: base of proximal phalanx of big toe.
Anatomical function:	Extends the big toe and three other toes.
Map:	Are found laterally on the top of the foot just in front of the ankle joint.
Is contracted by:	Lifting the toes off the floor/mat.
Character structure(s):	PUBERTY
Ego function:	GROUNDING AND REALITY TESTING, (b) relationship between reality and fantasy/imagination.
Psychological function:	To be rooted in one's individuality (stand by one's personality).
Ego function:	COGNITIVE SKILLS, (d) grasp of reality (ability to apply cognitive understanding to different situations).
Psychological function:	Ability to combine one abstract idea with another without losing the sense of grounding.
Child's developmental stage/age:	The child lifts up the toes, and the rest of the foot can stay on the ground. Fine adjustment of the different movements of the foot.

Bodymapping:

Client's position:	On the back.
Tester's position:	By the leg that is tested.
Activation in test position:	Extension of the four medial toes—just a small movement Support the foot.
Test location:	In the belly of the muscle.
Test direction:	Toward the ankle joint or toward the toes; choose which is best depending on the individual.

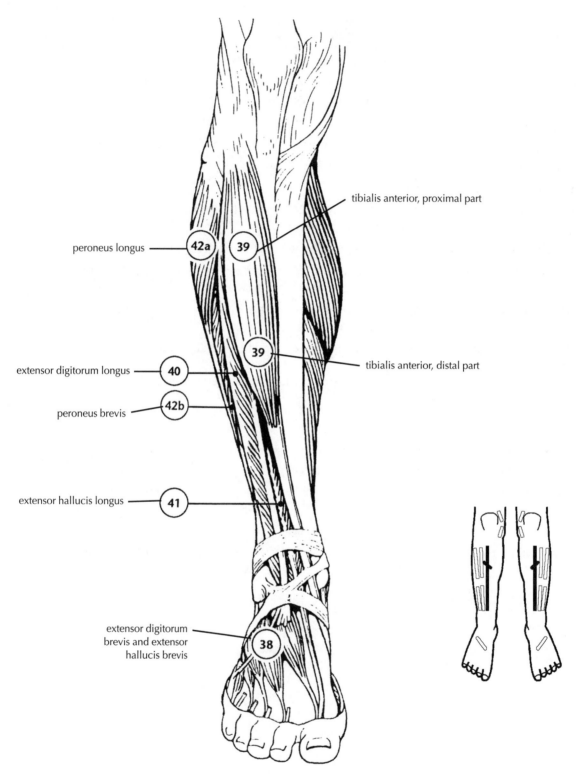

peroneus longus — 42a

tibialis anterior, proximal part — 39

39

tibialis anterior, distal part

extensor digitorum longus — 40

peroneus brevis — 42b

extensor hallucis longus — 41

extensor digitorum brevis and extensor hallucis brevis — 38

Right lower leg, ventral view

Name:	**Tibialis anterior**	**Number: 39**

Origin:	Lateral shaft of tibia; interosseous membrane.
Insertion:	Base of 1st metatarsal bone, first (medial) cuneiform bone.
Anatomical function:	Dorsiflexes, supinates, and pronates the foot.
Map:	Is found laterally along tibia.
Is contracted by:	Lifting the fore-foot with the heel on the floor/mat.
Character structure(s):	Proximal part: superficial: WILL deep: AUTONOMY Distal part: OPINIONS
Ego function:	GROUNDING AND REALITY TESTING, (b) relationship between reality and fantasy/imagination.
Psychological function:	WILL: comparing inner imagination and sensations to outer reality. AUT: sensing reality via a physical activity. OPINIONS: testing one's imaginings and thoughts.
Ego function:	COGNITIVE SKILLS, (d) grasp of reality (ability to apply cognitive understanding to different situations).
Psychological function:	WILL: ability to separate intentions from actions. AUT: ability to understand coherence through motor actions. OPINIONS: ability to "dance" between the abstract and the concrete; deduce abstract thinking from concrete thinking or vice versa.
Child's developmental stage/age:	WILL: The muscle takes part in push-off by stabilizing the arch of the foot so it can absorb the impact. AUT: The child lifts the foot while walking. OPINIONS: Bouncing on one or both feet without leaving the ground.

Bodymapping:

Client's position:	On the back.
Tester's position:	By the leg that is tested.
Activation in test position:	Dorsiflexion of the ankle joint.
Test location:	Proximally and distally on the muscle belly. Test both deeply and superficially at the proximal test location. Remember that the fascia is often very tight.
Test direction:	Distally.

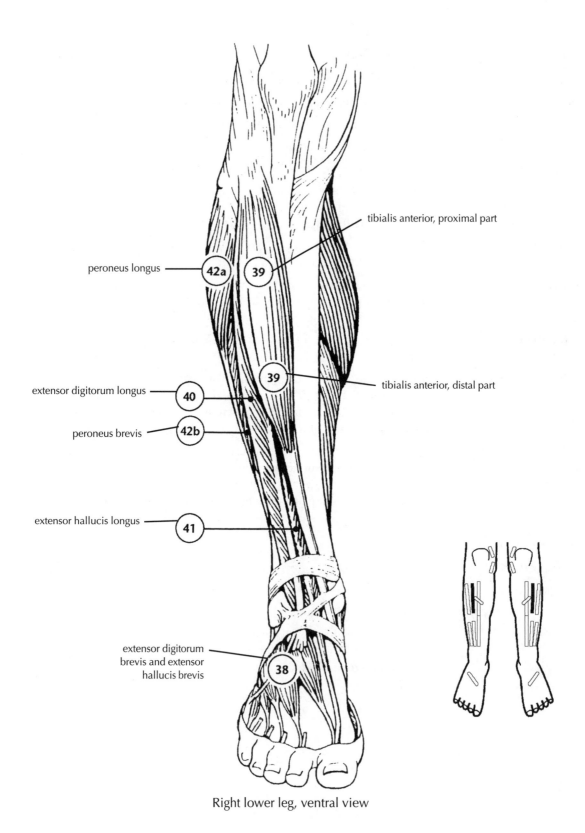

peroneus longus — **42a** **39** — tibialis anterior, proximal part

extensor digitorum longus — **40** **39** — tibialis anterior, distal part

peroneus brevis — **42b**

extensor hallucis longus — **41**

extensor digitorum brevis and extensor hallucis brevis — **38**

Right lower leg, ventral view

The Bodynamic Psycho-Motor Anatomy

Name:	**Extensor digitorum longus**	Number: 40

Origin:	Lateral condyle of tibia; proximal two-thirds of anterior shaft of fibula; interosseous membrane.
Insertion:	Extensor expansion of four lateral toes.
Anatomical function:	Toes: extension. Foot: assists dorsiflexion and pronation. Assists in tightening the plantar aponeurosis.
Map:	Is found laterally to tibialis anterior along tibia.
Is contracted by:	Lifting the four lateral toes away from the floor/mat.
Character structure(s):	LOVE/SEXUALITY
Ego function:	GROUNDING AND REALITY TESTING, (b) relationship between reality and fantasy/imagination.
Psychological function:	A realistic relationship with one's sex roles and alliances.
Ego function:	COGNITIVE SKILLS, (d) grasp of reality (ability to apply cognitive understanding to different situations).
Psychological function:	Ability to transfer cognitive understanding from one situation to a different but similar situation (through role-playing).
Child's developmental stage/age:	Takes part in walking. The child lifts the toes to be able to push off; at the same time aponeurosis plantaris is tightened so the foot becomes tight and steady, ready to roll through.

Bodymapping:

Client's position:	On the back.
Tester's position:	By the leg that is tested.
Activation in test position:	Extension of the four lateral toes, a small movement isolated from the ankle joint.
Test location:	Laterally to tibialis anterior, approximately at level with its distal test location.
Test direction:	Distally, medially.

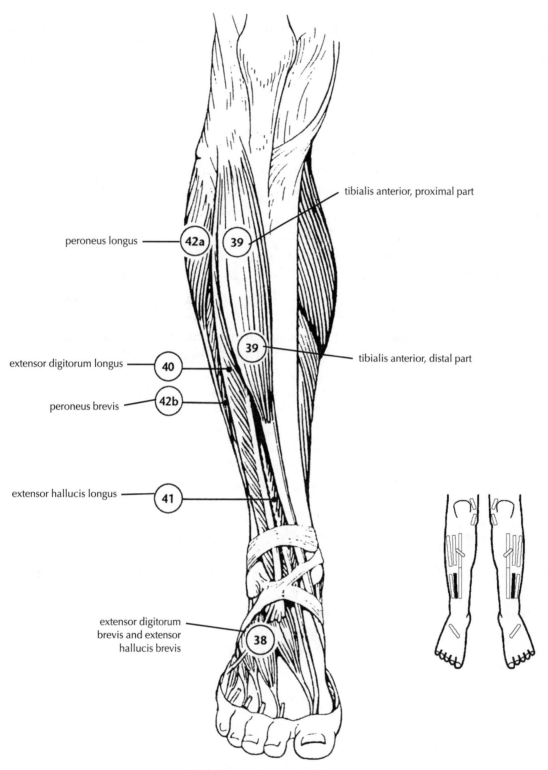

peroneus longus — **42a**

39 tibialis anterior, proximal part

39 tibialis anterior, distal part

extensor digitorum longus — **40**

peroneus brevis — **42b**

extensor hallucis longus — **41**

extensor digitorum brevis and extensor hallucis brevis — **38**

Right lower leg, ventral view

Name:	**Extensor hallucis longus**	**Number: 41**

Origin:	Anterior shaft of fibula; interosseous membrane.
Insertion:	Base of distal phalanx of big toe.
Anatomical function:	Big toe: extension. Foot: assists dorsiflexion. Assists in tightening the plantar aponeurosis.
Map:	Is found on anterolateral aspect of the lower leg deep to tibialis anterior and extensor digitorum longus. It becomes superficial distally in the leg.
Is contracted by:	Lifting the big toe away from the floor/mat.
Character structure(s):	OPINIONS
Ego function:	GROUNDING AND REALITY TESTING, (b) relationship between reality and fantasy/imagination.
Psychological function:	Ability to be rooted in one's values and test them in a group.
Ego function:	COGNITIVE SKILLS, (d) grasp of reality (ability to apply cognitive understanding to different situations).
Psychological function:	Thinking abstractly without letting go of the sense of reality.
Child's developmental stage/age:	Playing football, hopping on one foot, and triple jump (athletic sports). The child lifts the big toe (extension), tensing (or stretching) the plantar aponeurosis, and the foot becomes firm and steady, ready to roll through and then push off.

Bodymapping:

Client's position:	On the back.
Tester's position:	By the leg that is tested.
Activation in test position:	Extension of the big toe; just a small movement.
Test location:	Between the tendons of tibialis anterior and extensor digitorum longus.
Test direction:	Distally, medially.

Name:	**Tibialis posterior**	Number: *

Origin:	Intcrosseus membrane and adjacent posterolateral tibia and medial fibula.
Insertion:	Plantar surface of navicular and other carpal bones, bases of 2nd, 3rd, and 4th metatarsal bones.
Anatomical function:	Supinates the foot and assists plantar flexion of the ankle joint Forms a "stirrup" with peroneus longus and brevis.
Map:	Is found in the calf deep to the two toe flexors (flexor digitorum longus and flexor hallucis longus).
Is contracted by:	Lifting the inner edge of the foot while the heel, toes, and outer edge of the foot remain on the mat/floor.
Character structure(s):	NEED LOVE/SEXUALITY
Ego function:	SOCIAL BALANCE, (d) balancing sense of personal identity against being a group member.
Psychological function:	NEED: preserve own needs though others have different needs LOVE/SEX: love more than one person from the bottom of one's heart.
Ego function:	GENDER SKILLS, (e) manifestation of sensuality and sexuality.
Psychological function:	NEED: enjoy being touched. LOVE/SEX: manifesting one's joy ("jump for joy").
Child's developmental stage/age:	NEED: The child supinates the foot in enjoyment when being touched. LOVE/SEX: When the child is jumping up and down, he moves the ankle joint, and the foot is supported by the "stirrup."

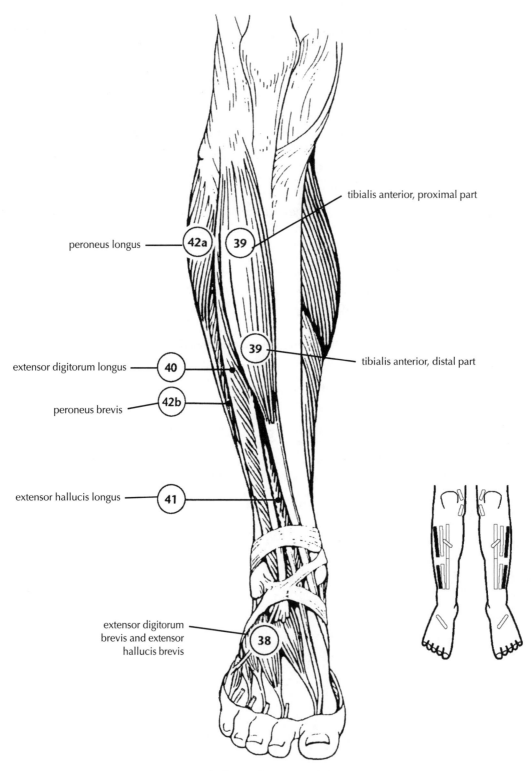

peroneus longus — 42a 39 — tibialis anterior, proximal part

extensor digitorum longus — 40 39 — tibialis anterior, distal part

peroneus brevis — 42b

extensor hallucis longus — 41

extensor digitorum
brevis and extensor
hallucis brevis — 38

Right lower leg, ventral view

Name:	**Peroneus longus and brevis**	Number: 42a, b

Origin:	Lateral surface of fibula.
Insertion:	(a) Longus: base of 1st metatarsal and cuneiform. (b) Brevis: base of 5th metatarsal.
Anatomical function:	Both muscles pronate the foot and assist plantarflexion of ankle.
Map:	Are found laterally to extensor digitorum, on the outside of the lower leg.
Is contracted by:	Lifting the outer edge of the foot away from the floor/mat.
Character structure(s):	(a) Longus: WILL (b) Brevis: SOLIDARITY/PERFORMANCE
Ego function:	SOCIAL BALANCE, (d) balancing sense of personal identity against being a group member.
Psychological function:	WILL: balancing what is best for oneself and best for the group. SOL/PERF: balancing being true to oneself, showing/feeling solidarity with those who are close, and those in the larger group.
Ego function:	GENDER SKILLS, (e) manifestation of sensuality and sexuality.
Psychological function:	WILL: manifest love and care. SOL/PERF: manifest one's attraction.
Child's developmental stage/age:	This muscle helps when balancing on one foot, i.e., when balancing on tree trunks (ages 3-4) and on beams and other narrow edges (ages 7-12).

Bodymapping:

Client's position:	On the back.
Tester's position:	By the leg that is tested.
Activation in test position:	Pronate the foot; if necessary put a hand on the outer edge (side) of the foot to guide the direction of the movement.
Test location:	(a) Longus: where the belly of the muscle is full. (b) Brevis: on the muscle on either side of the tendon of longus.
Test direction:	Distally.

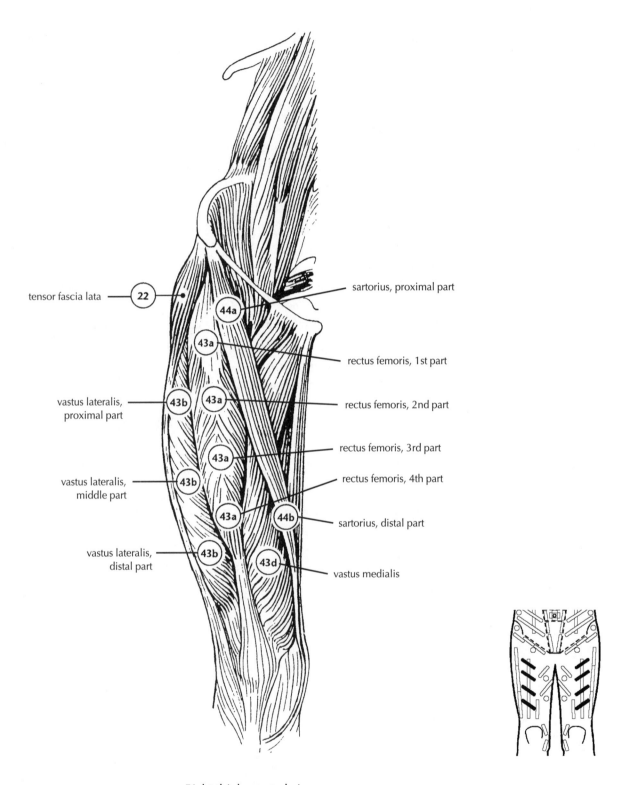

tensor fascia lata — 22

sartorius, proximal part

44a

43a

rectus femoris, 1st part

vastus lateralis,
proximal part — 43b 43a

rectus femoris, 2nd part

43a

rectus femoris, 3rd part

vastus lateralis,
middle part — 43b

rectus femoris, 4th part

43a 44b

sartorius, distal part

vastus lateralis,
distal part — 43b 43d

vastus medialis

Right thigh, ventral view

Name:	**Rectus femoris**	Number: 43a

Origin:	Anterior inferior iliac spine, just above the rim of the acetabulum.
Insertion:	Patella, tibial tuberosity via patellar ligament.
Anatomical function:	Flexes the thigh at the hip joint and extends the leg at the knee joint.
Map:	Is found in the middle of the front part of the thigh. One of the four muscles of quadriceps femoris.
Is contracted by:	Flexing/bending the hip joint by lifting the leg forward (upper part) and/or extending/stretching out the knee joint (lower part).
Character structure(s):	1st part: LOVE/SEXUALITY 2nd part: OPINIONS 3rd part: SOLIDARITY/PERFORMANCE 4th part: PUBERTY
Ego function:	BOUNDARIES, (d) boundaries of social space.
Psychological function:	LOVE/SEX: ability to create constructive alliances; make them visible and stand by them. OPINIONS: ability to share attitudes; attracted to those who have similar social norms, e.g., boy/girl scouts, sports fans. SOL/PERF: show solidarity with one group while being in another group; ability to preserve group connection to both groups. PUB: show solidarity with a larger group and at the same time be able to accept other norms.
Child's developmental stage/age:	Contracting the muscle from the knee allows a more powerful kick. These actions apply to quadriceps femoris as a whole: jumping/hopping (away-toward), maintaining balance, running, riding a bicycle.

Bodymapping:

Client's position:	On the back.
Tester's position:	By the leg that is tested.
Activation in test position:	Lift the extended leg; palpate the whole shape of the muscle.
Test location:	Test in four different locations along the length of the muscle.
Test direction:	Distally, pulling slightly laterally.

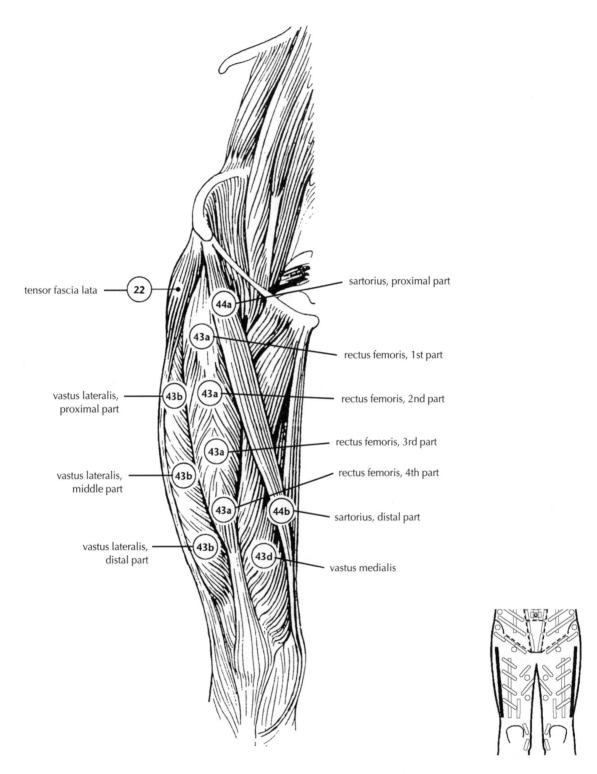

tensor fascia lata — (22)

sartorius, proximal part

(44a)

(43a)

rectus femoris, 1st part

vastus lateralis,
proximal part — (43b) (43a)

rectus femoris, 2nd part

(43a)

rectus femoris, 3rd part

vastus lateralis,
middle part — (43b)

rectus femoris, 4th part

(43a) (44b)

sartorius, distal part

vastus lateralis,
distal part — (43b) (43d)

vastus medialis

Right thigh, ventral view

142   **The Bodynamic Psycho-Motor Anatomy**

Name:	**Vastus lateralis**	Number: 43b

Origin:	Posterior shaft of femur, proximal half (linea aspera).
Insertion:	Patella, tibial tuberosity via patellar ligament.
Anatomical function:	Extends the leg at the knee joint.
Map:	Is found on the lateral side of the thigh. One of the four muscles of quadriceps femoris.
Is contracted by:	Extending/stretching out the knee joint.
Character structure(s):	Proximal part: WILL Middle part: LOVE/SEXUALITY Distal part: SOLIDARITY/PERFORMANCE
Ego function:	BOUNDARIES, (c) boundaries of territorial space.
Psychological function:	WILL: create and posses one's territory. LOVE/SEX: preserve and extend one's territorial space; one's own room for privacy. SOL/PERF: create territorial space that is convenient for the group.
Child's developmental stage/age:	Power in standing, walking, kicking, stamping the floor. WILL: my corner; my part of the table; creating a working place/cozy corner. LOVE/SEX: closing the door to one's own room, "doctor" games–practicing role play. SOL/PERF: arranging one's room and inviting friends–arranging and having secret dens, my street, your street; my town, your town.

Bodymapping:

Client's position:	On the back.
Tester's position:	By the leg that is tested.
Activation in test position:	Lift the extended leg; palpate the whole shape of the muscle.
Test location:	Test in three different locations along the muscle between iliotibial tract and rectus femoris.
Test direction:	Distally, pulling slightly laterally.

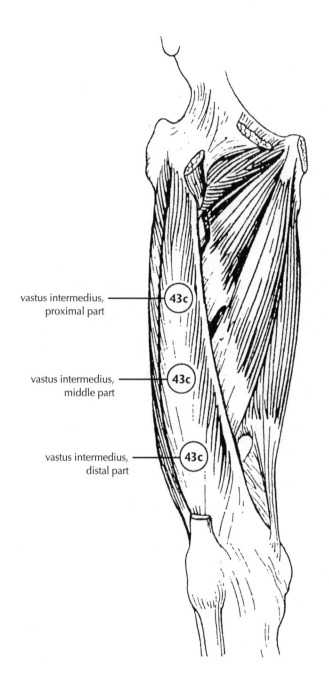

vastus intermedius,
proximal part — **43c**

vastus intermedius,
middle part — **43c**

vastus intermedius,
distal part — **43c**

Deep muscles of the right thigh,
ventral view

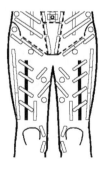

Name:	Vastus intermedius	Number: 43c

Origin:	Anterior and lateral shaft of femur.
Insertion:	Patella, tibial tuberosity via patellar ligament.
Anatomical function:	Extends the leg at the knee joint.
Map:	Is found in the middle of the thigh deep to rectus femoris. One of the four muscles of quadriceps femoris.
Is contracted by:	Hold the kneecap; if necessary pull the kneecap slightly distally, then pull the kneecap toward the stomach.
Character structure(s):	Proximal part: NEED Middle part: WILL Distal part: AUTONOMY
Ego function:	BOUNDARIES, (b) boundaries of personal space (energetic boundaries).
Psychological function:	NEED: being touched—ability to defend one's skin boundaries. WILL: ability to defend one's personal space and stay in contact. AUT: creating personal space; releasing energy without losing connection.
Child's developmental stage/age:	NEED: the child extends the leg when she rolls over and senses the skin against the floor/mat. WILL: stands with good posture, with slightly bent knees and hips (as if ready to carry/lift something); stands on one leg and kicks with the other leg. AUT: crawls, stands with feet turned out, and walks in the same way. Crawls away from safe person with a secure feeling that he/she will be there when returning.
Bodymapping:	
Client's position:	On the back.
Tester's position:	By the leg that is tested.
Activation in test position:	The tester supports the kneecap, and if necessary pulls it slightly distally; the client pulls the kneecap proximally (a small movement).
Test location:	Test in three locations along the muscle. First testing location is level with the belly of adductor longus.
Test direction:	Distally, medially.

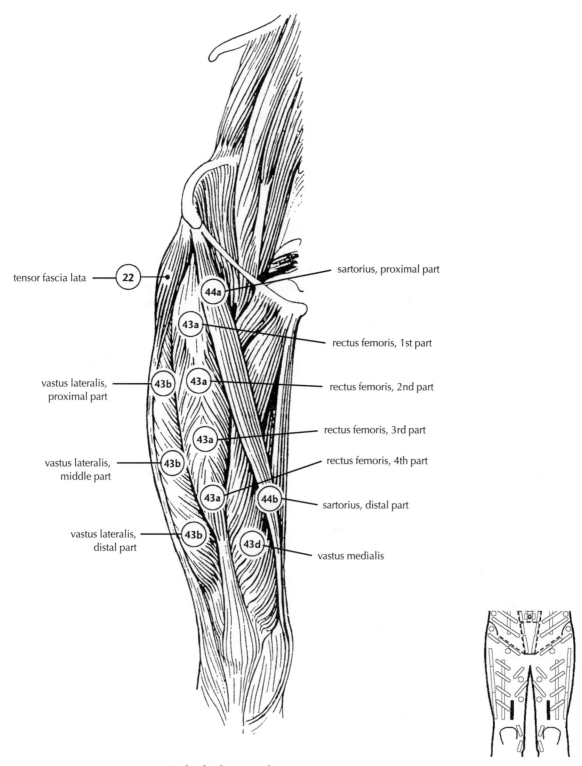

tensor fascia lata — **22**

sartorius, proximal part

44a

43a — rectus femoris, 1st part

vastus lateralis, proximal part — **43b**   **43a** — rectus femoris, 2nd part

43a — rectus femoris, 3rd part

rectus femoris, 4th part

vastus lateralis, middle part — **43b**

43a   **44b** — sartorius, distal part

vastus lateralis, distal part — **43b**

43d — vastus medialis

Right thigh, ventral view

Name:	Vastus medialis	Number: 43d

Origin:	Proximal, anterior, medial femur and intermuscular septum.
Insertion:	Patella, tibial tuberosity via patellar ligament.
Anatomical function:	Extends the leg at the knee joint, locking the knee.
Map:	Is found medially on the thigh, between rectus femoris and sartorius One of the four muscles of quadriceps femoris.
Is contracted by:	Extending the knee completely.
Character structure(s):	LOVE/SEXUALITY-PUBERTY
Ego function:	BOUNDARIES, (b) boundaries of personal space (energetic boundaries).
Psychological function:	LOVE/SEX: experiencing sensuality and maintaining choice over one's private areas of the body (where to be touched, how much, if one wants to be tickled, and so on). PUB: ability to be close together in an erotic way and experience the ability to decide one's sexual boundaries (where to be touched and how).
Ego function:	SOCIAL BALANCE, (e) balance of managing stress and resolving it.
Psychological function:	LOVE/SEX: the balance of preserving and expressing one's own sensuality/sexuality in relation to social norms. PUB: the balance of preserving and releasing one's own eroticism/sensuality in relation to social norms.
Ego function:	MANAGEMENT OF ENERGY, (e) containment of sensuality.
Psychological function:	LOVE/SEX: able to contain one's own sexual/sensual energy PUB: sensuality/sexuality/eroticism.
Ego function:	GENDER SKILLS, (d) containment of sensuality and sexuality.
Psychological function:	LOVE/SEX and PUB: as in Management of Energy.
Child's developmental stage/age:	More power and accuracy in kicking: able to tackle for a ball; kick ball away.

Bodymapping:

Client's position:	On the back.
Tester's position:	By the leg that is tested.
Activation in test position:	Extend the knee joint with slight lateral rotation of the hip joint; if necessary, lift the leg.
Test location:	Between rectus femoris and sartorius where the belly of the muscle is full.
Test direction:	In the direction of the fibers diagonally toward the knee.

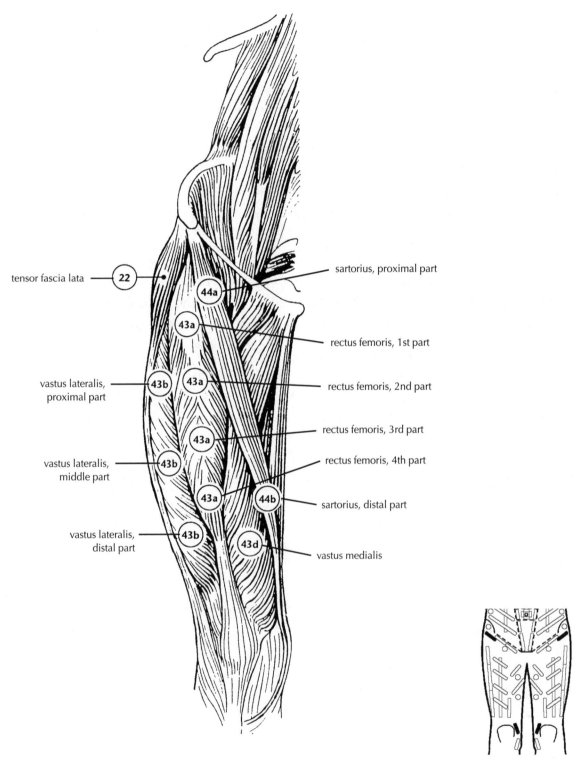

tensor fascia lata — **22**

sartorius, proximal part — **44a**

rectus femoris, 1st part — **43a**

vastus lateralis, proximal part — **43b**   **43a** — rectus femoris, 2nd part

rectus femoris, 3rd part — **43a**

vastus lateralis, middle part — **43b**

rectus femoris, 4th part — **43a**   **44b** — sartorius, distal part

vastus lateralis, distal part — **43b**   **43d** — vastus medialis

Right thigh, ventral view

Name:	Sartorius	Number: 44a, b

Origin:	Anterior, superior iliac spine.
Insertion:	Upper medial shaft of tibia.
Anatomical function:	Flexes, abducts, and laterally rotates the thigh at the hip joint. Flexes and assists medial rotation of knee joint, i.e., the big toe is turned toward the other leg.
Map:	Is found superficially crossing over the front of the thigh.
Is contracted by:	Lifting the leg from the floor/mat with slightly outwardly rotated hip joint and moving it into a cross-legged position.
Character structure(s):	(a) Proximal part: WILL (b) Distal part: OPINIONS
Ego function:	SOCIAL BALANCE, (e) balance of managing stress and resolving it.
Psychological function:	WILL: having drive; ability to meet challenges with a high level of energy. OPINIONS: having (maintaining) flexible opinions under conditions of high stress.
Ego function:	MANAGEMENT OF ENERGY, (b) containment of high-level energy.
Psychological function:	WILL: contain one's power in one's choices. OPINIONS: preserve direction and ethics (at a high energy level under conditions of stress).
Ego function:	44 (b) Distal part: GENDER SKILLS. (d) containment of sensuality and sexuality. (e) manifestation of sensuality and sexuality.
Psychological function:	OPINIONS: form and express one's opinions about sensuality and sexuality.
Child's developmental stage/age:	The child is able to sit in a cross-legged position (lotus position). The muscle helps with stabilizing the knee when standing on one leg; used to direct both the knee and the foot in walking, running, skipping, etc. WILL: walking on logs. OPINIONS: walking on a beam.
Shock:	This muscle is commonly impacted by shock.

Bodymapping:

Client's position:	On the back.
Tester's position:	By the leg that is tested.
Activation in test position:	Bend the hip and knee slightly, externally rotate the hip, and lift the leg.
Test location:	(a) Proximal: medially to rectus femoris. (b) Distal: slightly proximally to the test location of vastus medialis.
Test direction:	In the direction of the muscle fibers.

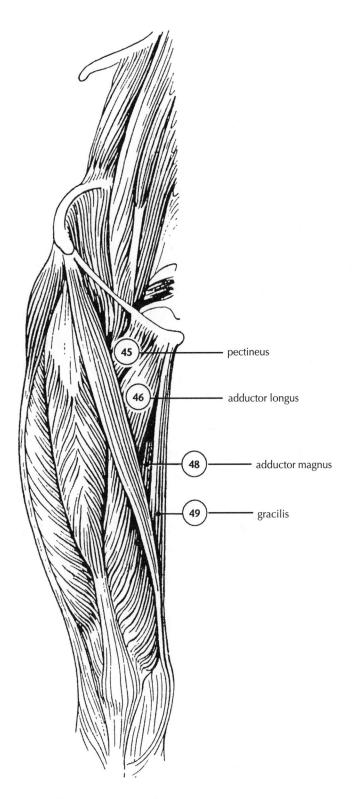

45 — pectineus

46 — adductor longus

48 — adductor magnus

49 — gracilis

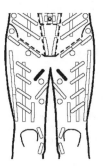

Right thigh, ventral view

Name:	**Pectineus**	**Number: 45**

Origin:	Anterior pubis.
Insertion:	Posterior femur between lesser trochanter and linea aspera.
Anatomical function:	Adducts and assists flexion and medial rotation of the thigh in the hip joint.
Map:	Is found superficially close to the groin on the inner side of the thigh.
Is contracted by:	Squeezing the legs together close to the genitals.
Character structure(s):	LOVE/SEXUALITY
Ego function:	MANAGEMENT OF ENERGY, (e) containment of sensuality.
Psychological function:	Containment of high energy while flirting, "fighting."
Ego function:	GENDER SKILLS, (d) containment of sensuality and sexuality.
Psychological function:	Declare attraction to the opposite sex.
Child's developmental stage/age:	The child pulls the leg medially in flirting, shyness—"hold on with the legs"; "doctor" games, desire to examine one's body and others' bodies, and ability to stop when it feels wrong.

Bodymapping:

Client's position:	On the back.
Tester's position:	By the leg that is tested.
Activation in test position:	Lift the leg from the floor/mat and adduct it.
Test location:	Find the depression below the inguinal ligament, medially to sartorius. Pectineus is found superficially between the depression and the tendon of adductor longus.
Test direction:	Distally, laterally.

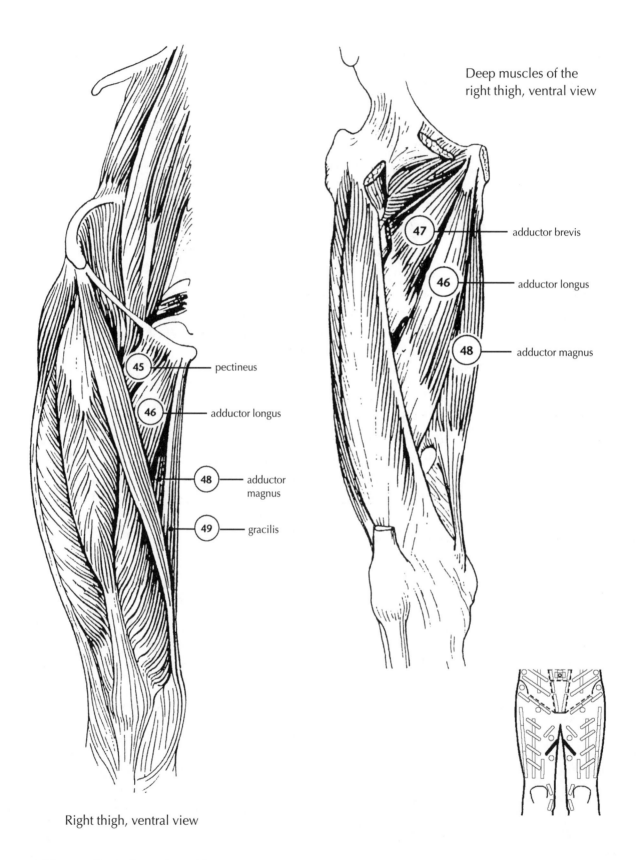

Deep muscles of the
right thigh, ventral view

47 — adductor brevis

46 — adductor longus

48 — adductor magnus

45 — pectineus

46 — adductor longus

48 — adductor
magnus

49 — gracilis

Right thigh, ventral view

Name:	**Adductor longus**	**Number: 46**

Origin:	Anterior pubis.
Insertion:	Linea aspera on posterior femur.
Anatomical function:	Adduction; assists flexion in the hip joint. The most important muscle of medial rotation along with the anterior fibers of adductor magnus.
Map:	Is found superficially on proximal, medial surface of the thigh from pubis to halfway down the thigh.
Is contracted by:	Squeezing the knees together with an inward rotation in the hip joint.
Character structure(s):	SOLIDARITY/PERFORMANCE
Ego function:	MANAGEMENT OF ENERGY, (e) containment of sensuality.
Psychological function:	Containment of shyness/modesty caused by awareness of one's own body.
Ego function:	GENDER SKILLS, (d) containment of sensuality and sexuality.
Psychological function:	Containment of sensual energy when talking with one's friends about an attraction one has to someone.
Child's developmental stage/age:	Ability to perform long jumps, climbing a rope, skipping rope/jumping rope, playing Chinese jump rope (similar to hopscotch with two holding the rope with their legs and the third hopping) in a threesome. Playing soccer/football: ability to kick the ball with a medial rotated movement with the top of the foot.

Bodymapping:

Client's position:	On the back.
Tester's position:	By the leg that is tested.
Activation in test position:	Medial rotation in the hip joint.
Test location:	The tendon of origin is found when the leg is lifted. Palpate the tendon and move the hand approximately one hand's width distally to the belly of the muscle between pectineus and gracilis.
Test direction:	Distally, laterally.

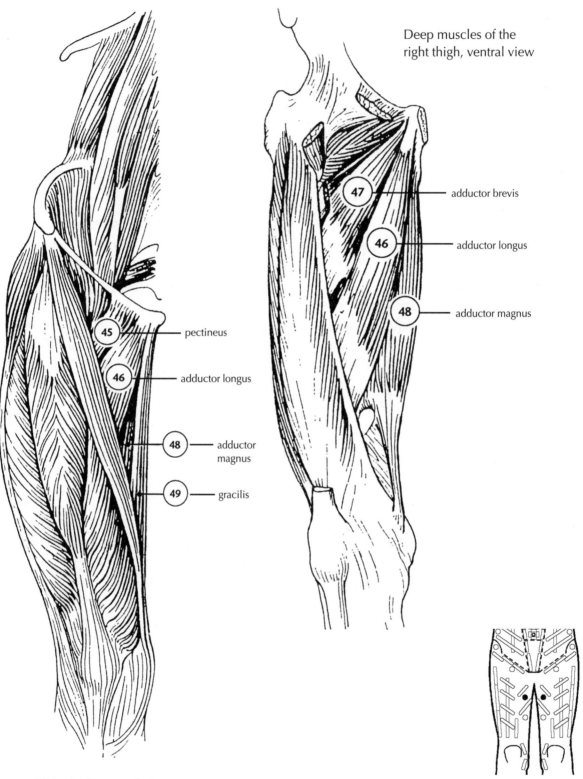

Deep muscles of the
right thigh, ventral view

47 — adductor brevis

46 — adductor longus

48 — adductor magnus

45 — pectineus

46 — adductor longus

48 — adductor magnus

49 — gracilis

Right thigh, ventral view

Name:	**Adductor brevis**	Number: 47

Origin:	Anterior pubis.
Insertion:	Linea aspera on posterior femur.
Anatomical function:	Adduction, flexion, extension, and lateral rotation in the hip joint.
Map:	Is found on the inner thigh distally to pectineus and deep to adductor longus.
Is contracted by:	Squeezing the legs together with a slight inward rotation, with focus on the upper thighs close to the genitals.
Character structure(s):	NEED
Ego function:	MANAGEMENT OF ENERGY, (e) containment of sensuality.
Psychological function:	Containment of enjoyment (caused by physical motion/movement).
Ego function:	GENDER SKILLS, (d) containment of sensuality and sexuality.
Psychological function:	Holding on to sensual energy while being in contact with others.
Child's developmental stage/age:	The child holds on to someone with the legs, like a young monkey. The muscle stabilizes the balance in broad-based walking (feet wide apart).

Bodymapping:	
Client's position:	On the back.
Tester's position:	By the leg that is tested.
Activation in test position:	Press the heel into the mat and adduct the thigh.
Test location:	Between pectineus and adductor longus, deep and slightly distal to adductor longus.
Test direction:	Distally.

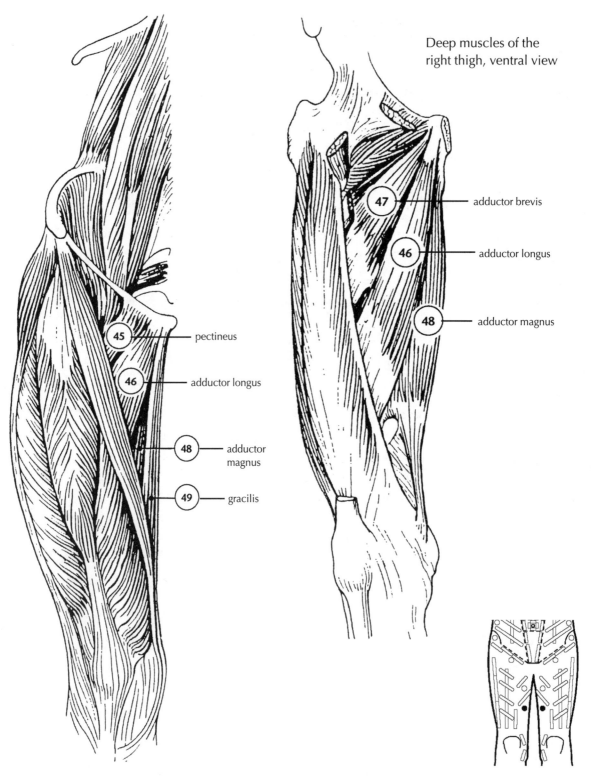

Deep muscles of the
right thigh, ventral view

47 adductor brevis

46 adductor longus

48 adductor magnus

45 pectineus

46 adductor longus

48 adductor
magnus

49 gracilis

Right thigh, ventral view

Name:	Adductor magnus	Number: 48

Origin:	Pubic ramus and ischial tuberosity.
Insertion:	Linea aspera and adductor tubercle of femur.
Anatomical function:	Adducts, extends, and medially rotates the thigh at the hip joint.
Map:	Big, thick triangular muscle found deep in the inner thigh The main adductor together with adductor longus.
Is contracted by:	Standing with feet wide apart and bringing the thighs together with a slight inward rotation without moving the feet. Kicking backward and adducting.
Character structure(s):	WILL
Ego function:	MANAGEMENT OF ENERGY, (e) containment of sensuality.
Psychological function:	Expands the ability for containment of all emotions and to change (switch) from one emotion to another (allowing the experience of having more than one emotion at the same time).
Ego function:	GENDER SKILLS, (d) containment of sensuality and sexuality.
Psychological function:	Expands the ability for containment of sensual and sexual energy.
Child's developmental stage/age:	The child is able to maintain balance while sitting on a potty. Lying down and stamping the floor in rage; the emotions expand out into the whole body, all the way out to the skin. Power in push-off while walking; included in the steering (directional) movements of the whole leg used during walking, changing direction, and stamping the floor; stabilizes the standing leg and helps the kicking leg move.

Bodymapping:

Client's position:	On the back.
Tester's position:	By the leg that is tested.
Activation in test position:	Adduct the leg and/or press the heel down into the floor/mat. (Take care not to contract semitendinosus instead). To isolate the adductor muscles from the quadriceps, extend the knee joint to tighten (contract) quadriceps.
Test location:	Test distally to adductor longus and proximally to where gracilis and sartorius meet; take care to separate from vastus medialis.
Test direction:	Medially, distally.

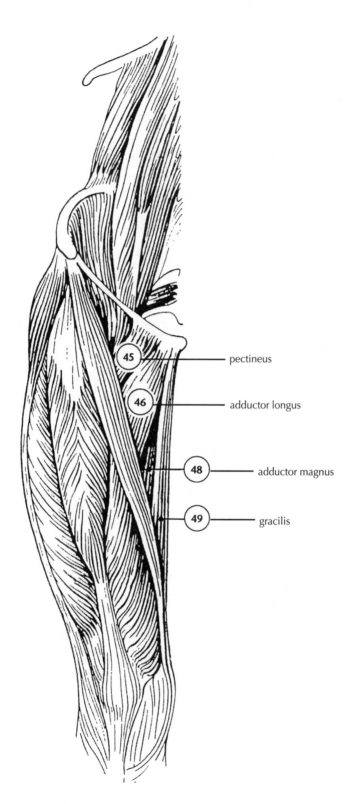

45 — pectineus

46 — adductor longus

48 — adductor magnus

49 — gracilis

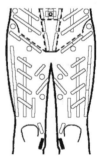

Right thigh, ventral view

Name:	**Gracilis**	**Number: 49**

Origin:	Anterior pubis.
Insertion:	Upper proximal shaft of tibia.
Anatomical function:	Hip joint: adducts, assists in flexion and extension. Knee joint: assists in flexion and medial rotation.
Map:	Long ribbon-shaped muscle that lies superficially on the medial edge of adductor longus.
Is contracted by:	Sitting: move the knees toward each other without moving the feet from the floor/mat.
Character structure(s):	AUTONOMY
Ego function:	SOCIAL BALANCE, (e) balance of managing stress and resolving it.
Psychological function:	Balancing stress, releasing it, and acting; having impulses to move with the stress energy and/or away from the stress energy.
Ego function:	MANAGEMENT OF ENERGY, (b) containment of high-level energy.
Psychological function:	Build up energy and preserve one's own impulses and curiosity at the same time.
Ego function:	GENDER SKILLS, (d) containment of sensuality and sexuality.
Psychological function:	Contain and keep one's lust and sensual impulses.
Child's developmental stage/age:	The child has an impulse and a desire to crawl out into the world (discover it); the muscle is used in crawling. The muscle stabilizes the knee when walking and moving to a standing position. Children at this age often bounce up and down at the knees when they are very eager.
Shock:	This muscle is commonly impacted by shock.

Bodymapping:	
Client's position:	On the back.
Tester's position:	By the leg that is tested.
Activation in test position:	Bend the knee and medially rotate it by turning the big toe toward the other leg while the heel is on the floor/mat.
Test location:	Approximately in the middle of the length of the muscle. Be careful: if you test too distally, it is difficult to distinguish sartorius, gracilis, and semitendinosus from each other.
Test direction:	In the direction of the fibers, distally.

Name:	**Connective tissue around the knee and ankle**	**Number: ***

Origin:	
Insertion:	
Anatomical function:	
Map:	Is found close to the knee and ankle.
Is contracted by:	
Character structure(s):	PERINATAL
Ego function:	MANAGEMENT OF ENERGY, (b) containment of high-level energy.
Psychological function:	Containment of high-level energy under pressure/strain.
Ego function:	SELF-ASSERTION, (a) self-assertion (manifesting one's power).
Psychological function:	Manifestation of power (instincts).
Child's developmental stage/age:	During birth, the connective tissue is part of the stretching reflex during second-stage labor, when the child pushes from the heels.

Name:	**Connective tissue of medial lateral rotators of the hip joint** **Number: ***

Origin:

Insertion:

Anatomical function:

Map: Is found close to the hip joint.

Is contracted by:

Character structure(s):   PERINATAL–EXISTENCE

Ego function: MANAGEMENT OF ENERGY, (b) containment of high-level energy.

Psychological function: Containment of high-level energy under pressure.

Ego function: SELF-ASSERTION, (a) self-assertion (manifesting one's power).

Psychological function: Assert one's power (instinct).

Child's developmental stage/age: PERINATAL: during birth, the child initially flexes the whole body and the limbs rotate inward during first-stage labor. When adrenaline is secreted during second-stage labor, the child starts to rotate the limbs outward and pushes to get through the birth canal with her own power/strength.
EXISTENCE: is part of the reflex system that is active when the child is moving around in the uterus.

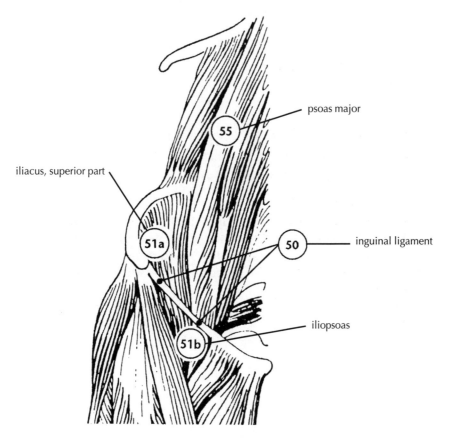

psoas major

iliacus, superior part

inguinal ligament

iliopsoas

Iliopsoas, ventral view

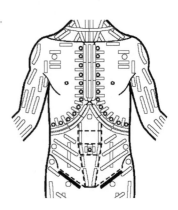

Name:	**Inguinal ligament**	Number: 50

Origin:	Anterior superior iliac spine.
Insertion:	Pubic tubercle.
Anatomical function:	Is a reinforcement of the lower edge of obliquus externus aponeurosis.
Map:	Is found in the groin; separates the trunk from the legs.
Is contracted by:	
Character structure(s):	Medial part: EXISTENCE Lateral part: NEED
Ego function:	CONNECTEDNESS, (a) bonding.
Psychological function:	EX: bonding (early connectedness). NEED: bonding (early connectedness).
Ego function:	CENTERING, (a) awareness of one's own center.
Psychological function:	EX: sensation/feeling of center. NEED: sense perception of one's own center.
Ego function:	MANAGEMENT OF ENERGY, (a) containment of emotions.
Psychological function:	EX: ability to be in a heightened energy state. NEED: recognition of one's emotions (grasp a name for them).
Child's developmental stage/age:	Stabilizes the muscles of the stomach area and thus stabilizes emotions.

Bodymapping:

Client's position:	On the back.
Tester's position:	By the leg that is tested.
Activation in test position:	
Test location:	Test in two locations, medially and laterally.
Test direction:	Test in a direction away from the genitals.

Name:	**Origin of iliacus**	Number: *

Origin:	Iliac fossa.
Insertion:	
Anatomical function:	Flexes the leg at the hip joint. Expands the sacroiliac joint (pelvis loosening).
Map:	Is found on the anterior surface of the edge of the iliac crest.
Is contracted by:	
Character structure(s):	PERINATAL
Ego function:	CONNECTEDNESS, (a) bonding.
Psychological function:	The ability to maintain oneself in bonding.
Ego function:	GENDER SKILLS, (a) awareness of gender.
Psychological function:	Awareness of one's gender.
Child's developmental stage/age:	The origin of iliacus is active when the fetus contracts itself during first-stage labor. When the child is lying alone after being born, he pulls himself into a fetal position.

Name:	**Insertion of iliopsoas**	Number: *

Origin:

Insertion: Lesser trochanter of femur.

Anatomical function: Flexes in the hip joint and rotates inward/medially.

Map: Is found in the hollow (with a pulse) under ligamentum inguinal, very close to the femur.

Is contracted by:

Character structure(s): PERINATAL

Ego function: CONNECTEDNESS, (a) bonding.

Psychological function: The ability to maintain oneself in bonding.

Child's developmental stage/age: The insertion of iliopsoas is active when the fetus contracts itself during first-stage labor. When the child is lying alone after being born, she pulls herself into a fetal position.

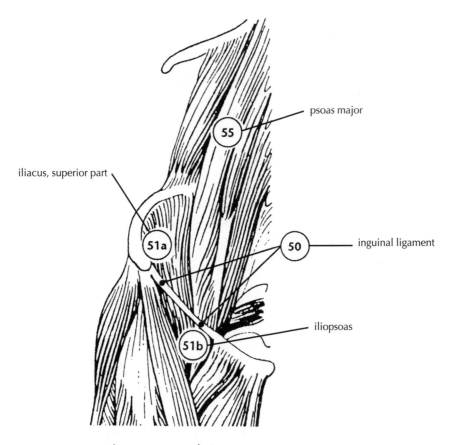

iliacus, superior part

psoas major

inguinal ligament

iliopsoas

Iliopsoas, ventral view

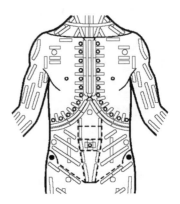

Name:	Iliacus	Number: 51a

Origin:	Upper two-thirds of the concavity of iliac fossa.
Insertion:	Onto tendon of psoas major and into lesser trochanter of femur.
Anatomical function:	Flexes thigh at the hip joint; assists in inward and outward rotation of the hip joint. Iliacus and psoas major together form the iliopsoas.
Map:	Is found deep on the anterior aspect of the hip bone (ilium). Iliacus is a thick flat muscle that blends together with the tendon of psoas major.
Is contracted by:	Balance on one foot; lift the other leg off the floor/mat and move it forward (flex the hip joint); tilt the pelvis slightly. Iliacus is active in the movement of the pelvis when it moves forward and backward.
Character structure(s):	Inferior part: EXISTENCE (is not tested separately) Superior part: LOVE/SEXUALITY
Ego function:	CONNECTEDNESS, (a) bonding.
Psychological function:	EX: early bonding. LOVE/SEX: preserving the sense of sexuality in contact.
Ego function:	CENTERING, (a) awareness of one's own center.
Psychological function:	EX: sensation of center. LOVE/SEX: preserve the sensation of one's own center and sensation of sexuality at the same time.
Ego function:	Superior part: GENDER SKILLS, (b) experience of gender. (e) manifestation of sensuality and sexuality.
Psychological function:	LOVE/SEX: (b) sensation of one's gender. LOVE/SEX: (e) able to manifest sensation of one's gender (both hide it, bring it forward, and the range between).
Child's developmental stage/age:	EX: the muscle takes part in the expression of all kinds of emotions when the child adds power to them and moves the pelvis and the legs; adds power in kicking. LOVE/SEX: the muscle tilts the pelvis back and forth, e.g., when the child swings/rocks, stands on one foot, and maintains its balance at the same time.
Bodymapping:	
Client's position:	On the back.
Tester's position:	On the side that is tested.
Activation in test position:	Lift the leg slightly off the floor/mat with knee extended.
Test location:	Place one hand on iliac crest most anterior. Push the skin up slightly, follow the curve of the hip bone, test into the muscle; move slowly, follow the exhalation.
Test direction:	Distally along iliac crest.

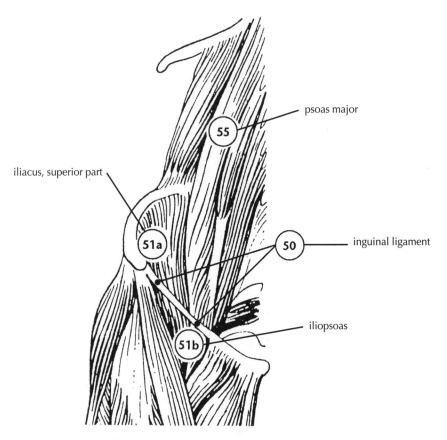

psoas major

iliacus, superior part

inguinal ligament

iliopsoas

Iliopsoas, ventral view

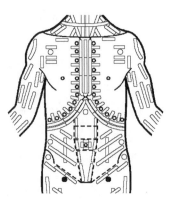

The Bodynamic Psycho-Motor Anatomy

Name:	**Iliopsoas**	**Number: 51b**

Origin:	Consists of the muscles psoas and iliacus.
Insertion:	Lesser trochanter of femur.
Anatomical function:	Flexes; inwardly and outwardly rotates the hip joint.
Map:	Is found in the hollow (with a pulse) under the inguinal ligament; deep to sartorius and rectus femoris.
Is contracted by:	Slight flexion in the hip joint and/or rotation of the leg medially in the hip joint.
Character structure(s):	NEED
Ego function:	CONNECTEDNESS, (a) bonding.
Psychological function:	Keep the bonding.
Ego function:	CENTERING, (a) awareness of one's own center.
Psychological function:	Experience of one's own center.
Child's developmental stage/age:	Holding on tight to the parent while sitting on their hip, like a young monkey does. This muscle is active when crossing one leg over the body to initiate rolling.

Bodymapping:	
Client's position:	On the back; the client bends his leg with the heel on the mat.
Tester's position:	On the side that is tested.
Activation in test position:	Rotate the leg medially; this isolates it from rectus femoris.
Test location:	Find the muscle in the hollow under the inguinal ligament (it has a pulse). Test deeply into femoral triangle and laterally.
Test direction:	Distally.

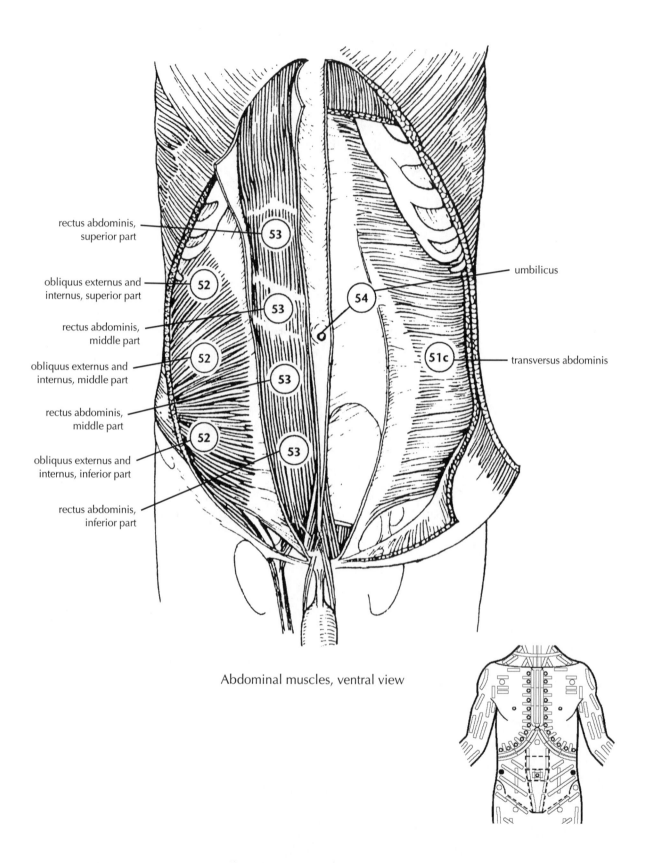

rectus abdominis,
superior part

obliquus externus and
internus, superior part

rectus abdominis,
middle part

obliquus externus and
internus, middle part

rectus abdominis,
middle part

obliquus externus and
internus, inferior part

rectus abdominis,
inferior part

umbilicus

transversus abdominis

Abdominal muscles, ventral view

Name:	Transversus abdominis	Number: 51c

Origin:	Lateral part of inguinal ligament; iliac crest; thoracolumbar fascia; cartilage of lower six ribs.
Insertion:	Abdominal aponeurosis to linea alba.
Anatomical function:	Pulls in the belly; part of the front of the abdominal wall; contraction of transversus abdominis restricts diaphragmatic breathing. If this muscle is tight/contracted, it forms a "wasp waist." The fascial layer connected to the muscle inserts on the front of the spine and is involved in the reflex system that keeps the spine straight.
Map:	Is found between the chest and the hip; the deepest layer of the abdominal muscles.
Is contracted by:	Pulling in the belly, as when you zip up your pants.
Character structure(s):	LOVE/SEXUALITY
Ego function:	MANAGEMENT OF ENERGY, (a) containment of emotions.
Psychological function:	Thoracolumbar fascia: containing high-level energy (instinct). Muscle: containing emotions concerning alliances.
Ego function:	GENDER SKILLS, (d) containment of sensuality and sexuality.
Psychological function:	Containment of sensuality and sexuality. When balanced you are able to sense sexuality and heart energy (love) at the same time.
Child's developmental stage/age:	The muscle connects the upper and lower parts of the body, stabilizes the trunk, e.g., maintaining balance while kicking a ball; bracing the belly to receive a punch in "boy's play"; to shut one's mind to emotions. The child is able to practice and master using a hula hoop.

Bodymapping:

Client's position:	On the back.
Tester's position:	Opposite the side that is tested.
Activation in test position:	Pull the stomach in as if zipping up a pair of tight jeans.
Test location:	In the waist deeply to obliquus externus and internus.
Test direction:	Slightly diagonally toward the central part of the body/and inferiorly (caudally).

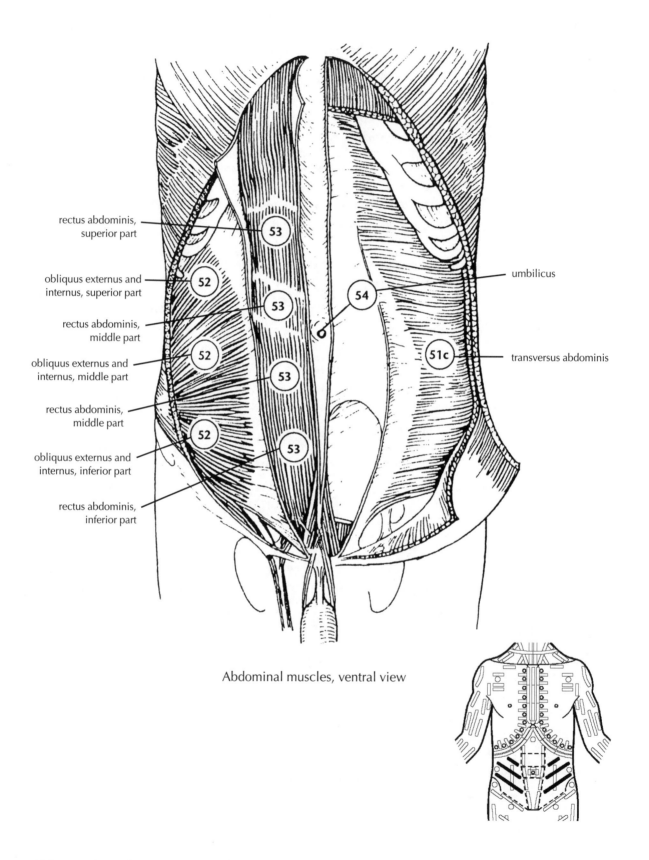

rectus abdominis,
superior part

obliquus externus and
internus, superior part

rectus abdominis,
middle part

obliquus externus and
internus, middle part

rectus abdominis,
middle part

obliquus externus and
internus, inferior part

rectus abdominis,
inferior part

umbilicus

transversus abdominis

53

52

53

52

53

52

53

54

51c

Abdominal muscles, ventral view

Name:	Obliquus externus and internus	Number: 52

Origin:	Externus: lower eight ribs. Internus: inguinal ligament; anterior iliac crest; thoracolumbar fascia.
Insertion:	Externus: abdominal aponeurosis, iliac crest. Internus: cartilages of bottom four ribs, abdominal aponeurosis.
Anatomical function:	Externus: lowers the ribs, rotates and laterally flexes the trunk. Internus: lowers the ribs, bends trunk forward and laterally. Forms the front of the abdominal wall with rectus abdominis and transversus abdominis; compresses the abdominal contents. These muscles provide stability so the diaphragm can contract powerfully.
Map:	Are found between the chest and the crest of the hip bone. In front of the abdomen they lie deep to rectus abdominis, and laterally they are superficial.
Is contracted by:	Rotating the trunk/spinal column; moving the left shoulder toward the right knee and vice versa.
Character structure(s):	Superior part: OPINIONS Middle part: SOLIDARITY/PERFORMANCE Inferior part: AUTONOMY
Ego function:	MANAGEMENT OF ENERGY, (a) containment of emotions.
Psychological function:	OPINIONS: sensing one's emotions in positioning and in giving care/support. SOL/PERF: be aware of emotions/feelings behind decisions/goal directions and visions; breadth of view. AUT: sense, name, and express one's emotions; own one's emotions/feelings.
Child's developmental stage/age:	OPINIONS: running in a jumping way with left arm toward right knee and vice versa; high jumps. The child starts reasoning. SOL/PERF: change of direction at high speed, twisting. AUT: crawling.

Bodymapping:	
Client's position:	On the back.
Tester's position:	Opposite the side that is tested.
Activation in test position:	The client lifts the head and shoulders and rotates, e.g., left shoulder toward right knee/foot.
Test location:	Is tested separately from rectus abdominis. Test with a flat hand in order not to reach into the inner organs. Test in three different locations on the muscle from the chest to the hip. Be careful not to get too close to the genital area. There might be scar tissue left by an operation.
Test direction:	Toward yourself in the direction of the fibers of externus. The most caudal test location is perpendicular to the other two in order to avoid the genital area.

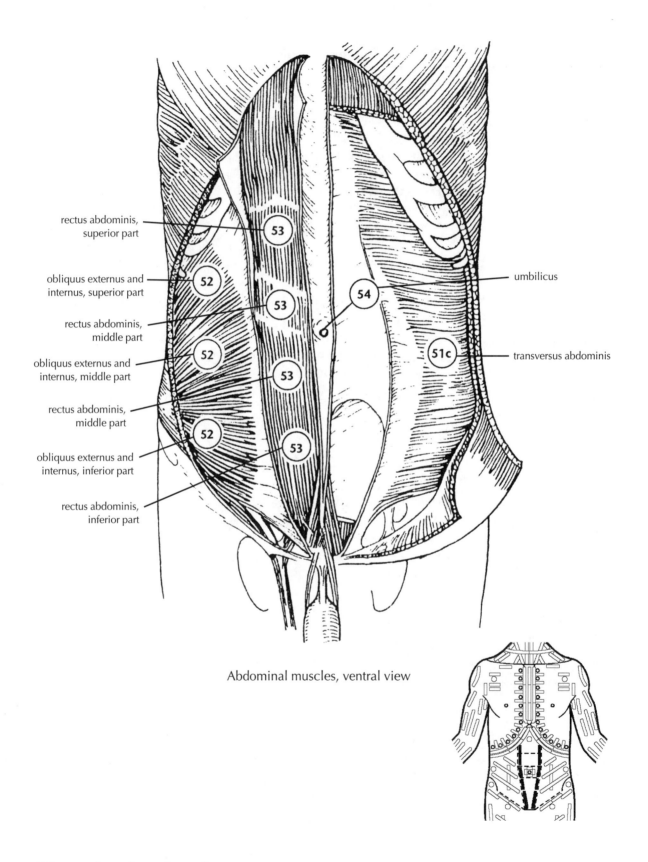

rectus abdominis, superior part

obliquus externus and internus, superior part

rectus abdominis, middle part

obliquus externus and internus, middle part

rectus abdominis, middle part

obliquus externus and internus, inferior part

rectus abdominis, inferior part

umbilicus

transversus abdominis

Abdominal muscles, ventral view

Name:	**Rectus abdominis**	Number: 53

Origin:	Cartilage of ribs 5, 6, and 7.
Insertion:	Crest of pubis, pubic symphysis.
Anatomical function:	The rectus lifts the body from a lying position, working against gravity. Flexing the lumbar spine by bringing the rib cage toward the pubic symphysis; lifts the pelvis.
Map:	Is found superficially on the front of the belly.
Is contracted by:	Bringing the sternum and lower ribs toward the pubis and vice versa.
Character structure(s):	Superior and inferior parts of the four parts: NEED The two middle parts: AUTONOMY
Ego function:	MANAGEMENT OF ENERGY, (a) containment of emotions.
Psychological function:	NEED: express needs through emotions. AUT: owning your own emotions.
Child's developmental stage/age:	NEED: the muscle stabilizes the rib cage to support power of the emotional expression of need. Active in rolling and creeping; the child is able to come from a lying to a sitting position. AUT: the muscle is active in rolling and crawling.

Bodymapping:	
Client's position:	On the back.
Tester's position:	Both right and left side can be tested from the same side.
Activation in test position:	Lift the head and look down at the toes.
Test location:	In four different locations along the muscle, number 2 approximately level with the umbilicus.
Test direction:	Distally; but it is a good idea to test the most inferior location in a superior direction.

Name:	**Pyramidalis**	Number: *

Origin:	Pubic bone and crest of pubic symphysis.
Insertion:	Linea alba (a strong fascial band between the two bellies of rectus abdominis).
Anatomical function:	Tightens linea alba.
Map:	Is placed in a sulcus of the front part of the rectus sheath (fascial system of rectus abdominis) in the lower ventral part just above the symphysis. Is variable and sometimes missing.
Is contracted by:	Active in lifting pubis toward sternum.
Character structure(s):	PUBERTY
Ego function:	GENDER SKILLS, (e) manifestation of sensuality and sexuality.
Psychological function:	Manifestation of sensuality and sexuality.
Child's developmental stage/age:	The muscle is active in sexual contact.

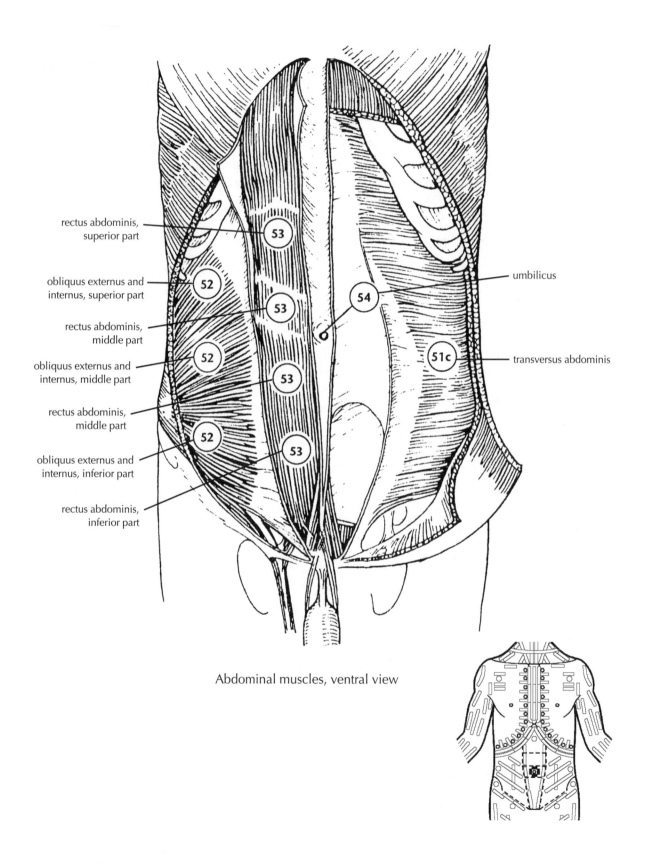

rectus abdominis,
superior part

obliquus externus and
internus, superior part

rectus abdominis,
middle part

obliquus externus and
internus, middle part

rectus abdominis,
middle part

obliquus externus and
internus, inferior part

rectus abdominis,
inferior part

umbilicus

transversus abdominis

53 **52** **54** **51c**

Abdominal muscles, ventral view

Name:	Umbilicus	Number: 54

Origin:	
Insertion:	Circular fibers in linea alba around the umbilicus.
Anatomical function:	Affects the flow through the navel cord.
Map:	Is found on the front of the abdomen, in the middle, just below the waist.
Is contracted by:	Slightly tightening the abdominal muscles around the umbilicus.
Character structure(s):	PERINATAL-EXISTENCE
Ego function:	BOUNDARIES, (a) the physical boundary.
Psychological function:	PERINATAL-EX: the earliest kind of boundary.
Ego function:	PATTERNS OF INTERPERSONAL SKILLS, (d) receiving and giving from one's core.
Psychological function:	PERINATAL-EX: relate to what you internalize; the first experience of accepting (taking in) or rejecting (pushing away).
Child's developmental stage/age:	The child takes in nourishment through the navel.

Bodymapping:

Client's position:	On the back.
Tester's position:	On either side of the client.
Activation in test position:	
Test location:	Test four locations on the circular fibers.
Test direction:	Around and along umbilicus.

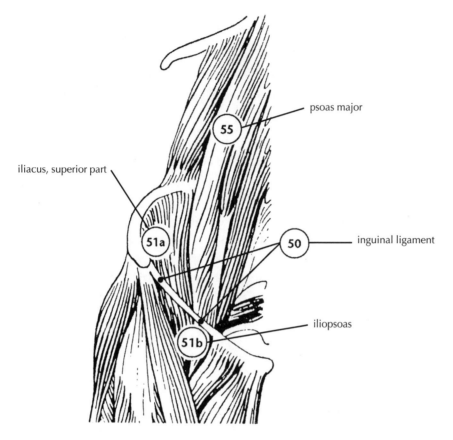

psoas major

iliacus, superior part

inguinal ligament

iliopsoas

Iliopsoas, ventral view

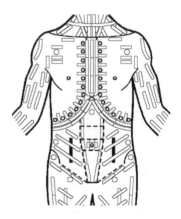

The Bodynamic Psycho-Motor Anatomy

Name:	**Psoas major**	Number: 55

Origin:	Bodies and transverse processes of lumbar vertebrae 1-4.
Insertion:	Lesser trochanter of femur.
Anatomical function:	Flexes the thigh and rotates the leg inward and outward in hip joint; flexes the lumbar spine.
Map:	Lies deep along the lumbar spinal column; deep to the intestines.
Is contracted by:	Lift the leg two inches from the floor/mat; make sure that you make room for a sway in your back.
Character structure(s):	AUTONOMY
Ego function:	CONNECTEDNESS, (a) bonding.
Psychological function:	Being oneself in connectedness.
Ego function:	CENTERING, (a) awareness of one's own center.
Psychological function:	Consciousness of one's own center.
Child's developmental stage/age:	The muscle is active in crawling and walking; stabilizes the spinal column.

Bodymapping:

Client's position:	On the back, with knees bent.
Tester's position:	On the side that is tested.
Activation in test position:	Lift the leg slightly.
Test location:	Ask the client to lift the head so you can locate rectus abdominis. Move your hand laterally from rectus abdominis. Move your fingers slowly and gently, sink into the client's belly following the client's exhalation. Ask the client to lift the leg. Test deeply close to the spine.
Test direction:	Inferiorly, slightly diagonally toward you or in the direction of the fibers.

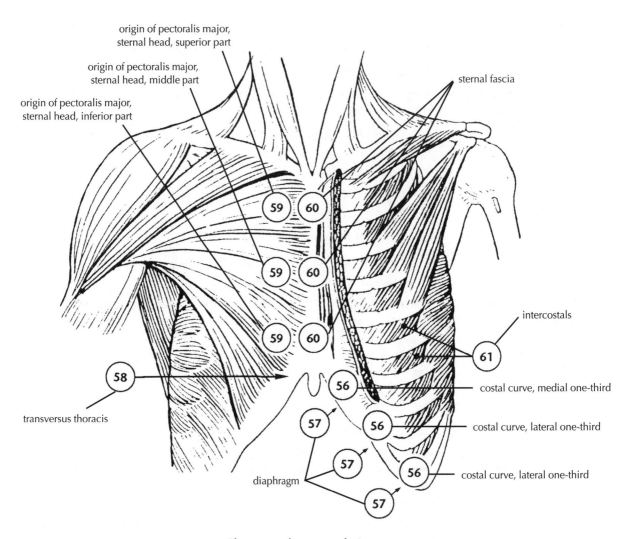

origin of pectoralis major,
sternal head, superior part

origin of pectoralis major,
sternal head, middle part

origin of pectoralis major,
sternal head, inferior part

sternal fascia

intercostals

costal curve, medial one-third

costal curve, lateral one-third

costal curve, lateral one-third

transversus thoracis

diaphragm

Chest muscles, ventral view

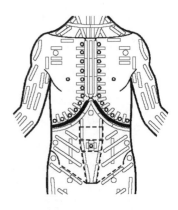

Name:	Costal curve	Number: 56

Origin:

Insertion:

Anatomical function: Forms the lower opening in the chest; is elastic in different movements of the torso, e.g., respiration; is origin for muscles, e.g., diaphragm on the inner side, and obliquus externus and internus on the outer side of the costal curve.

Map: Is formed by the cartilages on the lower ribs and creates the boundary between the chest and the abdomen.

Is contracted by:

Character structure(s): Medial one-third: LOVE/SEXUALITY
Middle one-third: OPINIONS
Lateral one-third: SOLIDARITY/PERFORMANCE

Ego function: MANAGEMENT OF ENERGY, (b) containment of high-level energy.

Psychological function: LOVE/SEX: containment of attraction/ecstasy/excitement.
OPINIONS: preserving one's own opinions in an open discussion.
SOL/PERF: preserving one's own energy and being part of building the group's energy at the same time.

Child's developmental stage/age: The costal curve is flexible in all twisting and turning movements.

Bodymapping:

Client's position: On the back.

Tester's position: On the side that is tested.

Activation in test position:

Test location: Start testing at the sternum and move laterally between the sternum to the "corner," mapping a general impression of muscle and connective tissue. Test in three different locations along the curve.

Test direction: Along the curve, medially-laterally.

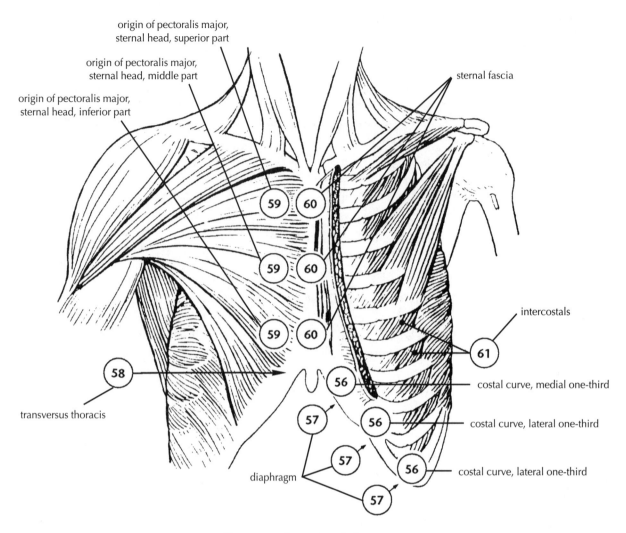

origin of pectoralis major,
sternal head, superior part

origin of pectoralis major,
sternal head, middle part

origin of pectoralis major,
sternal head, inferior part

sternal fascia

intercostals

transversus thoracis

costal curve, medial one-third

costal curve, lateral one-third

costal curve, lateral one-third

diaphragm

Chest muscles, ventral view

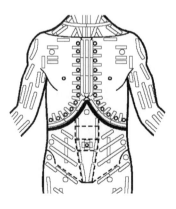

Name:	Diaphragm	Number: 57

Origin:	Sternal part: inner part of lower sternum. Costal part: inner surface of ribs 7-12. Lumbar part: lumbar vertebrae 1-3.
Insertion:	Central tendon.
Anatomical function:	Important in movement of respiration.
Map:	Dome-shaped muscular wall between the thoracic cavity and the abdominal cavity.
Is contracted by:	Inhalation, both reflex and voluntary movement. Expanding the lower chest anteriorly and laterally (obliquely), using resistance if needed, activates the diaphragm.
Character structure(s):	WILL
Ego function:	MANAGEMENT OF ENERGY, (a) containment of emotions.
Psychological function:	Master powerful emotions, and at the same time ability to accept additional emotions and sudden changes in emotions.
Child's developmental stage/age:	The muscle becomes active when the child's body has grown relatively large, so there is more room for the intestines. This happens at age 2-4, and the child is now capable of using the diaphragm to the fullest.

Bodymapping:

Client's position:	On the back, with knees bent.
Tester's position:	On the side that is tested.
Activation in test position:	Fill the lungs with air.
Test location:	Push up the skin; go as far in under the curve as possible. Test in three different locations.
Test direction:	Pull laterally along the curve.

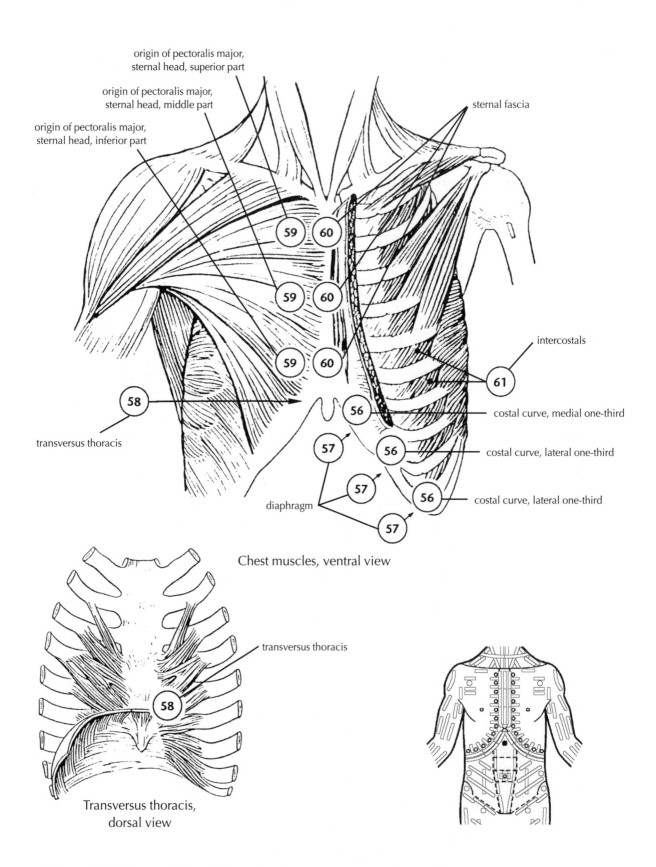

origin of pectoralis major,
sternal head, superior part

origin of pectoralis major,
sternal head, middle part

origin of pectoralis major,
sternal head, inferior part

sternal fascia

intercostals

costal curve, medial one-third

costal curve, lateral one-third

costal curve, lateral one-third

transversus thoracis

diaphragm

Chest muscles, ventral view

transversus thoracis

Transversus thoracis,
dorsal view

Name:	**Transversus thoracis**	**Number: 58**

Origin:	Inner surface of lower sternum and costal cartilages.
Insertion:	Inner surfaces of costal cartilages of ribs 2-6.
Anatomical function:	Exhalation. This muscle is already active in utero.
Map:	Is found on the inside surface of the frontal wall of the chest behind sternum (spider-shaped).
Is contracted by:	Exhaling—emptying the lungs as much as possible. Hold the breath as long as you can until the reflex kicks in and the muscle releases the voluntary tension.
Character structure(s):	1st part (superior): PERINATAL-EXISTENCE (is not tested separately) 2nd part: NEED (is not tested separately) 3rd part (inferior): AUTONOMY
Ego function:	CONNECTEDNESS, (a) bonding.
Psychological function:	Sensation of having inner space, life energy. PERINATAL-EX: surrendering to the breathing reflex, the experience of life energy/power. NEED: preserving life energy in connection. AUT: preserving one's own life energy in bonding.
Child's developmental stage/age:	The fetus starts to use this muscle in utero. Primary respiratory muscle in the first years.

Bodymapping:

Client's position:	On the back, with knees bent; this helps to relax the abdominal wall.
Tester's position:	On either side of the client.
Activation in test position:	Exhalation.
Test location:	The two upper locations: get an impression of the elasticity of the chest by firm pressure on sternum, knowing that ossification takes place over the years (is not tested). The lower location: palpate as far up as you can under the sternum; the location might be tender. Follow the breathing; test after exhalation.
Test direction:	Pull distally, or slightly obliquely.

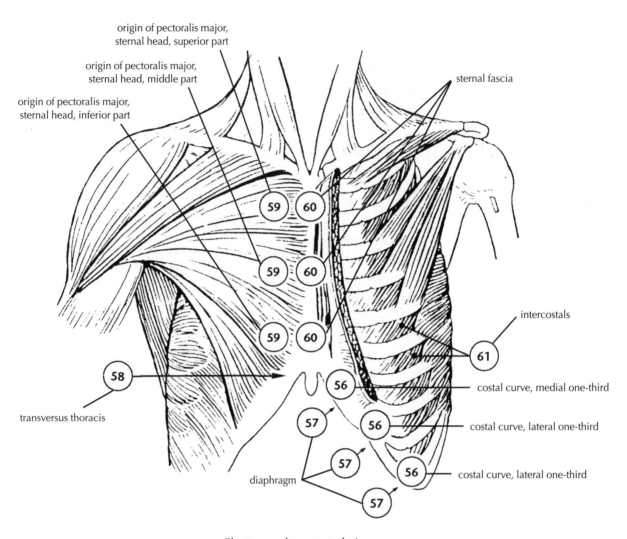

origin of pectoralis major,
sternal head, superior part

origin of pectoralis major,
sternal head, middle part

origin of pectoralis major,
sternal head, inferior part

sternal fascia

intercostals

costal curve, medial one-third

costal curve, lateral one-third

transversus thoracis

costal curve, lateral one-third

diaphragm

Chest muscles, ventral view

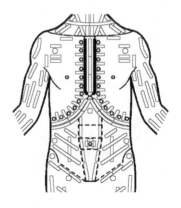

Name:	Origin of pectoralis major–sternal head	Number: 59

Origin:

Insertion:

Anatomical function:

Map:	Is found along the edges of the sternum.
Is contracted by:	Moving the arm across the front of the chest. Use the arm to pull hard toward the chest, and move the chest/sternum forward at the same time.
Character structure(s):	Superior part: EXISTENCE Middle part: NEED Inferior part: AUTONOMY
Ego function:	CONNECTEDNESS, (a) bonding.
Psychological function:	EX: maintain/preserve the bonding. NEED: maintain/preserve confidence in bonding. AUT: maintain/preserve the experience of one's self in bonding (one's inner space).
Child's developmental stage/age:	EX: the child pulls herself into contact by a reflex action (similar to the reflex action of hanging from a clothesline). NEED: hold on to someone like a young monkey (pull oneself close to the other). AUT: pull somebody close to oneself in contact.

Bodymapping:

Client's position:	On the back.
Tester's position:	On one of the sides.
Activation in test position:	Move the arm into a position in front of the chest.
Test location:	Test where the sternum and the cartilage of the ribs meet. Test in three different locations along the sternum.
Test direction:	Laterally.

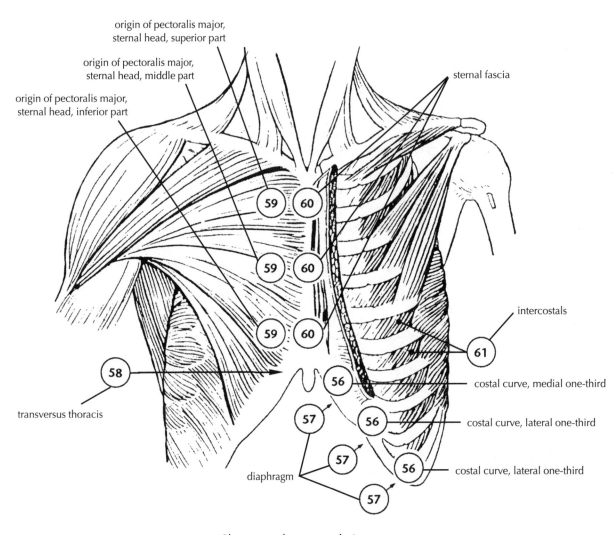

origin of pectoralis major,
sternal head, superior part

origin of pectoralis major,
sternal head, middle part

origin of pectoralis major,
sternal head, inferior part

sternal fascia

59 60

59 60

59 60

intercostals

58

56 61

57

56

costal curve, medial one-third

57

56

costal curve, lateral one-third

transversus thoracis

diaphragm

57

56

costal curve, lateral one-third

57

Chest muscles, ventral view

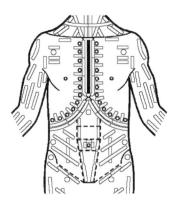

| **Name:** | **Sternal fascia** | **Number: 60** |

Origin:

Insertion:

| **Anatomical function:** | Is periosteum (a fascia) on the sternum, where pectoralis major also has its origin. |

| **Map:** | Is found in the central part of the sternum. |

Is contracted by:

| **Character structure(s):** | PERINATAL-EXISTENCE |

| **Ego function:** | CONNECTEDNESS, (a) bonding. |

| **Psychological function:** | PERINATAL-EX: sensation of connection
(The right to experience one's spirituality, one's self, and human contact at the same time). |

| **Child's developmental stage/age:** | The child has sensations of energy in contact. |

Bodymapping:

| **Client's position:** | On the back. |

| **Tester's position:** | On one of the sides. |

Activation in test position:

| **Test location:** | Test on location on the manubrium of the sternum and two locations on the body of the sternum. |

| **Test direction:** | Distally. |

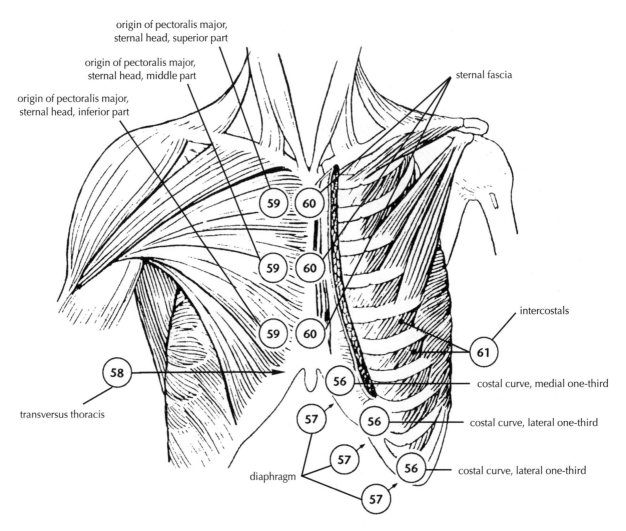

origin of pectoralis major,
sternal head, superior part

origin of pectoralis major,
sternal head, middle part

origin of pectoralis major,
sternal head, inferior part

sternal fascia

59 **60**

59 **60**

59 **60**

58

transversus thoracis

56

57

57

57

57

diaphragm

intercostals

61

costal curve, medial one-third

costal curve, lateral one-third

costal curve, lateral one-third

Chest muscles, ventral view

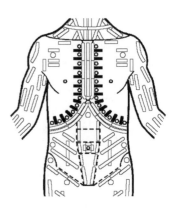

Name:	Intercostals	Number: 61

Origin:	Between adjacent ribs.
Insertion:	
Anatomical function:	Respiratory muscles.
Map:	Is found in the spaces between the ribs.
Is contracted by:	During breathing.
Character structure(s):	Between ribs 2-5: PERINATAL Between ribs 3-7: NEED Between ribs 6-9: AUTONOMY Between ribs 9-10: LOVE/SEXUALITY Between ribs 1-2 and 10-12: OPINIONS-SOLIDARITY/PERFORMANCE
Ego function:	MANAGEMENT OF ENERGY, (a) containment of emotions.
Psychological function:	PERINATAL rhythm of life, being, and receiving. NEED: regulating need impulses by regulating respiration. AUT: regulating impulses of desire by changing respiration. LOVE/SEX: regulating sensual/sexual energy. OPINIONS-SOL/PERF: regulating the space of attention in relation to oneself, the other, or the group.
Child's developmental stage/age:	Respiration; the efficiency of the muscles is increased as the child grows up.

Bodymapping:

Client's position:	On the back.
Tester's position:	On the side that is tested.
Activation in test position:	Follow the respiration; do not stay too long in each location.
Test location:	Test between the ribs lateral to the costal cartilage. Start at the top under the clavicle and follow the curve down the sternum and further.
Test direction:	Follow the ribs.

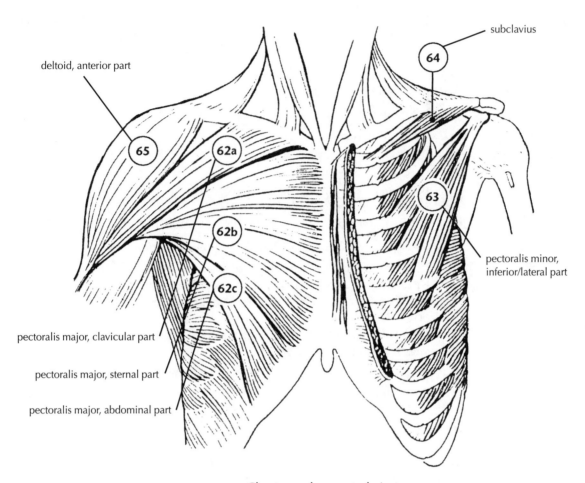

deltoid, anterior part

subclavius

64

65

62a

62b

62c

63

pectoralis minor,
inferior/lateral part

pectoralis major, clavicular part

pectoralis major, sternal part

pectoralis major, abdominal part

Chest muscles, ventral view

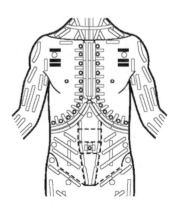

Name:	Pectoralis major	Number: 62a, b, c

Origin:	(a) Clavicular part: medial half of clavicle. (b) Sternal part: sternum, cartilages of upper six ribs. (c) Abdominal part: aponeurosis of external oblique.
Insertion:	Bicipital groove of humerus, lateral lip.
Anatomical function:	Adducts, medially rotates, and flexes the arm at the shoulder joint.
Map:	A flat, triangular fan-shaped muscle on the front of the chest.
Is contracted by:	From a position where the arm is stretched out horizontally and laterally from the body, move the arm into a position in front of the body.
Character structure(s):	(a) Clavicular part: LOVE/SEXUALITY (b) Sternal part: OPINIONS-SOLIDARITY/PERFORMANCE (c) Abdominal part: WILL
Ego function:	CENTERING, (d) feelings of self-esteem.
Psychological function:	LOVE/SEX: self-worth concerning sensuality/sexuality. OPINIONS-SOL/PERF: self-worth concerning opinions and group positions. WILL: self-worth concerning actions.
Ego function:	SELF-ASSERTION, (b) asserting oneself in one's roles.
Psychological function:	LOVE/SEX: manifest sensuality/sexuality (flirting). OPINIONS-SOL/PERF: manifest opinions and make one's mark in groups WILL: manifest power and emotions.
Ego function:	GENDER SKILLS, (c) experience of gender role.
Psychological function:	LOVE/SEX: integrate the family pattern of sex roles (flirting). OPINIONS-SOL/PERF: integrate the social sex-role patterns. WILL: imitate sex-role patterns.
Ego function:	62a, b: Clavicular and sternal part: GENDER SKILLS. (e) manifestation of sensuality and sexuality.
Psychological function:	LOVE/SEX: manifest sensuality and love (falling in love). OPINIONS-SOL/PERF: manifest sexuality.
Child's developmental stage/age:	The muscle lifts and enlarges the chest, as seen in boasting. WILL: lifting heavy things, throwing a ball, hugging. LOVE/SEX: throwing balls underhand and overhand; making flirting movements with the shoulder. OPINIONS-SOL/PERF: in many games and sports, e.g., pole vaulting, shot put, discus; beating one's breast like Tarzan.

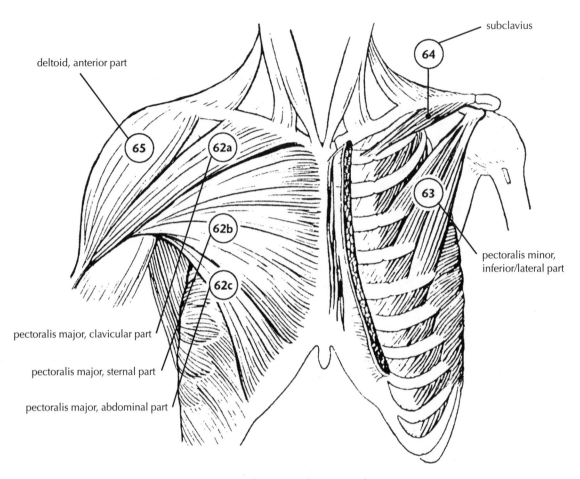

Chest muscles, ventral view

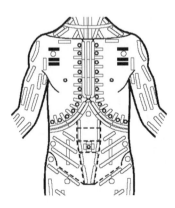

Name: **Pectoralis major**   **Number: 62a, b, c**

Bodymapping:

Client's position:	On the back.
Tester's position:	Opposite the side that is tested.
Activation in test position:	(a) Clavicular part: arm over head, lift the arm slightly. (b) Sternal part: arm out horizontally, lift the arm slightly. (c) Abdominal part: arm along the body, lift the arm slightly.
Test location:	(a) Clavicular part: below the clavicle where the muscle is full. (b) Sternal part: level with sternum where the muscle is full. (c) Abdominal part: find the muscle belly in the armpit, move the hand slightly medially along the muscle, and test there.
Test direction:	(a) Medially, slightly cranially. (b) Medially. (c) Medially, slightly caudally.

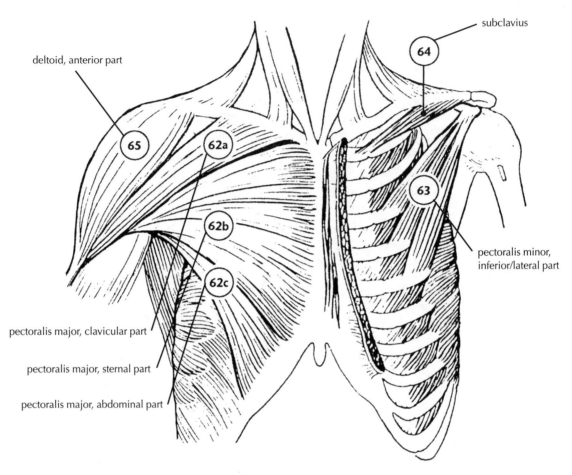

deltoid, anterior part

subclavius

pectoralis minor, inferior/lateral part

pectoralis major, clavicular part

pectoralis major, sternal part

pectoralis major, abdominal part

Chest muscles, ventral view

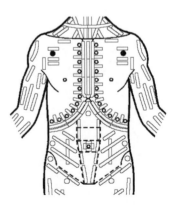

Name:	**Pectoralis minor**	Number: 63

Origin:	Anterior ribs 3, 4, and 5.
Insertion:	Coracoid process of the scapula.
Anatomical function:	Pulls the scapula forward, downward, and lifts the ribs Auxiliary muscle of respiration with the arm fixed.
Map:	Is found deep to pectoralis major.
Is contracted by:	Moving the shoulder slightly down and forward.
Character structure(s):	Superior part: NEED (is not tested separately) Inferior/lateral part: AUTONOMY
Ego function:	CENTERING, (d) feelings of self-esteem.
Psychological function:	NEED: self-worth concerning one's needs. AUT: self-worth concerning one's curiosity and enthusiasm.
Ego function:	SELF-ASSERTION, (b) asserting oneself in one's roles.
Psychological function:	NEED: express one's needs (reaching out for what you want). AUT: being enthusiastic and curious; experimenting.
Child's developmental stage/age:	The muscle stabilizes the shoulder area so the arms can reach out. The child points and says "What is that?" The child pulls himself forward in creeping and crawling and pulls himself to a standing position (both active and stabilizing).

Bodymapping:	
Client's position:	On the back.
Tester's position:	Opposite the side that is tested.
Activation in test position:	Push forward slightly with the shoulder; a small movement is most effective. Reaching toward the feet may also be effective.
Test location:	Where the muscle is full.
Test direction:	Caudally, slightly medially.

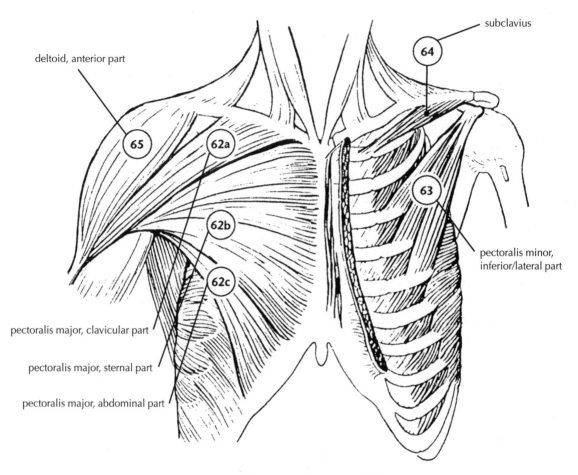

deltoid, anterior part

subclavius

pectoralis minor, inferior/lateral part

pectoralis major, clavicular part

pectoralis major, sternal part

pectoralis major, abdominal part

Chest muscles, ventral view

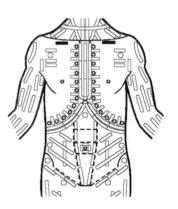

Name:	Subclavius	Number: 64

Origin:	1st rib.
Insertion:	Inferior shaft of clavicle.
Anatomical function:	Protects the clavicular joint; accessory muscle of respiration.
Map:	Is found between the 1st rib and the clavicle.
Is contracted by:	Moving the shoulder area down toward the chest.
Character structure(s):	WILL
Ego function:	GROUNDING AND REALITY TESTING, (c) experience and grounding of extrasensory perceptions.
Psychological function:	Becoming aware of the difference between extrasensory sensation and physical reality.
Child's developmental stage/age:	The muscle stabilizes the shoulder area in all movements where the arm is used with strength/power. The child lifts heavy things.

Bodymapping:

Client's position:	On the back.
Tester's position:	Opposite the side that is tested.
Activation in test position:	Move the shoulder area down toward the chest.
Test location:	Where the muscle is full, under the clavicle.
Test direction:	Medially along the clavicle.

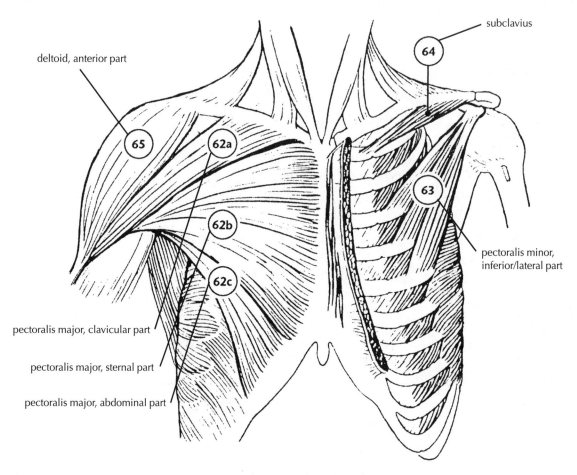

deltoid, anterior part

subclavius

pectoralis major, clavicular part

pectoralis major, sternal part

pectoralis major, abdominal part

pectoralis minor, inferior/lateral part

Chest muscles, ventral view

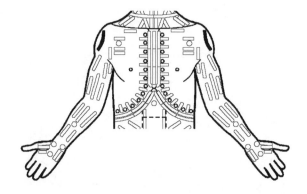

Name:	**Deltoid, anterior**	Number: 65

Origin:	Lateral third of clavicle.
Insertion:	Deltoid tuberosity of humerus.
Anatomical function:	Flexion, horizontal adduction, medial rotation in the shoulder joint.
Map:	Is found on the front of the shoulder; forms the front of the roundness of the shoulder.
Is contracted by:	Moving the arm slightly forward in the shoulder joint.
Character structure(s):	NEED
Ego function:	BOUNDARIES, (e) making space for oneself in social contact.
Psychological function:	Make space for one's needs.
Ego function:	PATTERNS OF INTERPERSONAL SKILLS, (a) reaching out.
Psychological function:	Insist on having one's needs fulfilled.
Child's developmental stage/age:	The muscle stabilizes the shoulder joint so the arms can be held in a reaching-out gesture. The child lifts the arms forward ("Lift me up"). The muscle is active during play, e.g., when the child is scribbling and when playing with toy cars.

Bodymapping:

Client's position:	On the back.
Tester's position:	On the side that is tested.
Activation in test position:	Lift the arm slightly, palm upward.
Test location:	Test where the muscle is full.
Test direction:	Distally, laterally.

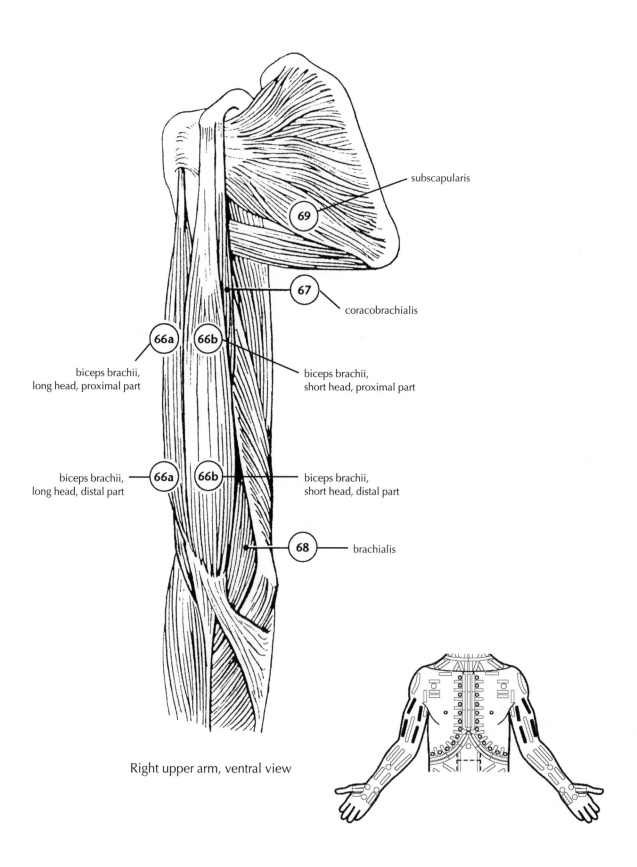

subscapularis

69

67

coracobrachialis

66a

66b

biceps brachii,
long head, proximal part

biceps brachii,
short head, proximal part

66a

66b

biceps brachii,
long head, distal part

biceps brachii,
short head, distal part

68

brachialis

Right upper arm, ventral view

| Name: | Biceps brachii | Number: 66a, b |

Origin:	(a) Long head: supraglenoid tubercle of the scapula. (b) Short head: coracoid process of the scapula.
Insertion:	Tuberosity of radius.
Anatomical function:	(a) Long head: flexes elbow and supinates the forearm; assists with abduction of shoulder joint. (b) Short head: flexes elbow and supinates the forearm (radio-ulnar joint); flexes shoulder joint.
Map:	Is found superficially on the front of the upper arm.
Is contracted by:	Bending the elbow joint with palm upward ("ripple one's muscles").

Character structure(s):	(a) Long head, proximal part: LOVE/SEXUALITY
	                    distal part: SOLIDARITY/PERFORMANCE
	(b) Short head, proximal part: NEED
	                    distal part: AUTONOMY

Ego function:	PATTERNS OF INTERPERSONAL SKILLS, (c) drawing toward oneself and holding on closely.
Psychological function:	LOVE/SEX: form alliances. SOL/PERF: make acquaintance with others. NEED: go into close contact/pull oneself into close contact. AUTONOMY: create close contact because of their own enthusiasm and interest.
Child's developmental stage/age:	LOVE/SEX: swinging, turning/dancing while holding hands, throwing a ball (underhand). SOL/PERF: drawing things toward oneself, reaching out for things and people, doing pull-ups. NEED: pulling oneself toward someone and drawing things toward oneself. AUTONOMY: taking in something or someone and drawing it/them toward oneself; pulling oneself up to a standing position.

Bodymapping:	
Client's position:	On the back.
Tester's position:	By the arm that is tested.
Activation in test position:	With the palm upward, flex the elbow joint.
Test location:	Test in two different locations on each belly of the muscle.
Test direction:	Distally.

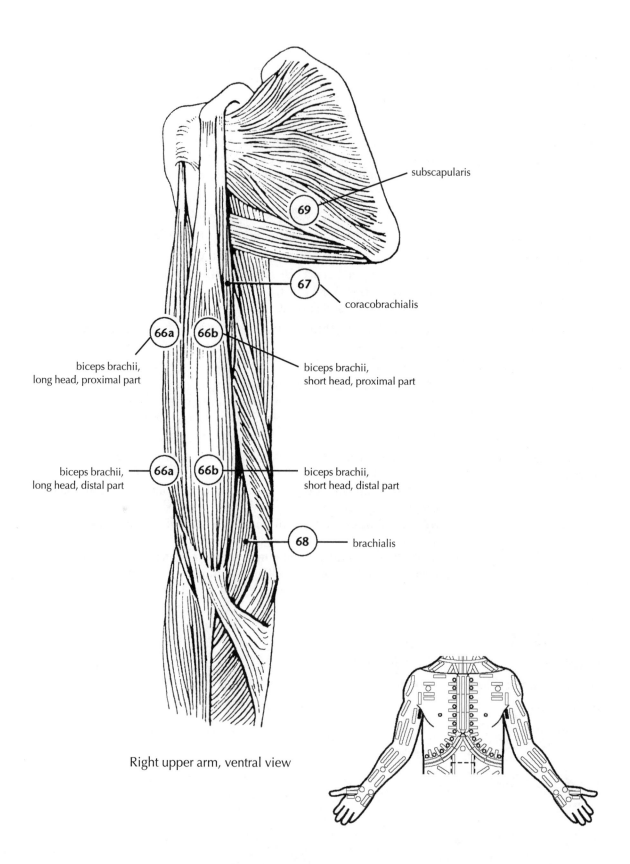

subscapularis

69

67

coracobrachialis

66a

66b

biceps brachii,
long head, proximal part

biceps brachii,
short head, proximal part

66a

66b

biceps brachii,
long head, distal part

biceps brachii,
short head, distal part

68

brachialis

Right upper arm, ventral view

Name:	**Coracobrachialis**	**Number: 67**

Origin:	Coracoid process.
Insertion:	Medial surface and border of humerus.
Anatomical function:	Flexes, rotates medially, and adducts in the shoulder joint.
Map:	Is found deep to deltoid and pectoralis major on the front and medial side of the upper arm.
Is contracted by:	Moving the arm slightly forward and into a position in front of the body (in the shoulder joint).
Character structure(s):	AUTONOMY
Ego function:	PATTERNS OF INTERPERSONAL SKILLS, (a) reaching out. (c) drawing toward oneself and holding on closely.
Psychological function:	Reach out, receive, and maintain contact (with people and objects).
Child's developmental stage/age:	The muscle stabilizes the arm when the child reaches out for something it wants and when the child points at things, "naming the world." The child catches a big ball underarm by bringing the arms together in front of the body.

Bodymapping:

Client's position:	On the back.
Tester's position:	By the arm that is tested.
Activation in test position:	Elbow joint is bent passively; the hand hangs loose. By lifting the elbow, the muscle is activated separately from biceps.
Test location:	Test where the belly of the muscle can be palpated.
Test direction:	Distally, along the arm.

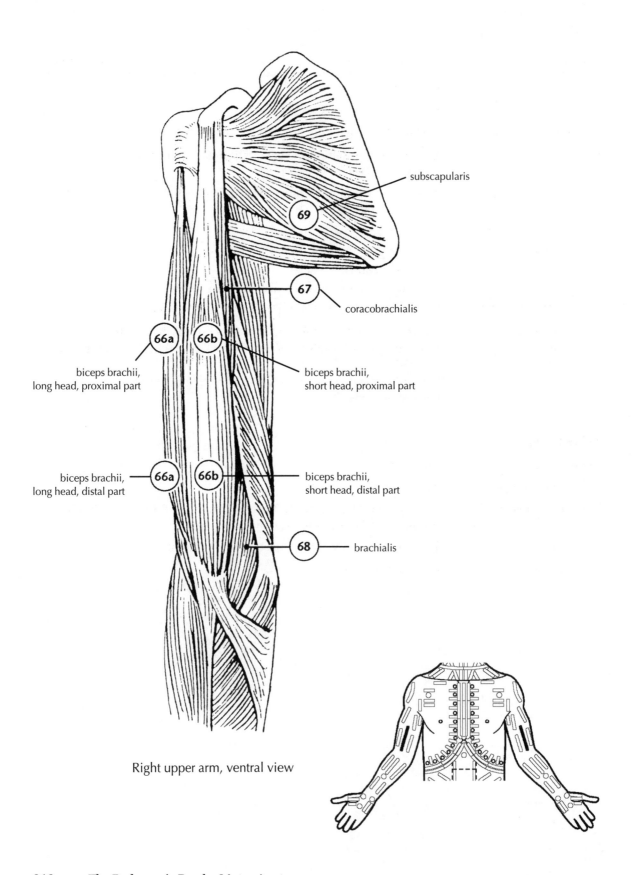

subscapularis

69

67 coracobrachialis

66a **66b**

biceps brachii,
long head, proximal part

biceps brachii,
short head, proximal part

66a **66b**

biceps brachii,
long head, distal part

biceps brachii,
short head, distal part

68 brachialis

Right upper arm, ventral view

The Bodynamic Psycho-Motor Anatomy

Name:	**Brachialis**	Number: 68

Origin:	Lower half of anterior shaft of humerus.
Insertion:	Tuberosity of ulna.
Anatomical function:	Flexes the elbow joint.
Map:	Is found distally on the upper arm covered almost completely by biceps.
Is contracted by:	Bending the elbow joint.
Character structure(s):	WILL
Ego function:	PATTERNS OF INTERPERSONAL SKILLS, (c) drawing toward oneself and holding on closely.
Psychological function:	Drawing in; holding on to close contact.
Child's developmental stage/age:	The child is able to hold and lift heavy things. The muscle is active in hugging.

Bodymapping:

Client's position:	On the back.
Tester's position:	By the arm that is tested.
Activation in test position:	Flex elbow joint; if necessary give resistance.
Test location:	Test deep to biceps from the medial side of the arm.
Test direction:	Distally.

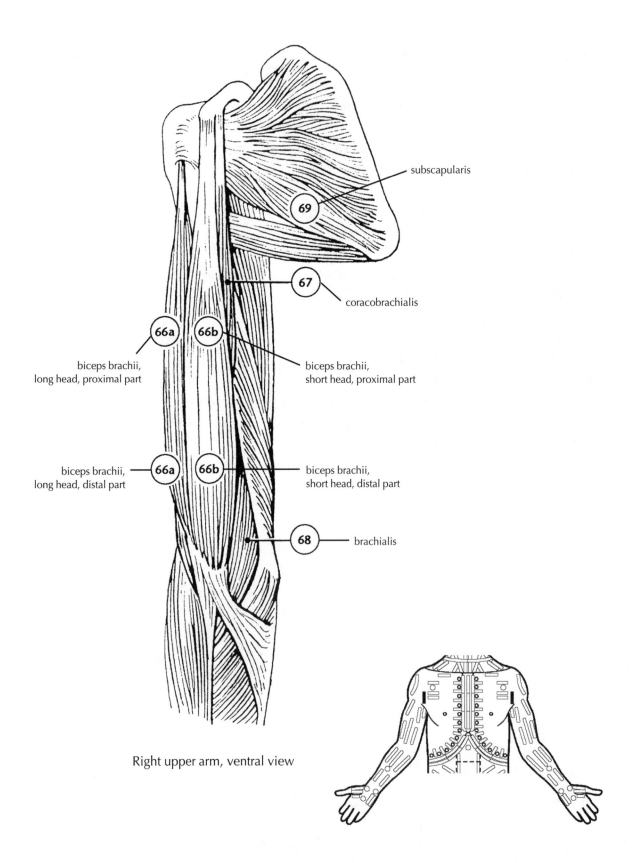

subscapularis

coracobrachialis

biceps brachii,
long head, proximal part

biceps brachii,
short head, proximal part

biceps brachii,
long head, distal part

biceps brachii,
short head, distal part

brachialis

Right upper arm, ventral view

Name:	**Subscapularis**	Number: 69

Origin:	Subscapula fossa of scapula (on anterior surface next to chest wall).
Insertion:	Lesser tubercle of humerus.
Anatomical function:	Rotates the arm medially in the shoulder joint Is part of the rotator cuff.
Map:	The muscle emerges from the lateral border of scapula and forms a large part of the posterior wall of the armpit.
Is contracted by:	Turning the upper arm inward in the shoulder joint.
Character structure(s):	NEED
Ego function:	SOCIAL BALANCE, (c) degree of "facade" and maintaining one's front.
Psychological function:	Flexibility in following immediate need impulses.
Child's developmental stage/age:	The muscle is active when the child reaches out for something and when rolling from belly to back. It stabilizes when the child pushes herself up from the floor/mat, and it stabilizes creeping.

Bodymapping:

Client's position:	On the back.
Tester's position:	On the side that is tested.
Activation in test position:	Pull the scapula laterally away from the spine to make the muscle more accessible as it lies between the scapula and the chest wall. Rotate the arm medially.
Test location:	Where the muscle is full on the anterior surface of the scapula.
Test direction:	Any way possible.

| Name: | **Connective tissue of medial and lateral rotators of the shoulder joint** | Number: * |

Origin:

Insertion:

Anatomical function:

Map: Is found close to the shoulder joint.

Is contracted by:

Character structure(s):   PERINATAL
EXISTENCE

Ego function: MANAGEMENT OF ENERGY, (b) containment of high-level energy.

Psychological function: Containing high-level energy under pressure.

Ego function: SELF-ASSERTION, (a) self assertion (manifesting one's power).

Psychological function: Manifesting one's power (instinct).

Child's developmental stage/age: PERINATAL: The connective tissue is part of the reflex system, and during second-stage labor it assists in stabilizing the throat and neck so the power/strength can get through when the child pushes from the heels. EXISTENCE: The connective tissue is part of the reflex system that is active when the child is moving around in utero.

Name:	**Connective tissue around elbow and wrist**	Number *

Origin:

Insertion:

Anatomical function:

Map: Is found close to the elbow joint and the wrist.

Is contracted by:

Character structure(s):   PERINATAL

Ego function: MANAGEMENT OF ENERGY, (b) containment of high-level energy.

Psychological function: Containing high-level energy under pressure/stress.

Ego function: SELF-ASSERTION, (a) self-assertion (manifesting one's power).

Psychological function: Manifesting one's power/strength (instinct).

Child's developmental stage/age: During birth, the child rotates outward from the shoulder down through the elbow joint and the wrist during second-stage labor to stabilize the head and neck so the power/strength can get through when the child pushes from the heels.

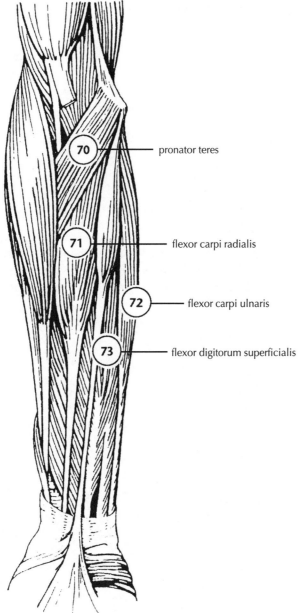

70 — pronator teres

71 — flexor carpi radialis

72 — flexor carpi ulnaris

73 — flexor digitorum superficialis

Right forearm, ventral view

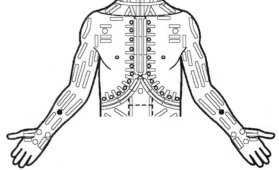

The Bodynamic Psycho-Motor Anatomy

Name:	Pronator teres	Number: 70

Origin:	Above the medial condyle of humerus; coronoid process of ulna.
Insertion:	Middle, lateral shaft of radius.
Anatomical function:	Pronates the forearm and assists flexion of the elbow joint.
Map:	Is found radially (on the thumb side) on the front of the forearm in the superficial layer.
Is contracted by:	Forearm rotates so the palm is turned down to the floor/mat; the back of the hand is turned upward.
Character structure(s):	AUTONOMY
Ego function:	PATTERNS OF INTERPERSONAL SKILLS, (d) receiving and giving from one's core.
Psychological function:	Give from one's sense of core and from one's emotions.
Child's developmental stage/age:	The child plays "give-and-take" games, lets things fall, lets go. The muscle is active in top-grip, which later develops into cross-thumb grasp.

Bodymapping:

Client's position:	On the back.
Tester's position:	By the arm that is tested.
Activation in test position:	Palm toward the ceiling; support the forearm with one hand underneath it and use the other hand for testing. Find biceps insertion and pronator teres in relation to this. Client turns palm toward the mat.
Test location:	Distal to biceps insertion where the belly of the muscle is full.
Test direction:	In the direction of the muscle fibers.

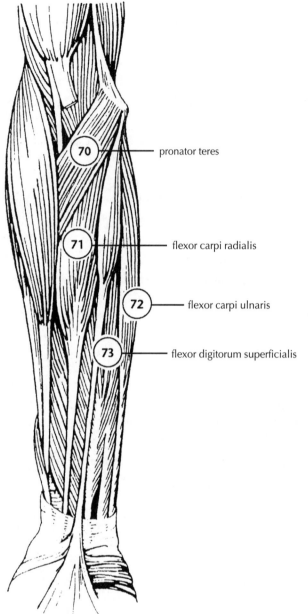

70 — pronator teres

71 — flexor carpi radialis

72 — flexor carpi ulnaris

73 — flexor digitorum superficialis

Right forearm, ventral view

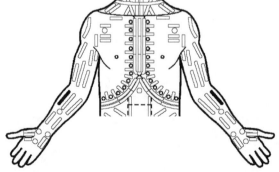

Name:	**Flexor carpi radialis**	Number: 71

Origin:	Medial epicondyle of humerus.
Insertion:	Base of 2nd and 3rd metacarpal bones.
Anatomical function:	Flexes and radially flexes the wrist; assists in pronation.
Map:	Is found distally to pronator teres on the ulnar side (little finger side), approximately two inches distal to the elbow joint on the anterior surface of the forearm.
Is contracted by:	Flexing the wrist, mostly toward the thumb side, as if trying to touch the elbow with the thumb.
Character structure(s):	WILL
Ego function:	PATTERNS OF INTERPERSONAL SKILLS, (c) drawing toward oneself and holding on closely.
Psychological function:	Pull in toward oneself, hold firmly, and pull toward one's core/heart.
Child's developmental stage/age:	The child piles bricks on top of each other; catches a small ball close to its body; throws underhand; throws/bounces a big ball on the floor several times.

Bodymapping:

Client's position:	On the back.
Tester's position:	By the arm that is tested.
Activation in test position:	Give resistance to radial flexion of the hand, i.e., flex the wrist toward the thumb side.
Test location:	Locate the belly of the muscle distally to pronator teres; find the tendon at the wrist if necessary. Test where the muscle is full, i.e., proximally on the forearm.
Test direction:	Distally.

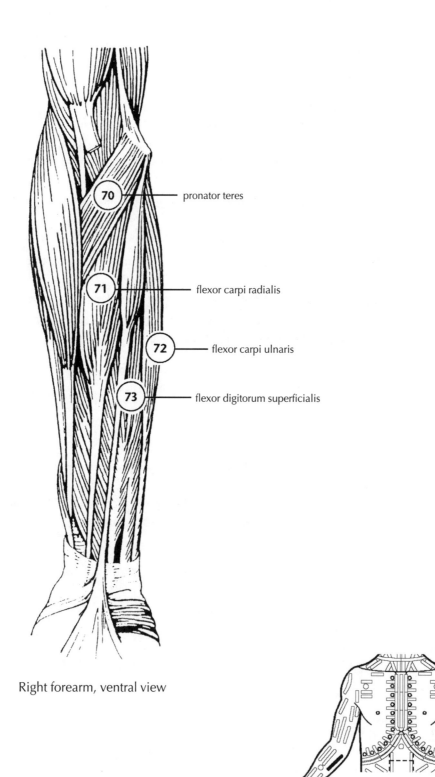

70 — pronator teres

71 — flexor carpi radialis

72 — flexor carpi ulnaris

73 — flexor digitorum superficialis

Right forearm, ventral view

Name:	Flexor carpi ulnaris	Number: 72

Origin:	Medial epicondyle humerus; proximal posterior ulna.
Insertion:	Pisiform, hamate, base of 5th metacarpal.
Anatomical function:	Flexes and ulnar flexes the wrist.
Map:	Is found on the anterior medial side on the forearm (anteroulnar).
Is contracted by:	Flexing the wrist mostly toward the little finger as if trying to reach the elbow.
Character structure(s):	LOVE/SEXUALITY
Ego function:	PATTERNS OF INTERPERSONAL SKILLS, (c) drawing toward oneself and holding on closely.
Psychological function:	Surrounding the contact sensually and drawing the contact toward oneself.
Child's developmental stage/age:	The child is able to tip/tilt the hand when drinking, wave like royalty, and catch and throw a ball with one hand. The child is starting to play ball games against the wall and to further develop the grasp, starting with the little finger and thumb when holding a pencil.

Bodymapping:

Client's position:	On the back.
Tester's position:	By the arm that is tested.
Activation in test position:	With the hand in a supinated position (palm upward), flex the wrist forward and toward the little-finger side. Give resistance to the hand if necessary.
Test location:	Find the muscle on the forearm along the medial edge of the ulna. Find the tendon at the wrist. Test where the muscle is full, i.e., proximally on the forearm.
Test direction:	Distally.

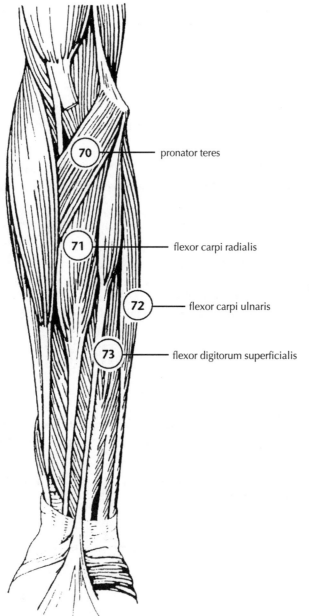

70 — pronator teres

71 — flexor carpi radialis

72 — flexor carpi ulnaris

73 — flexor digitorum superficialis

Right forearm, ventral view

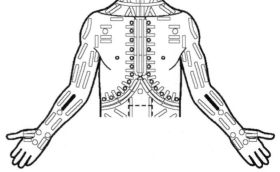

The Bodynamic Psycho-Motor Anatomy

Name:	**Flexor digitorum superficialis**	**Number: 73**

Origin:	Medial epicondyle humerus; coronoid process ulna; anterior surface of radius.
Insertion:	Sides of shaft of middle phalanges of the four lateral fingers.
Anatomical function:	Flexes the proximal interphalangeal joints (PIP) and metacarpophalangeal joints (MCP), and assists wrist flexion.
Map:	A broad muscle that forms the middle layer on the front of the forearm.
Is contracted by:	Flexing the first (proximal interphalangeal) joints of the fingers.
Character structure(s):	AUTONOMY
Ego function:	COGNITIVE SKILLS, (b) cognitive grasp.
Psychological function:	To concretize/make more specific.
Ego function:	PATTERNS OF INTERPERSONAL SKILLS, (b) gripping and holding on.
Psychological function:	Grasping for contact and holding on to it.
Child's developmental stage/age:	From the age of eight months, the muscle is active in scrape-grip, developing into a top-grip, a cross-grip, and a supinated grip. The child takes hold of everything and anything for closer examination; rolls a ball, initially not directionally, later directionally. Piles bricks on top of each other; draws; holds on to a big ball together with flexor pollicis longus.

Bodymapping:

Client's position:	On the back.
Tester's position:	By the arm that is tested.
Activation in test position:	Resist flexion at the middle phalanges of the fingers. If it is difficult to find/feel, clench the fist.
Test location:	Test on the lower half of the forearm deeply to the long tendons (slightly ulnarly).
Test direction:	Distally.

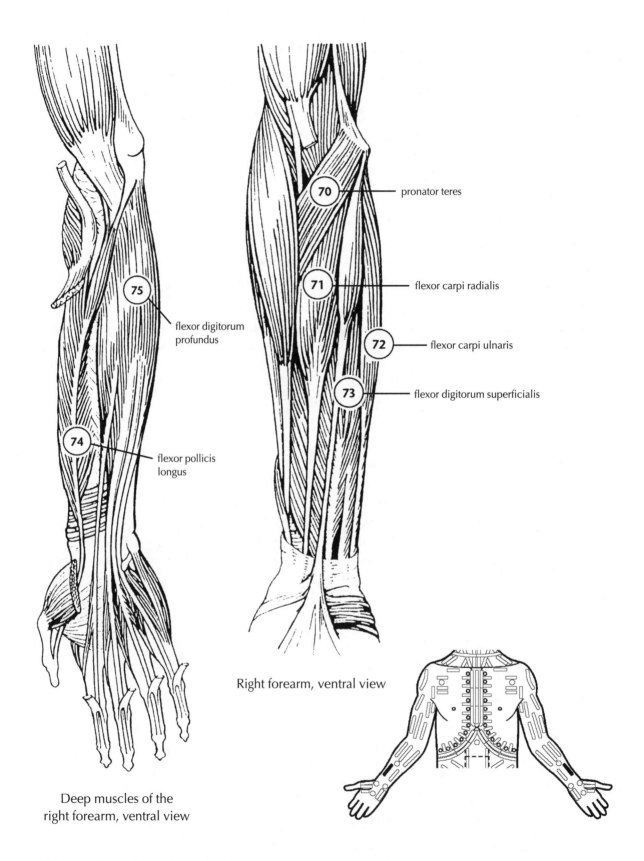

70 — pronator teres

71 — flexor carpi radialis

72 — flexor carpi ulnaris

73 — flexor digitorum superficialis

75 flexor digitorum profundus

74 flexor pollicis longus

Right forearm, ventral view

Deep muscles of the
right forearm, ventral view

Name:	**Flexor pollicis longus**	Number: 74

Origin:	Middle of anterior radius; interosseous membrane.
Insertion:	Distal phalanx of thumb.
Anatomical function:	Flexes thumb at interphalangeal (IP) joint and assists flexion of wrist.
Map:	Is found radial (thumb side) over the radius on the lower part of the anterior surface of the forearm.
Is contracted by:	Flexing the distal joint of thumb.
Character structure(s):	AUTONOMY
Ego function:	COGNITIVE SKILLS, (b) cognitive grasp.
Psychological function:	Put things together, make coherent/see things as parts of a greater whole (operative thinking).
Ego function:	PATTERNS OF INTERPERSONAL SKILLS, (b) gripping and holding on.
Psychological function:	Hold on to and/or maintain contact around an activity.
Child's developmental stage/age:	The muscle is active in tweezers grip. The child examines little things, sees things as parts of a greater whole, lays things in a bowl, and is able to do a jigsaw puzzle.

Bodymapping:

Client's position:	On the back.
Tester's position:	By the arm that is tested.
Activation in test position:	Flex distal joint of the thumb.
Test location:	Radial to the tendon of flexor carpi radialis.
Test direction:	Distally.

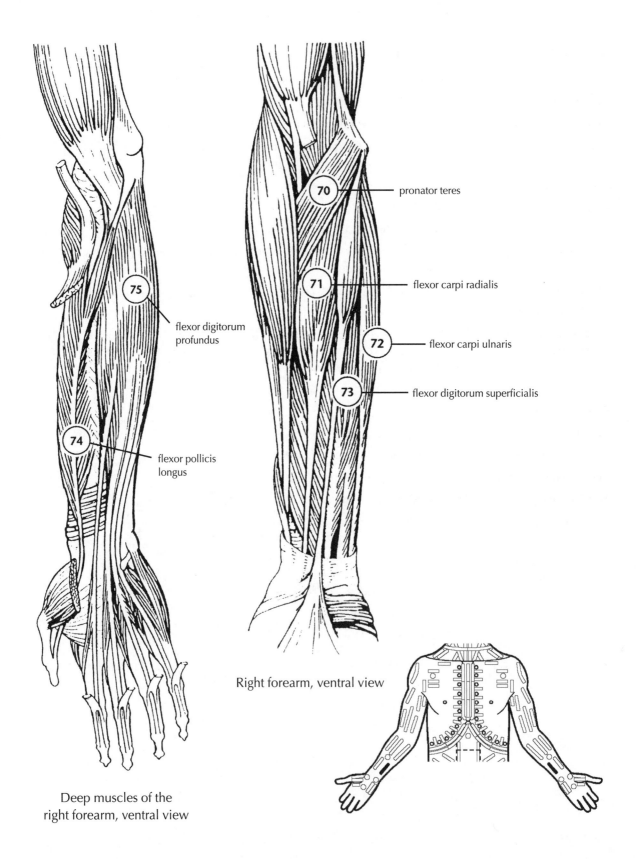

70 — pronator teres

71 — flexor carpi radialis

72 — flexor carpi ulnaris

73 — flexor digitorum superficialis

75 — flexor digitorum profundus

74 — flexor pollicis longus

Right forearm, ventral view

Deep muscles of the
right forearm, ventral view

230   **The Bodynamic Psycho-Motor Anatomy**

Name:	**Flexor digitorum profundus**	**Number: 75**

Origin:	Middle of anterior surface ulna; interosseous membrane.
Insertion:	Base of distal phalanges of the four lateral fingers.
Anatomical function:	Flexes all the joints of the fingers and assists with wrist flexion.
Map:	Is found on little-finger (ulnar) side in the deep group of muscles.
Is contracted by:	Flexing the joints of the fingers, especially the distal ones.
Character structure(s):	NEED
Ego function:	COGNITIVE SKILLS, (b) cognitive grasp.
Psychological function:	To grasp/understand the words describing both the world at hand and emotions.
Ego function:	PATTERNS OF INTERPERSONAL SKILLS, (b) gripping and holding on.
Psychological function:	Maintain/"stick to" close contact and hold on to what one wants.
Child's developmental stage/age:	The child is able to grasp things and hold on to them. Can keep things in the hand and take them to the mouth, even if, in the beginning, it takes time to reach the mouth.

Bodymapping:

Client's position:	On the back.
Tester's position:	By the arm that is tested.
Activation in test position:	Flex the distal joints of the fingers.
Test location:	Is tested between medial border of ulna and flexor carpi ulnaris. Test deeply slightly proximal to the middle of the forearm.
Test direction:	Distally.

Name:	**Lumbricals**	**Number:** *

Origin:	Flexor digitorum profundus tendons.
Insertion:	Extensor expansion associated with interphalangeal joints of 2nd to 5th finger.
Anatomical function:	Flexes the metacarpophalangeal joints and extends the interphalangeal joints.
Map:	Are found in the palm between the tendons of flexor digitorum profundus.
Is contracted by:	Balancing/holding playing cards in one hand, i.e., bending the hand so the knuckles become visible with the fingers extended at the same time.
Character structure(s):	SOLIDARITY/PERFORMANCE
Ego function:	COGNITIVE SKILLS, (b) cognitive grasp.
Psychological function:	Grasp scientific and mathematical thinking, logical thinking, linguistic thinking.
Child's developmental stage/age:	The child is able to think/understand mathematics and physics, do experiments, take small things apart.

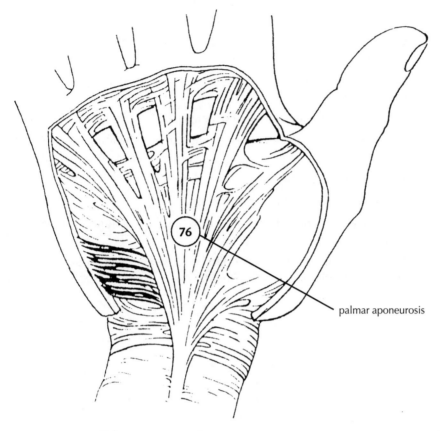

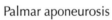

Palmar aponeurosis

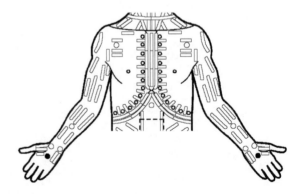

Name:	**Palmar aponeurosis**	Number: 76

Origin:	Triangular shape with apex from flexor retinaculum in center of the wrist.
Insertion:	Superficial fibers to the skin of the palm and fingers; deep fibers to flexor tendons and deep ligaments to MCP joints and proximal phalanges of fingers.
Anatomical function:	Stabilizes palm, e.g., when the hand is used to grasp.
Map:	Is found in the hollow of the palm.
Is contracted by:	Stretching out the fingers, and then the whole system of fibers is tightened so the skin becomes firm. It is also tightened when the wrist is bent backward.
Character structure(s):	NEED
Ego function:	COGNITIVE SKILLS, (b) cognitive grasp.
Psychological function:	Grasping shapes of objects. Consistency in contact with people and things; "sensing and feeling the world," understanding the difference between soft and hard etc.
Ego function:	PATTERNS OF INTERPERSONAL SKILLS, (b) gripping and holding on.
Psychological function:	Grasp the world, hold on to it.
Child's developmental stage/age:	The child is able to grasp so firmly that she is able to hang onto a clothesline, carrying her own weight in the same way that monkeys hang onto their mother's fur; this also allows her to make contact.

Bodymapping:

Client's position:	On the back.
Tester's position:	By the hand that is tested.
Activation in test position:	Stretch/extend the fingers.
Test location:	In the middle of the palm.
Test direction:	Toward the wrist.

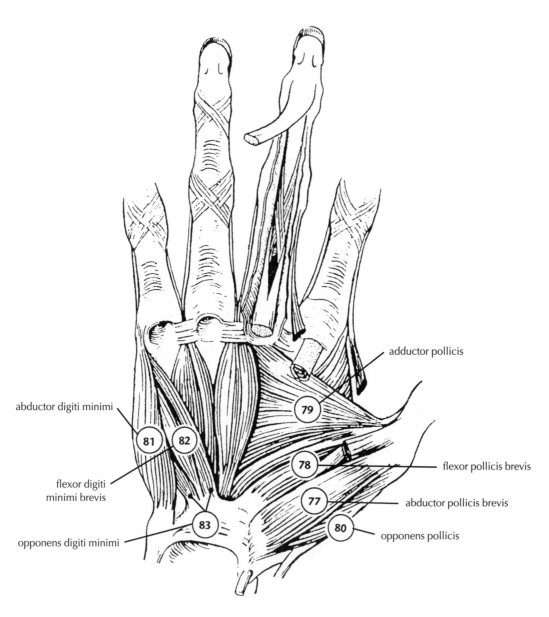

abductor digiti minimi

flexor digiti
minimi brevis

opponens digiti minimi

adductor pollicis

flexor pollicis brevis

abductor pollicis brevis

opponens pollicis

Muscles of the right palm

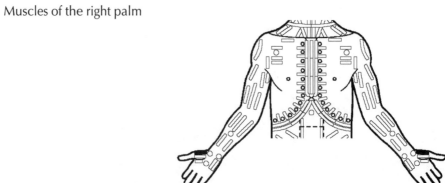

Name:	**Abductor pollicis brevis**	**Number: 77**

Origin:	Flexor retinaculum; trapezium and scaphoid bones.
Insertion:	Base of proximal phalanx of thumb.
Anatomical function:	Abducts, flexes, and assists in opposition of the thumb at carpometacarpal joint.
Map:	The most superficial muscle in the ball of the thumb, along the bone.
Is contracted by:	Spreading the fingers. Moving the thumb at a right angle to the palm, away from the other fingers.
Character structure(s):	SOLIDARITY/PERFORMANCE
Ego function:	COGNITIVE SKILLS, (b) cognitive grasp.
Psychological function:	To take in/survey a group and make room for new points of view.
Child's developmental stage/age:	The child is able to receive a ball, spreading the fingers and preparing to catch it. The muscle takes part in forming a broader surface as a starting point to prepare to catch the ball.

Bodymapping:

Client's position:	On the back.
Tester's position:	By the hand that is tested.
Activation in test position:	Spread the fingers.
Test location:	On the belly of the muscle.
Test direction:	Toward the wrist.

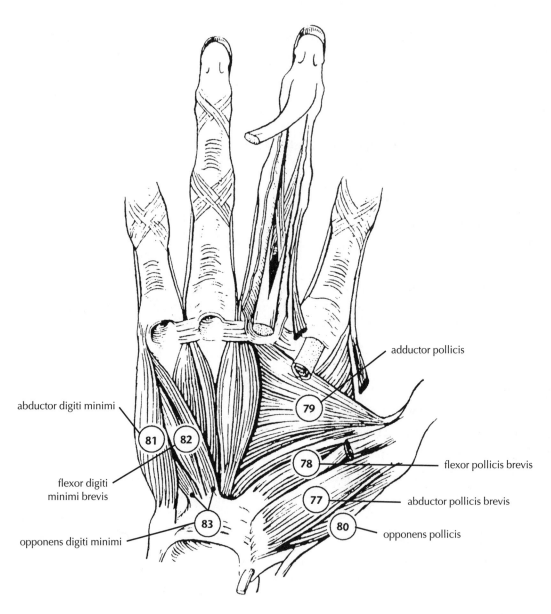

adductor pollicis

abductor digiti minimi

flexor digiti
minimi brevis

opponens digiti minimi

flexor pollicis brevis

abductor pollicis brevis

opponens pollicis

Muscles of the right palm

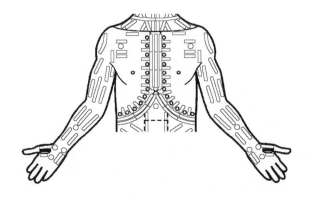

Name:	**Flexor pollicis brevis**	Number: 78

Origin:	Flexor retinaculum; trapezium; 1st metacarpal bone.
Insertion:	Base of proximal phalanx of the thumb (radial side).
Anatomical function:	Flexes the metacarpophalangeal joint of the thumb; assists in abduction and opposition of the thumb.
Map:	Is found on the ulnar side (little finger side) of abductor pollicis brevis, and is partly covered by it.
Is contracted by:	Flexing the thumb toward the palm.
Character structure(s):	WILL
Ego function:	COGNITIVE SKILLS, (b) cognitive grasp.
Psychological function:	Process thinking; expanding operative thinking to abstract thinking, e.g., "now we are going to hang a picture on the wall" means getting a hammer and searching for all the things that are necessary to do so.
Ego function:	PATTERNS OF INTERPERSONAL SKILLS, (b) gripping and holding on.
Psychological function:	Holding on to emotions and holding on to what one wants.
Child's developmental stage/age:	The child is able to catch a medium sized ball with his hands (he no longer needs to pull the ball towards his stomach); throws a small ball with precision.

Bodymapping:

Client's position:	On the back.
Tester's position:	By the hand that is tested.
Activation in test position:	Flex the thumb down toward the palm.
Test location:	Where the muscle is full.
Test direction:	Toward the wrist.

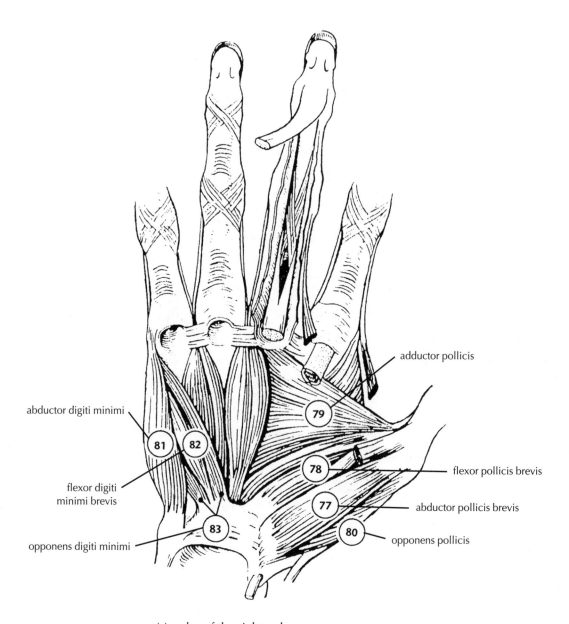

adductor pollicis

abductor digiti minimi

81 **82**

flexor digiti
minimi brevis

opponens digiti minimi

83

79

78 flexor pollicis brevis

77 abductor pollicis brevis

80 opponens pollicis

Muscles of the right palm

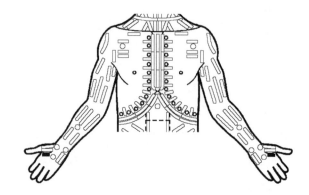

Name:	**Adductor pollicis**	Number: 79

Origin:	Shaft of 3rd metacarpal; capitate bone.
Insertion:	Base of proximal phalanx of the thumb.
Anatomical function:	Adducts and assists opposition of the thumb.
Map:	Is found in the palm, in the web space between the thumb and the index finger.
Is contracted by:	Moving the thumb toward the index finger.
Character structure(s):	WILL
Ego function:	COGNITIVE SKILLS, (b) cognitive grasp.
Psychological function:	Grasping the cause, reasons, and consequences.
Ego function:	PATTERNS OF INTERPERSONAL SKILLS, (b) gripping and holding on.
Psychological function:	Grasping and holding on to contacts (one can hold on to a game, a dialogue/talk, and things that can be done with someone else).
Child's developmental stage/age:	The child is able to build with bricks, making (building) tall towers; improves drawing, holds utensils for eating, and carries heavy things.

Bodymapping:

Client's position:	On the back.
Tester's position:	By the hand that is tested.
Activation in test position:	Move the thumb toward the index finger.
Test location:	Find the belly of the muscle in the palmar web space between the thumb and index finger.
Test direction:	Toward the center of the palm in the direction of the fibers.

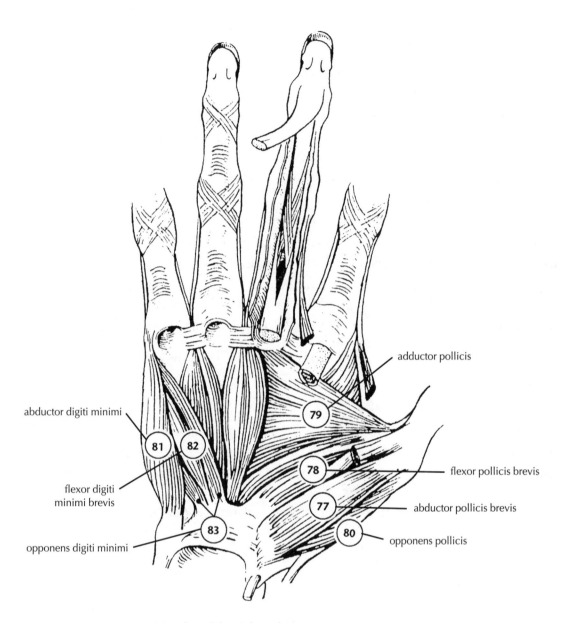

abductor digiti minimi

adductor pollicis

flexor digiti
minimi brevis

flexor pollicis brevis

abductor pollicis brevis

opponens digiti minimi

opponens pollicis

Muscles of the right palm

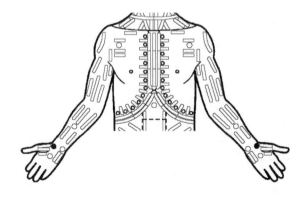

Name:	**Opponens pollicis**	Number: 80

Origin:	Flexor retinaculum; trapezium bone.
Insertion:	Lateral shaft of 1st metacarpal.
Anatomical function:	Opposes the thumb (opposition is a combination of flexion, abduction, and medial rotation; all muscles in the pad of the thumb are involved).
Map:	Is found deep between first metacarpal bone and the pad of the thumb.
Is contracted by:	Moving the thumb and little finger toward each other.
Character structure(s):	OPINIONS
Ego function:	COGNITIVE SKILLS, (b) cognitive grasp.
Psychological function:	Forming one's own opinions.
Ego function:	SELF-ASSERTION, (a) self-assertion (manifestation one's power).
Psychological function:	Manifest one's own opinions (oppose).
Ego function:	PATTERNS OF INTERPERSONAL SKILLS, (b) gripping and holding on.
Psychological function:	Holding on to one's own opinions and staying flexible in discussions.
Child's developmental stage/age:	The child has correct writing grip with more precise motor function/coordination; ability to put small things together and being precise when putting small marks on things.

Bodymapping:

Client's position:	On the back.
Tester's position:	By the hand that is tested.
Activation in test position:	Move thumb and little finger toward each other.
Test location:	Is tested deeply, between the first metacarpal bone and the pad of the thumb.
Test direction:	Along the bone toward the wrist.

Name:	**Insertions of flexors and extensors on the proximal phalanx of the little finger**	Number: *

Origin:

Insertion:

Anatomical function:

Map: Is found at the base of the proximal phalanx of the little finger.

Is contracted by:

Character structure(s):   EXISTENCE-NEED

Ego function: PATTERNS OF INTERPERSONAL SKILLS, (b) gripping and holding on.
                                                    (f) Releasing, letting go.

Psychological function: (b) Gripping/holding on/drawing in until satisfied/filled up with what one needs.
(f) Releasing when one is filled up and satisfied.

Child's developmental stage/age: This reflex movement is a remnant from animals' pumping action.
The child pumps the breast, sensing the breast and that there is food inside.
Flexor draws in and extensor lets go when it is satisfied.

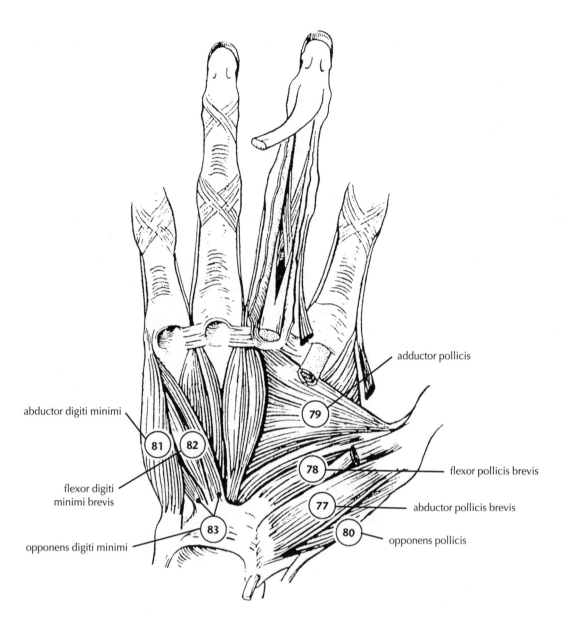

abductor digiti minimi

flexor digiti
minimi brevis

opponens digiti minimi

adductor pollicis

flexor pollicis brevis

abductor pollicis brevis

opponens pollicis

Muscles of the right palm

Name:	**Abductor digiti minimi**	**Number: 81**

Origin:	Pisiform.
Insertion:	Base of proximal phalanx of little finger.
Anatomical function:	Abducts the little finger at the metacarpophalangeal (MCP) joint and assists in opposition.
Map:	Is found superficially in the pad of the little finger.
Is contracted by:	Spreading the fingers, moving the little finger away from the others.
Character structure(s):	LOVE/SEXUALITY
Ego function:	COGNITIVE SKILLS, (b) cognitive grasp.
Psychological function:	Grasping one's own sensual and sexual appeal/effect.
Ego function:	PATTERNS OF INTERPERSONAL SKILLS, (f) releasing, letting go.
Psychological function:	Flexibility in alliances.
Ego function:	GENDER SKILLS, (e) manifestation of sensuality and sexuality.
Psychological function:	Flirting and showing one's sensuality and sexuality.
Child's developmental stage/age:	The muscle balances and administers the grip of objects where fine adjustment of movements is necessary, e.g., when the child drinks from a small cup.

Bodymapping:

Client's position:	On the back.
Tester's position:	By the hand that is tested.
Activation in test position:	Spread the fingers.
Test location:	On the belly of the muscle, laterally on the pad of the little finger.
Test direction:	Deeply along the bone toward the wrist.

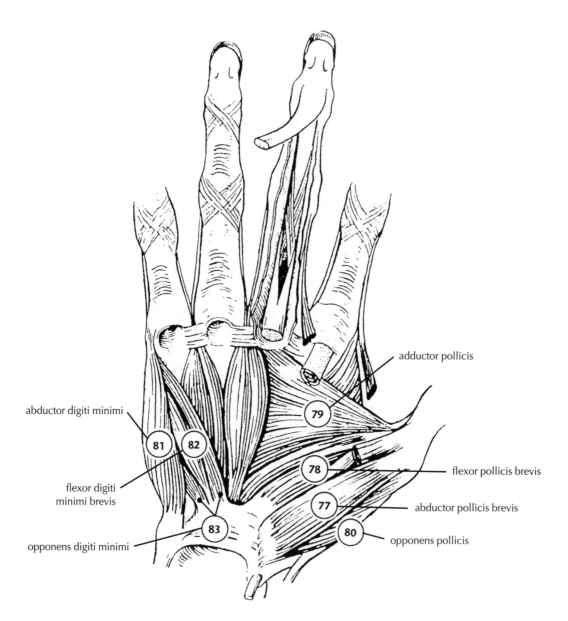

abductor digiti minimi

adductor pollicis

flexor digiti
minimi brevis

flexor pollicis brevis

abductor pollicis brevis

opponens digiti minimi

opponens pollicis

Muscles of the right palm

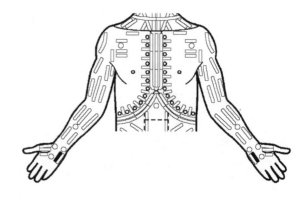

Name:	**Flexor digiti minimi brevis**	**Number: 82**

Origins:	Hamate bone and flexor retinaculum.
Insertions:	Base of proximal phalanx of little finger.
Anatomical function:	Flexes the little finger at metacarpophalangeal joint (MCP).
Map:	Is found superficially in the middle of the pad of the little finger.
Is contracted by:	Moving the little finger toward the wrist.
Character structure(s):	NEED
Ego function:	COGNITIVE SKILLS, (b) cognitive grasp.
Psychological function:	Connecting concrete words to people and things one touches.
Ego function:	PATTERNS OF INTERPERSONAL SKILLS, (b) gripping and holding on.
Psychological function:	Ability to fill oneself up with contact until satisfied.
Child's developmental stage/age:	First kind of finger grip/hand grip (ulnar-palmar grip). The child senses what she holds in her hands; pumping while breast- or bottle-feeding.

Bodymapping:

Client's position:	On the back.
Tester's position:	By the hand that is tested.
Activation in test position:	Move the little finger as far down toward the wrist as possible.
Test location:	On the belly of the muscle on the pad of the little finger.
Test direction:	Toward the wrist.

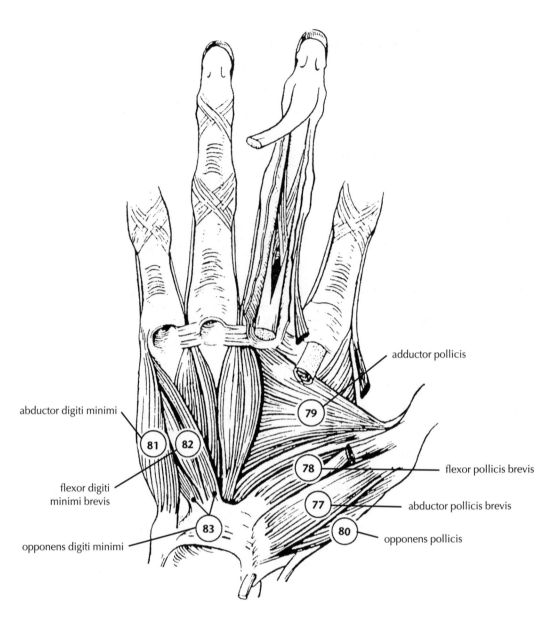

adductor pollicis

abductor digiti minimi

(81) (82)

(79)

flexor digiti
minimi brevis

(78)

flexor pollicis brevis

(77)

abductor pollicis brevis

opponens digiti minimi

(83)

(80)

opponens pollicis

Muscles of the right palm

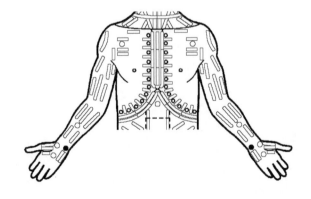

Name:	**Opponens digiti minimi**	**Number: 83**

Origin:	Hamate bone and flexor retinaculum.
Insertion:	Ulnar border of 5th metacarpal bone.
Anatomical function:	Moves the little finger toward the thumb.
Map:	Is found deep between the 5th metacarpal bone and the pad of the little finger.
Is contracted by:	Moving the little finger and the thumb toward each other.
Character structure(s):	OPINIONS
Ego function:	COGNITIVE SKILLS, (b) cognitive grasp.
Psychological function:	Forming opinions (forming opinions by comparing your own thoughts with something you have read or learned before). One can think about something in an abstract way and form an opinion on it.
Ego function:	SELF-ASSERTION, (a) self-assertion (manifesting one's power).
Psychological function:	Being flexible in discussions.
Ego function:	PATTERNS OF INTERPERSONAL SKILLS, (b) gripping and holding on.
Psychological function:	Beginning and maintaining a dialogue (cognitive exchange) with others.
Child's developmental stage/age:	The child has a normal adult grip; she is able to draw circles, straight lines, diagonal lines, zigzags, snakes, and spiral shapes. Ability to cut different shapes with scissors, straight lines, curves, etc. The child can draw, tie shoelaces in a bow, button small and special-shaped buttons, comb her hair, etc.

Bodymapping:

Client's position:	On the back.
Tester's position:	By the hand that is tested.
Activation in test position:	Move the little finger and the thumb toward each other.
Test location:	Between the bone and the pad of the little finger.
Test direction:	Along the bone toward the wrist.

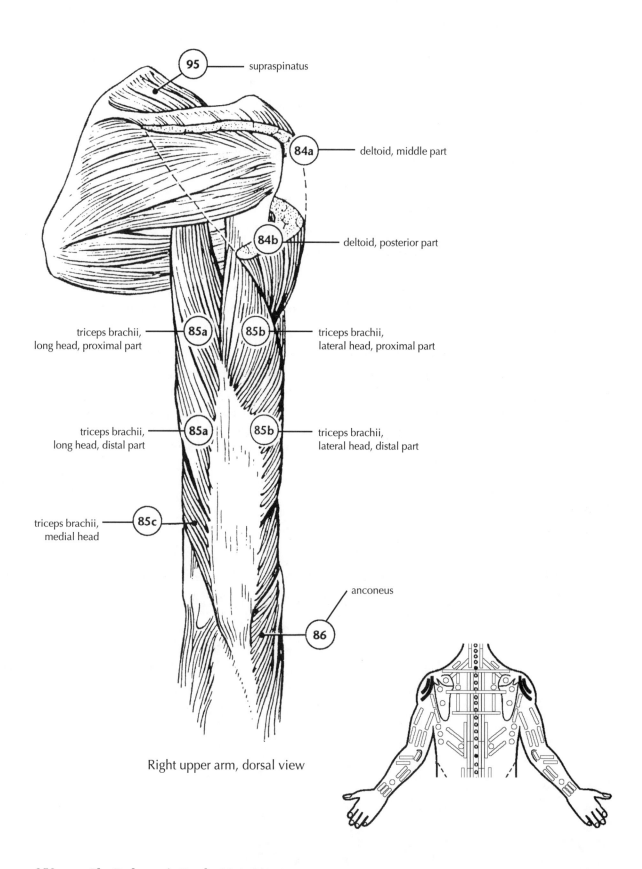

95 —— supraspinatus

84a —— deltoid, middle part

84b —— deltoid, posterior part

triceps brachii,
long head, proximal part —— 85a   85b —— triceps brachii,
lateral head, proximal part

triceps brachii,
long head, distal part —— 85a   85b —— triceps brachii,
lateral head, distal part

triceps brachii,
medial head —— 85c

anconeus
86

Right upper arm, dorsal view

Name:	Deltoid	Number: 84a, b

Origin:	(a) Middle part: lateral acromion process. (b) Posterior part: spine of scapula.
Insertion:	Deltoid tuberosity of humerus.
Anatomical function:	(a) Middle part: abducts the arm in the shoulder joint. (b) Posterior part: abducts and extends and laterally rotates the arm in the shoulder joint.
Map:	Is found on the top side and back side of the shoulder. Forms the back and the side of the roundness of the shoulder.
Is contracted by:	(a) Raising the arm up and out from the side. (b) Raising the arm backward, slightly rotated laterally.
Character structure(s):	(a) Middle part: AUTONOMY (b) Posterior part: WILL
Ego function:	BOUNDARIES, (e) making space for oneself in social contact.
Psychological function:	AUT: making room for your own impulses when in contact with other people. WILL: making room for your own choices and seeing the consequences.
Ego function:	PATTERNS OF INTERPERSONAL SKILLS, (g) taking on chores (assignments).
Psychological function:	AUT: doing assignments without losing one's own impulses and ideas WILL: doing assignments from one's own desire and will (not feeling "I ought to").
Child's developmental stage/age:	AUT: the child lifts the arms up and out so others have to move away. It lifts the arm when pointing at things; throws a ball without precision. WILL: the child moves the arm backward, carries things on the back, e.g., little sisters or brothers, backpacks (forms the shoulder yoke), throws a ball with more power and more precision.

Bodymapping:	
Client's position:	On the stomach.
Tester's position:	By the shoulder that is tested.
Activation in test position:	(a) Move the arm out from the side. (b) Lift the arm away from the mat.
Test location:	(a) On the top side of the shoulder, where the muscle is full (b) On the back side of the shoulder, where the muscle is full.
Test direction:	(a) Distally. (b) Distally, laterally.

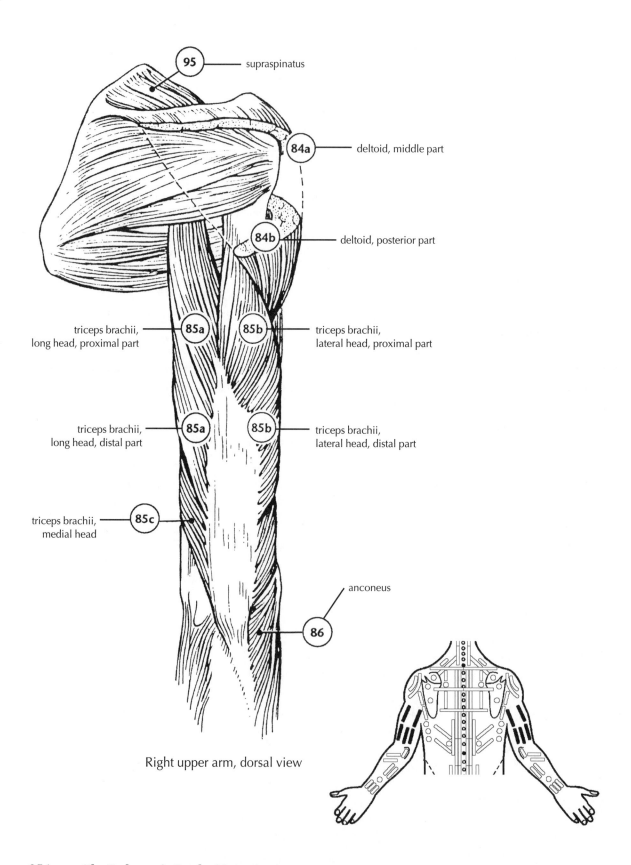

95 — supraspinatus

84a — deltoid, middle part

84b — deltoid, posterior part

triceps brachii, long head, proximal part — 85a   85b — triceps brachii, lateral head, proximal part

triceps brachii, long head, distal part — 85a   85b — triceps brachii, lateral head, distal part

triceps brachii, medial head — 85c

anconeus

86

Right upper arm, dorsal view

Name:	Triceps brachii	Number: 85a, b, c

Origin:	(a) Long head: infraglenoid tubercle of scapula. (b) Lateral head: posterior humerus above groove. (c) Medial head: below groove.
Insertion:	Olecranon process of ulna.
Anatomical function:	(a) Extends the elbow joint; assists adduction and extension of shoulder joint. (b) + (c) Extend the elbow joint.
Map:	Is found on the back of the upper arm.
Is contracted by:	Extending the elbow and moving the arm backward (long head).

Character structure(s):	(a) Long head: proximal part: NEED
	                 distal part: AUTONOMY
	(b) Lateral head: proximal part: LOVE/SEXUALITY
	                  distal part: OPINIONS
	(c) Medial head: WILL

Ego function:	PATTERNS OF INTERPERSONAL SKILLS, (e) pushing away and holding at a distance.
Psychological function:	NEED: pushes oneself away in relation to unwanted things and persons; saying "no" in close relationships. AUT: same as need. LOVE/SEX: saying "no" and pushing away in relation to sensuality and close contact (family and close friends). OPINIONS: saying "no" and pushing away from more superficial contacts and colleagues. WILL: holding on to one's "no."
Child's developmental stage/age:	NEED: push oneself away; lie on the stomach and lift oneself up. AUT: push oneself away in contact; crawl. LOVE/SEX: skip rope, ride a bicycle. OPINIONS: throw with power, e.g., shot put; walk on one's hands. WILL: push away and hold at a distance, push heavy things (wheel barrow); stubbornness in pushing.

Bodymapping:	
Client's position:	On the stomach.
Tester's position:	By the arm that is tested.
Activation in test position: Test location, test direction:	(a) Upper test location: lift arm (extension in shoulder joint). Lower test location: extension in elbow joint. Test-direction: distally, slightly laterally in relation to the body. (b) Extension in elbow joint. Test-direction: distally, slightly medially. Test in two locations. (c) Extension in elbow joint. Test-direction: distally, slightly laterally. Is marked as the middle line on the Bodymap.

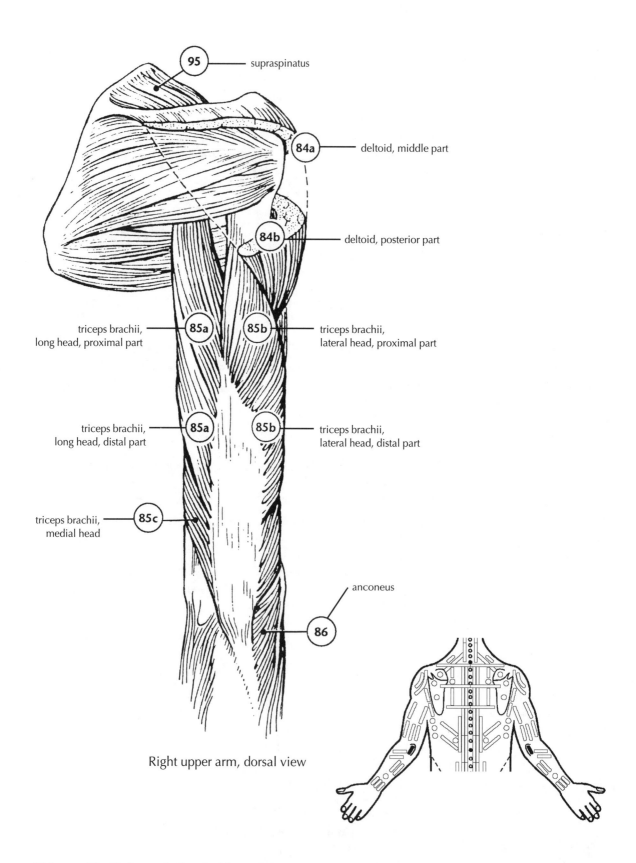

95 — supraspinatus

84a — deltoid, middle part

84b — deltoid, posterior part

triceps brachii,
long head, proximal part — 85a

85b — triceps brachii,
lateral head, proximal part

triceps brachii,
long head, distal part — 85a

85b — triceps brachii,
lateral head, distal part

triceps brachii,
medial head — 85c

anconeus — 86

Right upper arm, dorsal view

Name: **Anconeus**   **Number: 86**

Origin:	Lateral epicondyle of humerus.
Insertion:	Olecranon process of ulna.
Anatomical function:	Extends the elbow joint.
Map:	Is found posterolaterally and slightly distally to the elbow joint.
Is contracted by:	Full extension of the elbow joint.
Character structure(s):	SOLIDARITY/PERFORMANCE
Ego function:	PATTERNS OF INTERPERSONAL SKILLS, (e) pushing away and holding at a distance.
Psychological function:	Ability to say "no" in a group and hold on to it.
Child's developmental stage/age:	Precision and fine adjustment in activities of throwing, badminton, discus, tennis, etc.

Bodymapping:

Client's position:	On the stomach.
Tester's position:	By the arm that is tested.
Activation in test position:	Extend the elbow (almost an overextension).
Test location:	Distal to tip of elbow, lateral to ulna.
Test direction:	Distally, medially.

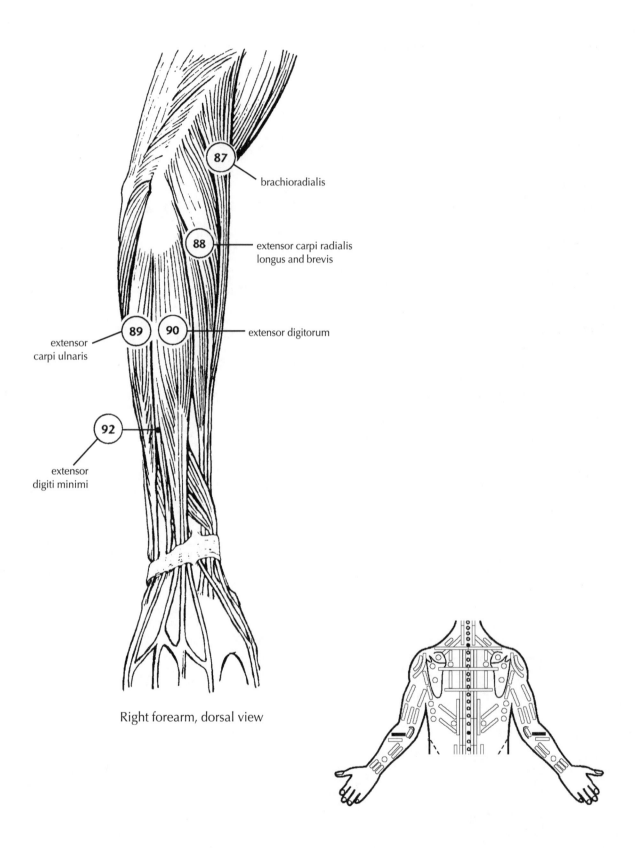

87 brachioradialis

88 extensor carpi radialis
longus and brevis

90 extensor digitorum

89 extensor
carpi ulnaris

92

extensor
digiti minimi

Right forearm, dorsal view

Name:	**Brachioradialis**	Number: 87

Origin:	Lateral supracondylar ridge of humerus.
Insertion:	Styloid process of radius.
Anatomical function:	Flexes the elbow joint with forearm in mid position between pronation and supination.
Map:	Is found on the radial side of the forearm (the thumb side) where it forms the round contour.
Is contracted by:	Flexing the elbow with forearm in mid position between pronation and supination.
Character structure(s):	LOVE/SEXUALITY
Ego function:	PATTERNS OF INTERPERSONAL SKILLS, (c) drawing toward oneself and holding on closely.
Psychological function:	Hold on to an alliance in a flexible way and stay in contact with others as well.
Child's developmental stage/age:	Ball games, throwing, skipping rope, carrying dolls, carrying heavy things, holding handlebars (of a bicycle), pulling on the handlebars when pedaling up hills.

Bodymapping:

Client's position:	On the back with a flexed elbow and the forearm in mid position.
Tester's position:	By the arm that is tested.
Activation in test position:	Flex the elbow joint; give slight resistance to the forearm if necessary.
Test location:	Where the belly of the muscle is full.
Test direction:	Distally.

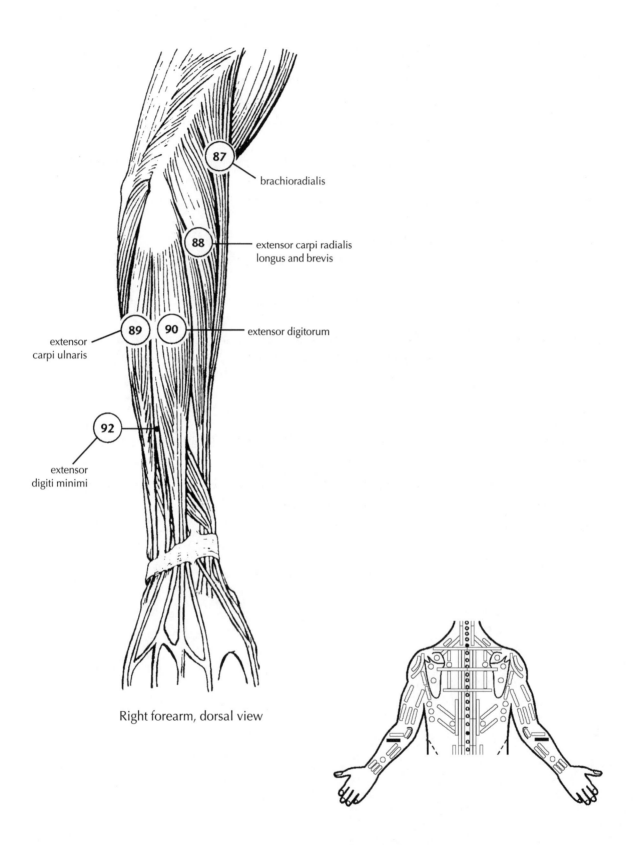

87 brachioradialis

88 extensor carpi radialis
    longus and brevis

extensor
carpi ulnaris 89 90 extensor digitorum

92

extensor
digiti minimi

Right forearm, dorsal view

The Bodynamic Psycho-Motor Anatomy

Name:	**Extensor carpi radialis longus and brevis**	**Number: 88**

Origin:	Lateral supracondylar ridge; lateral epicondyle of humerus (common extensor tendon).
Insertion:	Longus: base of 2nd metacarpal. Brevis: base of 3rd metacarpal.
Anatomical function:	Longus: extends and radially flexes the wrist; assists with flexion of the elbow. Brevis: extends and radially flexes the wrist.
Map:	Is found centrally on the back of the forearm (dorsal surface), next to brachioradialis.
Is contracted by:	Keeping the elbow slightly flexed extending the wrist, pulling toward the thumb side.
Character structure(s):	WILL
Ego function:	PATTERNS OF INTERPERSONAL SKILLS, (e) pushing away and holding at a distance.
Psychological function:	Saying absolutely "no" and saying "stop."
Child's developmental stage/age:	The child is able to hold the hands in a position to push, to catch a big ball when bouncing it against the ground, to throw a ball more accurately, and to push toy cars along the floor. The child is developing a firmer and yet more flexible grip, starting to be able to control the power used in grip, e.g., when fondling.

Bodymapping:

Client's position:	On the back.
Tester's position:	By the arm that is tested.
Activation in test position:	Extend the wrist backward and toward the thumb side. Keep the elbow slightly flexed. Give resistance to the back of the hand if necessary.
Test location:	Where the belly of the muscle is full.
Test direction:	Distally.

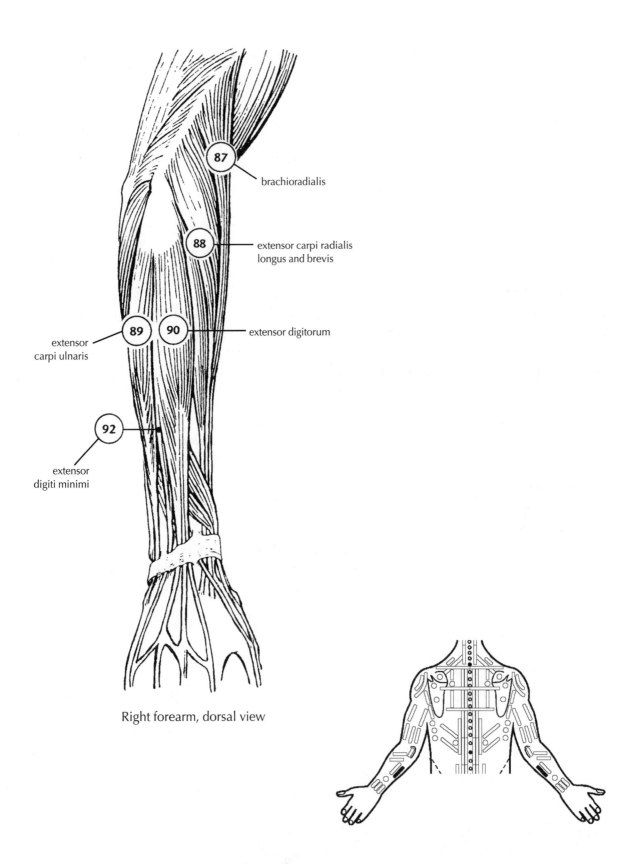

87 — brachioradialis

88 — extensor carpi radialis longus and brevis

89 — extensor carpi ulnaris

90 — extensor digitorum

92 — extensor digiti minimi

Right forearm, dorsal view

Name:	**Extensor carpi ulnaris**	**Number: 89**

Origin:	Lateral epicondyle of humerus (common extensor tendon); posterior proximal ulna.
Insertion:	Base of 5th metacarpal bone.
Anatomical function:	Extends and ulnar flexes the wrist (little finger side).
Map:	Is found close to ulna on the back of the forearm (dorsal surface).
Is contracted by:	Extending the wrist mostly toward the little finger side.
Character structure(s):	AUTONOMY
Ego function:	PATTERNS OF INTERPERSONAL SKILLS, (e) pushing away and holding at a distance.
Psychological function:	Make space for oneself and withdraw from contact; ability to say "no"/"stop."
Child's developmental stage/age:	The muscle is active in cross-palmar grasp (the turned-in primitive grasp) and waving to people. Scribbling becomes softer and drawing more rounded with looser forms and lines in different directions.

Bodymapping:

Client's position:	On the back.
Tester's position:	By the arm that is tested.
Activation in test position:	Extension of the wrist in ulnar direction (toward the little finger).
Test location:	Where the belly of the muscle is full.
Test direction:	Distally.

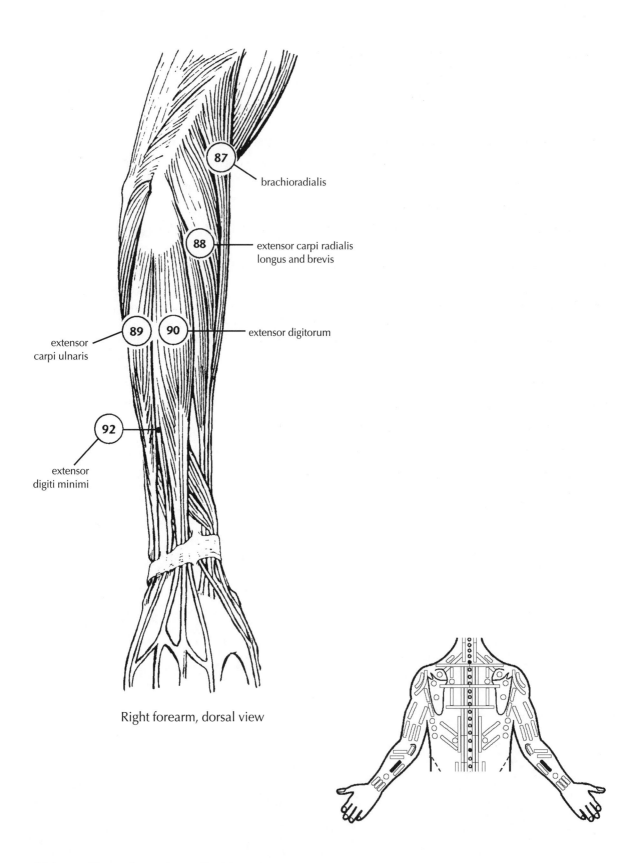

87 — brachioradialis

88 — extensor carpi radialis longus and brevis

89 — extensor carpi ulnaris

90 — extensor digitorum

92 — extensor digiti minimi

Right forearm, dorsal view

The Bodynamic Psycho-Motor Anatomy

Name:	**Extensor digitorum**	Number: 90

Origin:	Lateral epicondyle of humerus (common extensor tendon).
Insertion:	Base of middle and distal phalanges of four lateral fingers (dorsal surface).
Anatomical function:	Extends the fingers and assists in extension of wrist.
Map:	Is found centrally on the dorsal surface of the forearm.
Is contracted by:	Extending the fingers fully.
Character structure(s):	AUTONOMY
Ego function:	PATTERNS OF INTERPERSONAL SKILLS, (f) releasing, letting go.
Psychological function:	Releasing contact with people and things.
Child's developmental stage/age:	The child is able to let go of objects (toys) and experience the sensation of the space and form of things with their hands.

Bodymapping:

Client's position:	On the back.
Tester's position:	By the arm that is tested.
Activation in test position:	Extend the fingers fully.
Test location:	Where the belly of the muscle is full.
Test direction:	Distally.

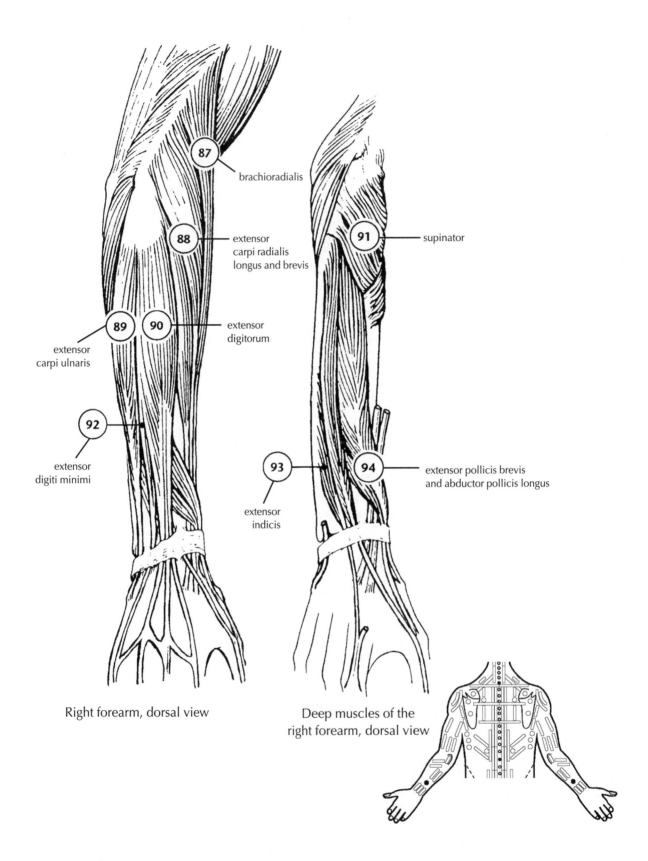

87 brachioradialis

88 extensor
carpi radialis
longus and brevis

89 90 extensor
digitorum

extensor
carpi ulnaris

92

extensor
digiti minimi

91 supinator

93 94 extensor pollicis brevis
and abductor pollicis longus

extensor
indicis

Right forearm, dorsal view

Deep muscles of the
right forearm, dorsal view

Name:	**Supinator**	Number: 91

Origin:	Lateral epicondyle of humerus; supinator crest of ulna.
Insertion:	Dorsal and lateral surfaces of upper third of radius.
Anatomical function:	Supinates the forearm.
Map:	Is found deep in the forearm just below the elbow joint line.
Is contracted by:	Rotating the forearm so the palm is turned upward and the back of the hand is turned downward.
Character structure(s):	AUTONOMY
Ego function:	PATTERNS OF INTERPERSONAL SKILLS, (d) receiving and giving from one's core.
Psychological function:	Deeply receive what is given to you.
Child's developmental stage/age:	The child plays "give and take" games. Is able to put things on top of each other as he can now supinate the hand; uses the tweezers grip, puts things inside other things, does little jigsaws.

Bodymapping:	
Client's position:	On the back, the arm in a supinated position, with a slightly flexed elbow joint.
Tester's position:	By the arm that is tested.
Activation in test position:	Supinate the arm slightly more and the muscle tightens.
Test location:	Test deeply, laterally to pronator teres and deep to brachioradialis.
Test direction:	Distally.

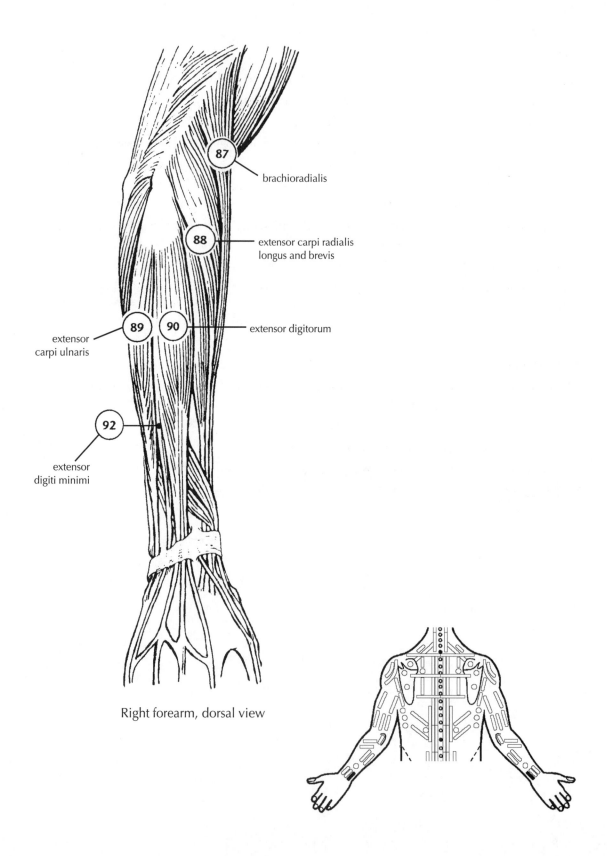

87 brachioradialis

88 extensor carpi radialis
longus and brevis

89 extensor
carpi ulnaris

90 extensor digitorum

92
extensor
digiti minimi

Right forearm, dorsal view

Name:	Extensor digiti minimi	Number: 92

Origin:	Common tendon attached to lateral epicondyle of humerus.
Insertion:	Dorsal surface of base of proximal phalanx of little finger.
Anatomical function:	Extends the little finger and assists in dorsal flexion of the wrist.
Map:	A small, slim muscle usually on the ulnar (little finger) side of extensor digitorum on back of the forearm.
Is contracted by:	Moving the little finger away from the palm.
Character structure(s):	NEED
Ego function:	PATTERNS OF INTERPERSONAL SKILLS, (f) releasing, letting go.
Psychological function:	Releasing contact when satisfied (with people and things); ability to postpone one need in order to satisfy another need.
Child's developmental stage/age:	The flexor reflex matures (four months) and is no longer dominant. Ability to let go of a grip (release) starts on the little finger side. The child is able to let go of things little by little.

Bodymapping:

Client's position:	On the back, the hand lying loose.
Tester's position:	By the arm that is tested.
Activation in test position:	Lift the little finger independently of the other fingers.
Test location:	On the belly of the muscle along ulna.
Test direction:	Distally.

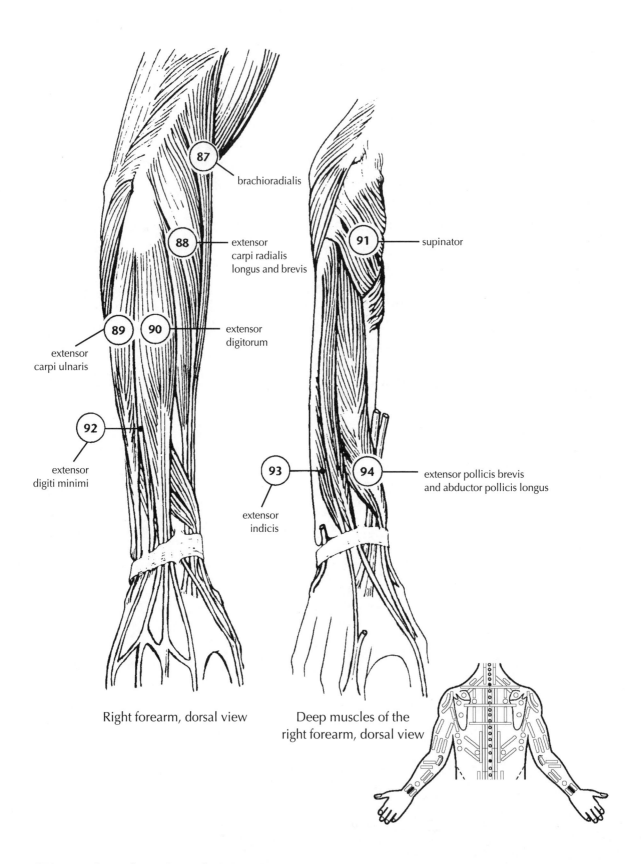

87 brachioradialis

88 extensor
carpi radialis
longus and brevis

89 extensor
carpi ulnaris

90 extensor
digitorum

91 supinator

92 extensor
digiti minimi

93 extensor
indicis

94 extensor pollicis brevis
and abductor pollicis longus

Right forearm, dorsal view

Deep muscles of the
right forearm, dorsal view

Name:	**Extensor indicis**	Number: 93

Origin:	Posterior ulna; interosseus membrane.
Insertion:	Extensor expansion of index finger.
Anatomical function:	Extends index finger and assists in extension of the wrist.
Map:	Is found deep on the back of the forearm, little finger side.
Is contracted by:	Extending the index finger in a pointing movement.
Character structure(s):	AUTONOMY
Ego function:	COGNITIVE SKILLS, (b) cognitive grasp.
Psychological function:	Put words to objects and causal connection thinking.
Ego function:	PATTERNS OF INTERPERSONAL SKILLS, (f) releasing, letting go.
Psychological function:	Is able to release things; can connect and disconnect, e.g., point at something else.
Child's developmental stage/age:	The child points at things "naming the world." It is able to release things completely and to control the grip with the index finger; 3-point grip. Cross-palmar-grasp (turned-in-primitive-grasp) with an extended index finger.

Bodymapping:

Client's position:	On the back.
Tester's position:	By the arm that is tested.
Activation in test position:	Lift the index finger.
Test location:	Deeply in the muscle belly on the posterior surface (back) of forearm just above the wrist, close to ulnar. Follow the tendon from the wrist to the muscle.
Test direction:	Distally.

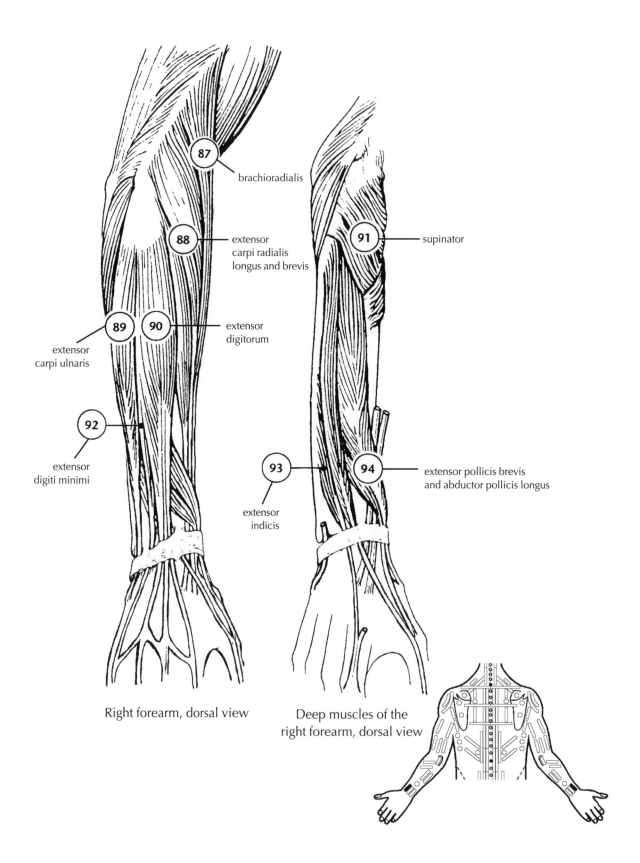

87 brachioradialis

88 extensor
carpi radialis
longus and brevis

89 90 extensor
digitorum

extensor
carpi ulnaris

91 supinator

92

extensor
digiti minimi

93 94 extensor pollicis brevis
and abductor pollicis longus

extensor
indicis

Right forearm, dorsal view

Deep muscles of the
right forearm, dorsal view

| **Name:** | **Extensor pollicis brevis and abductor pollicis longus** | **Number: 94** |

Origin:	Posterior radius; interosseus membrane and ulna.
Insertion:	Base of proximal phalanx of thumb and base of 1st metacarpal.
Anatomical function:	Extensor pollicis brevis: extends the base joint of the thumb (carpometacarpal) and assists in abduction of the wrist Abductor pollicis longus: abducts and extends the base joint of the thumb.
Map:	Are found deep on the back of the forearm. Lie superficially proximally to the place where they cross over radius.
Is contracted by:	Moving the thumb sideways away from the other fingers and slightly up and away from the palm.
Character structure(s):	LOVE/SEXUALITY
Ego function:	PATTERNS OF INTERPERSONAL SKILLS, (f) releasing, letting go.
Psychological function:	Release a contact completely and at the same time preserve the significance of the contact internally.
Child's developmental stage/age:	The child has a half-pronated adult grip; catches a bigger ball; catches and throws little balls. Develops more complex hand motor functions—draws pictures of people with head, face (eyes, nose, mouth), and arms with hands; uses a pair of scissors more at a tilt, paints with brushes, dresses and undresses herself, can get hold of hooks and little buttons, wipes herself.

Bodymapping:

Client's position:	On the back.
Tester's position:	By the arm that is tested.
Activation in test position:	Move the thumb away from the other fingers; in reality you test only the abductor.
Test location:	Proximally to the location where they cross the radius.
Test direction:	Distally.

Name: **Connective tissue on top of the shoulder**   **Number: ***
                    (shoulder plexus)

Origin:

Insertion:

Anatomical function:

Map: Shoulder plexus is found on top of the shoulder area between trapezius
                                  and supraspinatus.

Is contracted by:

Character structure(s):   PERINATAL

Ego function: MANAGEMENT OF ENERGY, (b) containment of high-level energy.

Psychological function: Physical integration of power or energy.

Child's developmental
stage/age: Part of the reflex of pushing out during birth.

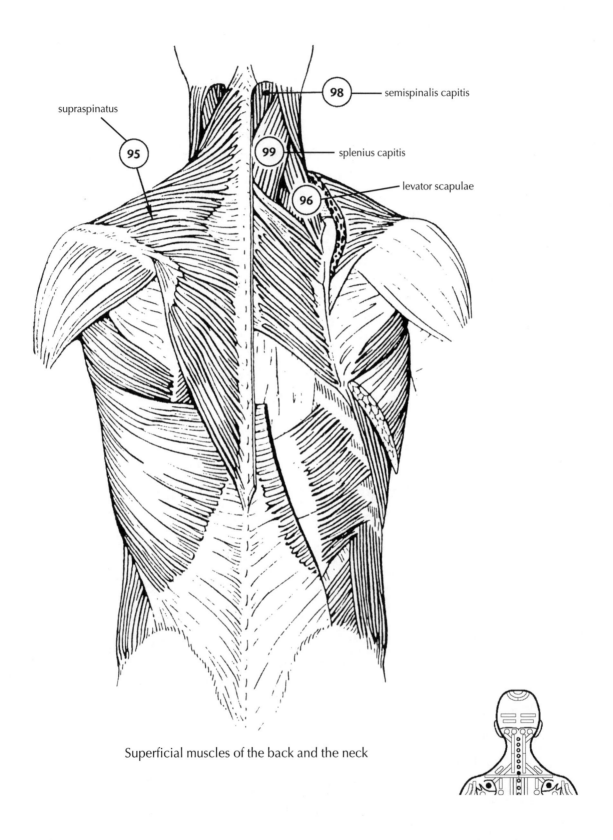

supraspinatus

95

98 — semispinalis capitis

99 — splenius capitis

96

levator scapulae

Superficial muscles of the back and the neck

Name:	**Supraspinatus**	Number: 95

Origin:	Supraspinous fossa of scapula.
Insertion:	Greater tubercle of humerus.
Anatomical function:	Abducts the arm and stabilizes the head of humerus; is part of the rotator cuff.
Map:	A small triangular muscle located at the top of the scapula (in supraspinous fossa), covered by trapezius.
Is contracted by:	Moving the arm slightly away from the body (abduction); the first five degrees are activated exclusively by supraspinatus.
Character structure(s):	AUTONOMY
Ego function:	GROUNDING AND REALITY TESTING, (c) experience and grounding of extrasensory perceptions.
Psychological function:	Ground extrasensory perception by sensing one's position/placement in the room/space.
Child's developmental stage/age:	The muscle stabilizes the shoulder joint so the arm can be lifted and moved in all positions. The child does "flying" movements.

Bodymapping:

Client's position:	On the stomach.
Tester's position:	Opposite the side that is tested.
Activation in test position:	Hold the head with the nose slightly in the air and turned to the opposite side, so the fibers of trapezius are tightened and out of action. Supraspinatus contracts when the arm is initially moved away from the body.
Test location:	Deep to trapezius, proximally to the spine of the scapula.
Test direction:	In the direction of the fibers (medially).

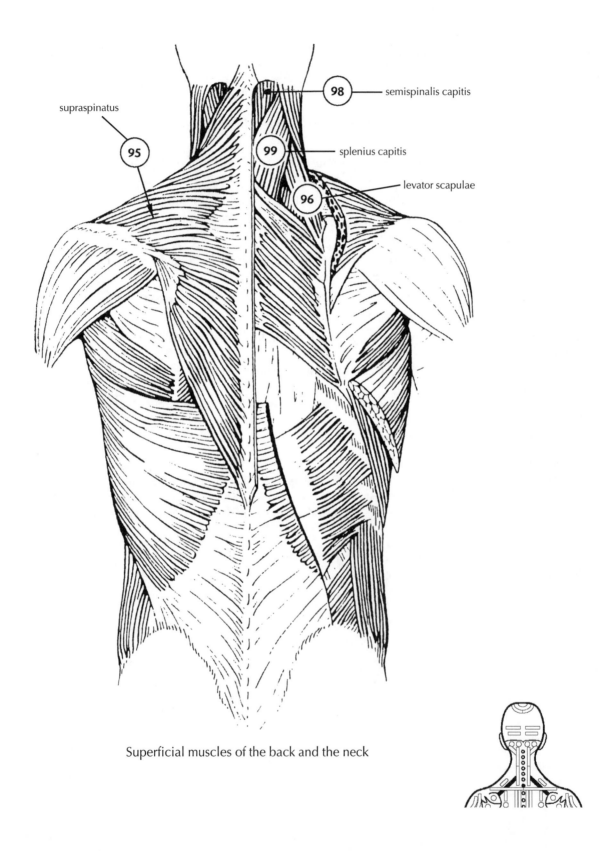

supraspinatus

95

semispinalis capitis

98

splenius capitis

99

levator scapulae

96

Superficial muscles of the back and the neck

Name:	**Levator scapulae**	Number: 96

Origin:	Transverse processes of C1-C4.
Insertion:	Medial border of scapula, at and above the spine of scapula.
Anatomical function:	Elevates the medial border of the scapula, rotates the scapula, and bends the neck laterally.
Map:	Is found superficially in the posterolateral neck. The origin is covered by sternocleidomastoid; the insertion is covered by trapezius.
Is contracted by:	Lifting scapula from the inner upper corner of the scapula.
Character structure(s):	WILL
Ego function:	MANAGEMENT OF ENERGY, (b) containment of high-level energy.
Psychological function:	Containing strong emotions for a short period of time so one can find suitable ways to express them.
Ego function:	PATTERNS OF INTERPERSONAL SKILLS, (g) taking on chores (assignments).
Psychological function:	Consciously choosing tasks, partly because of seeing the consequences.
Child's developmental stage/age:	The muscle expands the lungs, expands the physical space in the chest, and together with the diaphragm helps the child to have the full capacity of the lungs; in this way helps the child to express emotions with power. The muscle is used when the child carries heavy things and when using all his physical power doing different things.

Bodymapping:

Client's position:	On the stomach.
Tester's position:	On the side that is tested.
Activation in test position:	Find the insertion on the scapula. Ask the client to pull the scapula up toward the head to activate it.
Test location:	Test slightly superior to the superior angle of the scapula.
Test direction:	Distally, laterally.

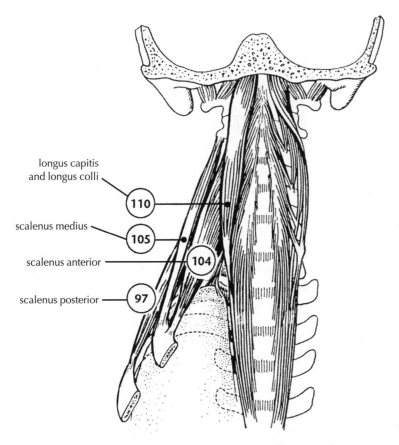

longus capitis
and longus colli
110

scalenus medius
105

scalenus anterior
104

scalenus posterior
97

Deep muscles of the neck, ventral view

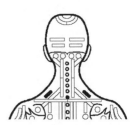

The Bodynamic Psycho-Motor Anatomy

Name:	**Scalenus posterior**	**Number: 97**

Origin:	Transverse processes of C4-C6.
Insertion:	2nd rib.
Anatomical function:	Raises 2nd rib (respiratory inspiration). Acting together, they flex the neck. Acting on one side, it laterally flexes and rotates the neck.
Map:	As a group, the scalene muscles are deep but lie more superficially in the lower anterolateral neck between trapezius, sternocleidomastoid, and the clavicle. Scalenus posterior commonly acts with scalenus medius.
Is contracted by:	Pulling the neck down toward the scapulas (making a short neck). Part of creating a "bull's neck," thus part of forming the "shoulder yoke" with levator scapulae.
Character structure(s):	WILL
Ego function:	POSITIONING, (e) orienting (keeping or losing one's head).
Psychological function:	Maintaining an orientation while changing direction.
Ego function:	COGNITIVE SKILLS, (a) orienting.
Psychological function:	Orienting oneself in time and space (fantasy and reality).
Ego function:	MANAGEMENT OF ENERGY, (b) containment of high-level energy.
Psychological function:	Containing strong/stressful/vigorous emotions.
Child's developmental stage/age:	The muscle is active in walking, maintaining the face in a forward position during the four phases of rotation; it rotates the neck and head and works as a stabilizer. The child is able to turn (rotate) the head further backward. The muscle takes part in creating "bull's neck" and thus the "shoulder yoke" together with levator scapulae.

Bodymapping:

Client's position:	On the back or on the stomach.
Tester's position:	By the top of the head.
Activation in test position:	Make the neck short.
Test location:	Find the area between trapezius, sternocleidomastoid, and the clavicle. Palpate the transverse processes on cervical vertebrae. Scalenus medius is often found slightly behind the transverse processes. Scalenus posterior is further back and is tested under the edge of trapezius. Contract levator scapulae to distinguish scalenus posterior.
Test direction:	However possible.

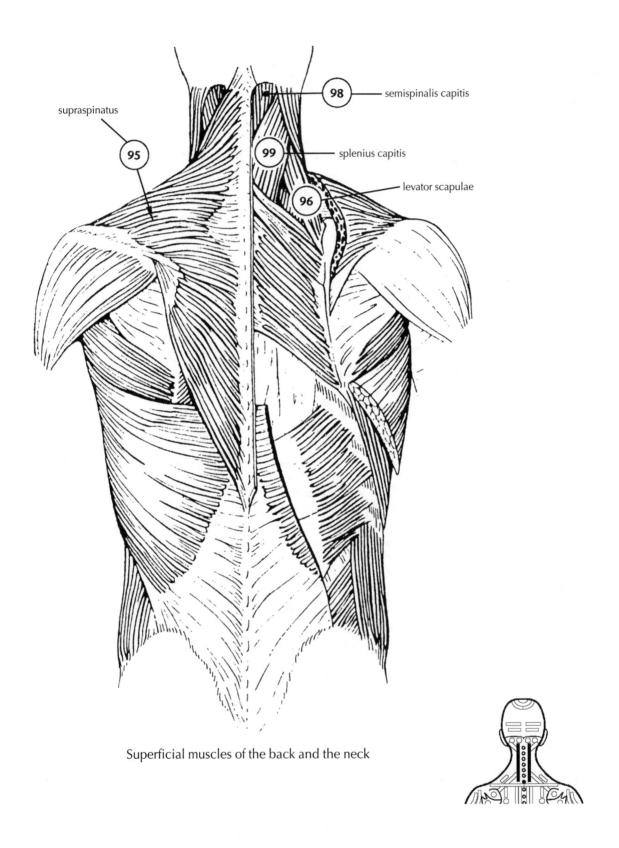

supraspinatus

95

98 semispinalis capitis

99 splenius capitis

96 levator scapulae

Superficial muscles of the back and the neck

The Bodynamic Psycho-Motor Anatomy

Name:	**Semispinalis capitis**	**Number: 98**

Origin:	Lower cervical C5-C7 and upper thoracic T1-T6 vertebrae.
Insertion:	Between superior and inferior nuchal lines of occipital bone.
Anatomical function:	Extends and rotates the head/neck.
Map:	Is found in the neck where it is visible as a vertical column under the skin on either side of the central line.
Is contracted by:	Extending the neck backward (gently). Pressing the head/neck backward against resistance.
Character structure(s):	NEED
Ego function:	POSITIONING, (e) orienting (keeping or losing one's head).
Psychological function:	Experience of oneself in the room/space.
Ego function:	COGNITIVE SKILLS, (a) orienting.
Psychological function:	Able to orient in the world with the help of vertical lines.
Child's developmental stage/age:	The child lifts its head while it is lying on its stomach, holds its head, and turns the head slightly from side to side.

Bodymapping:

Client's position:	On the back.
Tester's position:	By the top of the head.
Activation in test position:	Press the back of the head gently backward into the floor/mat.
Test location:	Palpate laterally to the spinous processes of T1 to C3 through the upper trapezius muscle. Test in two different locations along the muscle.
Test direction:	In the direction of the fibers.

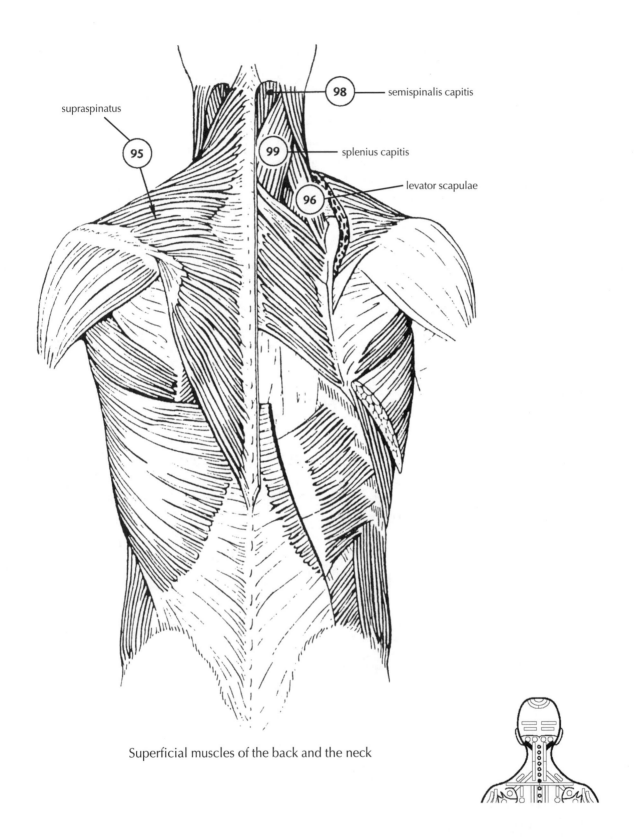

supraspinatus

95

98 — semispinalis capitis

99 — splenius capitis

levator scapulae

96

Superficial muscles of the back and the neck

Name:	**Splenius capitis**	Number: 99

Origin:	Ligamentum nuchae; spinous processes of C7, T1-T3.
Insertion:	Mastoid process, occipital bone.
Anatomical function:	Acting together, they extend, hyperextend head/neck. Acting on one side, they laterally flex, rotate head/neck.
Map:	Is found between spinous process and mastoid process, covered by trapezius and sternocleidomastoid.
Is contracted by:	Turning the head to the side (rotating the neck).
Character structure(s):	NEED
Ego function:	POSITIONING, (e) orienting (keeping or losing one's head).
Psychological function:	Maintaining the connection to oneself while perceiving the surroundings (mind and body connection).
Ego function:	COGNITIVE SKILLS, (a) orienting.
Psychological function:	Experiencing the world and obtaining words for it.
Child's developmental stage/age:	When lying on her stomach and sitting, the child turns her head from side to side and lifts it. The child turns her head to follow/look at things and people so she can form a meaning about the experience (perception). The child also turns her head away when she wants to move or get out of contact.
Shock:	This muscle is related to the reflex system and is therefore often influenced by/involved in shock and trauma.

Bodymapping:

Client's position:	On the back.
Tester's position:	By the top of the head.
Activation in test position:	Turn the head to the same side as is tested.
Test location:	Between spinous process C7 and mastoid process.
Test direction:	Cranially, laterally.

Name:	**Splenius cervicis**	Number: *

Origin:	Spinous processes of T3-T6.
Insertion:	Posterior tubercles of transverse processes of C1-C3.
Anatomical function:	Acting together, they extend and hyperextend the head/neck. Acting one side, it laterally flexes and rotates the head/neck.
Map:	Is found in the neck and upper back, covered by trapezius.
Is contracted by:	Turning the head/neck to the side.
Character structure(s):	LOVE/SEXUALITY
Ego function:	POSITIONING, (e) orienting (keeping or losing one's head).
Psychological function:	Maintaining dignity and sensuality/sexuality at the same time (i.e., in flirting).
Ego function:	COGNITIVE SKILLS, (a) orienting.
Psychological function:	Orienting in relation to the culturally accepted way of flirting (both from the family culture and that of the family's surroundings e.g., working class/middle class).
Ego function:	GENDER SKILLS, (c) experience of gender role.
Psychological function:	Orienting oneself and maintaining the dignity in one's sex roles.
Child's developmental stage/age:	Tilts and draws the head/neck backward.

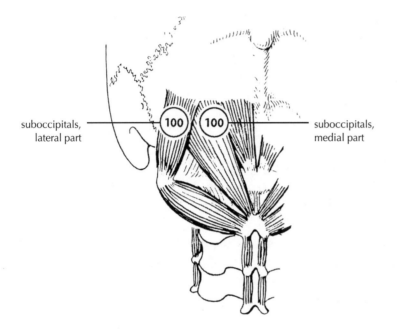

subccipitals,
lateral part

subccipitals,
medial part

Suboccipitals, left side

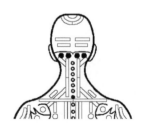

Name:	Suboccipitals	Number: 100

Origin:	Four small paired muscles between the cranium and the two upper vertebrae (atlas, axis).
Insertion:	
Anatomical function:	Turning the face laterally (rotating). Extending the head backward; nodding the head.
Map:	Are found deep between the head (cranium) and the spinous processes on atlas and axis.
Is contracted by:	Turning the head slightly to the side (rotating). Lifting the chin (extending the head backward).
Character structure(s):	Medial part: PERINATAL Lateral part: NEED Origins and insertions: EXISTENCE (is not tested separately)
Ego function:	COGNITIVE SKILLS, (a) orienting.
Psychological function:	PERINATAL: maintain the strength/power from the layer of instincts and the sensation of a right to have this strength/power. NEED: orient oneself in relation to one's needs (nod and turn, "yes" and "no"). EXISTENCE: orient oneself in relation to physical existence.
Child's developmental stage/age:	PERINATAL: the medial part is active in birth when the child squeezes/presses his way out in second-stage labor. Active in both the seeking and sucking reflexes. NEED: lateral part takes part in the first voluntary (will-determined) movement of the head. The child turns the head and nods ("yes" and "no"). EXISTENCE: origins and insertions are active in both the seeking and sucking reflexes and when the child holds the head. Activated in the falling reflex—holding the head back; and automatically activated if the head is dropping or is unsupported.
Bodymapping:	
Client's position:	On the back.
Tester's position:	By the top of the head.
Activation in test position:	Hold the head at the occipital bone; move it slightly so the upper muscles release and allow your fingers to go deeply. Hold the fingers passively and quietly in the deep layer. (1) Palpate the medial muscles through semispinalis laterally to spinous process (ligamentum nuchae). (2) Palpate the lateral muscles at the lateral edge of semispinalis. Sense the muscles extending (lifting the chin) and rotating slightly (turning the head).
Test location:	(1) Through semispinalis laterally to spinous process (ligamentum nuchae). (2) Laterally at the edge of semispinalis, push it slightly medially if necessary.
Test direction:	However possible.

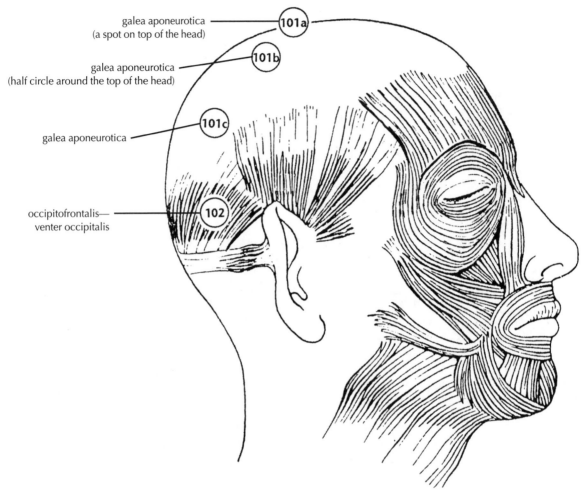

galea aponeurotica
(a spot on top of the head) — 101a

galea aponeurotica
(half circle around the top of the head) — 101b

galea aponeurotica — 101c

occipitofrontalis—
venter occipitalis — 102

Superficial muscles of the head,
right lateral view

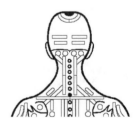

Name: **Galea aponeurotica (a spot on top of the head)**   **Number: 101a**

Origin:	A fibrous sheet covering the skull from the occipital nuchal lines to the eyebrows (skull cap).
Insertion:	
Anatomical function:	Functions as connective tissue to muscles, e.g., occipitofrontalis.
Map:	Is found where the newborn baby has a soft spot on top of the head.
Is contracted by:	
Character structure(s):	EXISTENCE
Ego function:	GROUNDING AND REALITY TESTING, (c) experience and grounding of extrasensory perceptions.
Psychological function:	Grounding one's spirituality in physical strength.
Ego function:	SELF-ASSERTION, (c) forward momentum and sense of direction.
Psychological function:	Own one's instinctive physical and visionary strength.
Child's developmental stage/age:	The place on the head that presses against the birth opening/cervix.

Bodymapping:

Client's position:	On the back.
Tester's position:	By the top of the head.
Activation in test position:	
Test location:	Level with the ears on the top of the head.
Test direction:	Inferiorly.

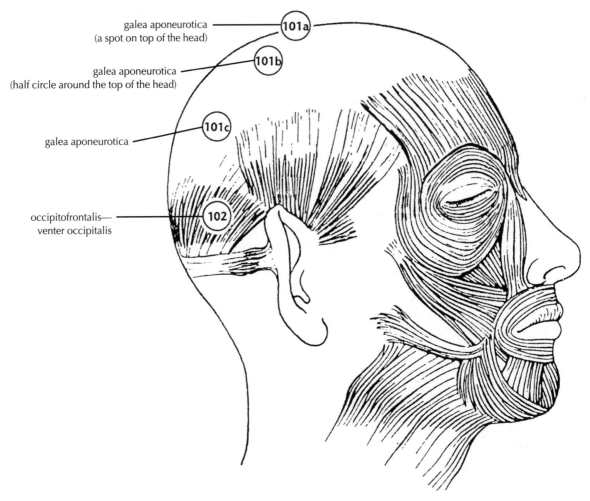

galea aponeurotica
(a spot on top of the head) — 101a

galea aponeurotica — 101b
(half circle around the top of the head)

galea aponeurotica — 101c

occipitofrontalis— — 102
venter occipitalis

Superficial muscles of the head,
right lateral view

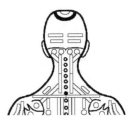

Name:	**Galea aponeurotica (half circle around the top of the head)**	**Number: 101b**

Origin:	A fibrous sheet covering the skull from the occipital nuchal lines to the eyebrows (skull cap).
Insertion:	
Anatomical function:	Functions as connective tissue to muscles, e.g., occipitofrontalis.
Map:	Is found on top of the head around the place where the newborn has a soft spot.
Is contracted by:	
Character structure(s):	PERINATAL
Ego function:	GROUNDING AND REALITY TESTING, (c) experience and grounding extrasensory perceptions.
Psychological function:	Grounding of extrasensory perceptions in stressful situations (high-stress situations).
Ego function:	MANAGEMENT OF ENERGY, (b) containment of high-level energy.
Psychological function:	Containing high level energy without losing the sensation of one's own body.
Ego function:	SELF-ASSERTION, (c) forward momentum and sense of direction.
Psychological function:	Maintaining one's strength in forward momentum and direction.
Child's developmental stage/age:	The area of the baby's head that is impacted during the second stage of labor contractions. Pressure at this time comes both from the birth canal and from inside the child (the child's own strength). This provides the basic ability to maintain direction and have confidence in the possibility of getting through stressful situations.

Bodymapping:	
Client's position:	On the back.
Tester's position:	By the top of the head.
Activation in test position:	
Test location:	Approximately 2-4 fingers distally from the top of the head.
Test direction:	Cranially.

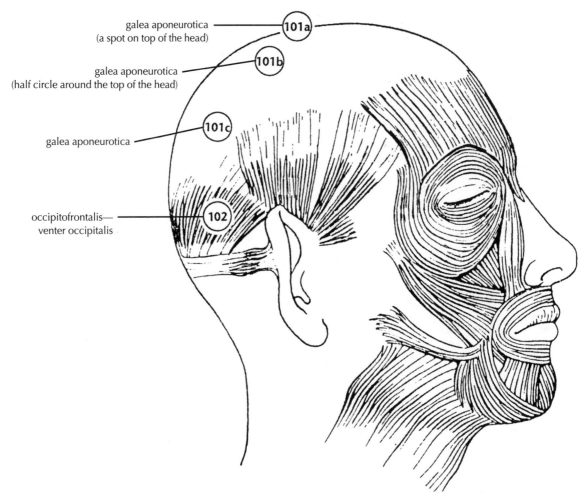

galea aponeurotica
(a spot on top of the head) — 101a

galea aponeurotica
(half circle around the top of the head) — 101b

galea aponeurotica — 101c

occipitofrontalis—
venter occipitalis — 102

Superficial muscles of the head,
right lateral view

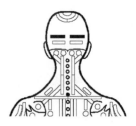

| Name: | **Galea aponeurotica** | **Number: 101c** |

Name: **Galea aponeurotica** **Number: 101c**

Origin:	A fibrous sheet covering the skull from occipital nuchal lines to the eyebrows (skull cap).
Insertion:	
Anatomical function:	Functions as connective tissue to muscles, e.g., occipitofrontalis.
Map:	Is found on the back of the head, approximately two finger widths above the ears.
Is contracted by:	
Character structure(s):	SOLIDARITY/PERFORMANCE
Ego function:	COGNITIVE SKILLS, (e) planning.
Psychological function:	Long-term planning; ability to keep an eye on the goal in relation to one's visions.
Ego function:	SELF-ASSERTION, (c) forward momentum and sense of direction.
Psychological function:	Flexibility in the present while preserving a sense of direction toward long-term purposes.
Child's developmental stage/age:	The center of vision is located posterior in the brain. Galea aponeurotica provides physical boundaries around this part of the brain; is activated when hitting a ball with the head.
Bodymapping:	
Client's position:	On the back.
Tester's position:	By the top of the head.
Activation in test position:	
Test location:	Above and posterior to the ear on the aponeurosis.
Test direction:	Cranially.

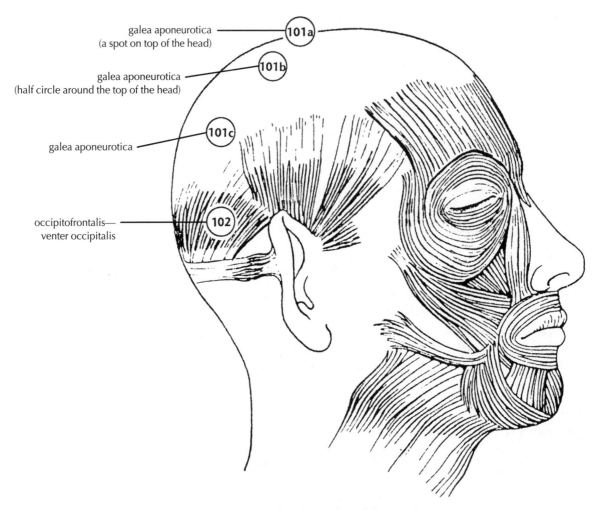

galea aponeurotica
(a spot on top of the head) — **101a**

galea aponeurotica
(half circle around the top of the head) — **101b**

galea aponeurotica — **101c**

occipitofrontalis—
venter occipitalis — **102**

Superficial muscles of the head,
right lateral view

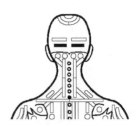

The Bodynamic Psycho-Motor Anatomy

Name:	Occipitofrontalis—venter occipitalis	Number: 102

Origin:	Lateral two-thirds of superior nuchal line of occipital bone and mastoid process.
Insertion:	Galea aponeurotica (skull cap).
Anatomical function:	Draws the scalp backward.
Map:	Is found on the back of the head level with the top of the ear.
Is contracted by:	Moving the scalp.
Character structure(s):	WILL
Ego function:	COGNITIVE SKILLS, (e) planning.
Psychological function:	Short-term planning.
Ego function:	SELF-ASSERTION, (c) forward momentum and sense of direction.
Psychological function:	Ability to maintain focus toward goals (short-term) even when disrupted.
Child's developmental stage/age:	The child is able to move the scalp. The muscle stabilizes when the child grimaces strongly.

Bodymapping:

Client's position:	On the back.
Tester's position:	By the top of the head.
Activation in test position:	
Test location:	Find the muscle in a small concavity on the back of the head behind the ear.
Test direction:	Cranially.

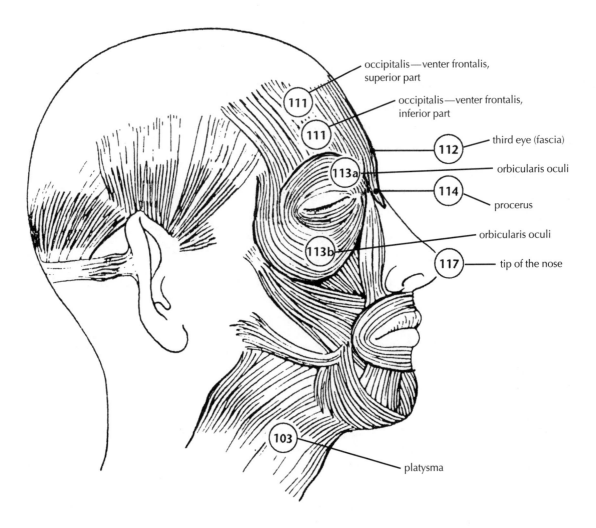

occipitalis—venter frontalis, superior part — 111

occipitalis—venter frontalis, inferior part — 111

third eye (fascia) — 112

orbicularis oculi — 113a

procerus — 114

orbicularis oculi — 113b

tip of the nose — 117

platysma — 103

Superficial muscles of the face, right lateral view

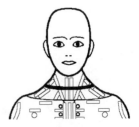

Name:	**Platysma**	**Number: 103**

Origin:	Subcutaneous fascia of upper one-fourth of chest.
Insertion:	Subcutaneous fascia and muscles of chin and jaw.
Anatomical function:	Depresses and draws lower lip laterally; draws up skin of chest.
Map:	Is found on the front and laterally (anterior-laterally) on the throat and down over the upper part of the chest; a flat superficial muscle connected to the skin.
Is contracted by:	Pulling the mouth outward and downward.
Character structure(s):	OPINIONS
Ego function:	SOCIAL BALANCE, (c) degree of "facade" and maintaining one's front.
Psychological function:	Ability to express oneself in a way that maintains one's role.
Ego function:	MANAGEMENT OF ENERGY, (b) containment of high-level energy.
Psychological function:	Containing high energy while exchanging opinions.
Ego function:	GENDER SKILLS, (e) manifestation of sensuality and sexuality.
Psychological function:	Making facial expressions with issues of sensuality and sexuality.
Child's developmental stage/age:	Forms a boundary around the upper part of the chest and throat in relation to having facial expressions for opinions and facial expressions about sensuality and sexuality.

Bodymapping:

Client's position:	On the back.
Tester's position:	By the top of the head.
Activation in test position:	Pull the mouth to the side and down.
Test location:	In the middle of the neck laterally to the throat.
Test direction:	Cranially.

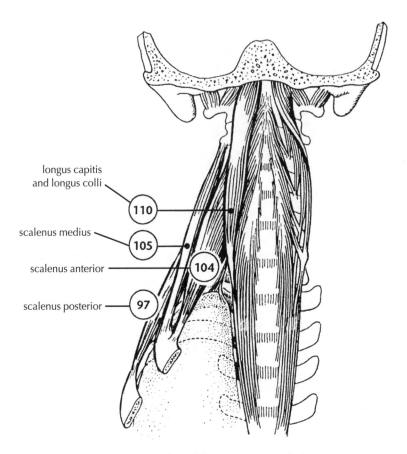

longus capitis
and longus colli — (110)

scalenus medius — (105)

scalenus anterior — (104)

scalenus posterior — (97)

Deep muscles of the neck, ventral view

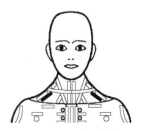

Name:	Scalenus anterior	Number: 104

Origin:	Transverse processes C3–C6.
Insertion:	Superior surface of 1st rib.
Anatomical function:	Raises 1st rib in inspiration Acting together, they flex the neck. Acting on one side, it laterally flexes and rotates the neck.
Map:	As a group the scalene muscles are deep but lie more superficially in the lower anterolateral neck between trapezius, sternocleidomastoid, and the clavicle. Scalenus anterior is often covered in part by sternocleidomastoid clavicular head.
Is contracted by:	Turning the head to side and flexing forward (tilting the head to the same side if necessary).
Character structure(s):	NEED
Ego function:	POSITIONING, (e) orienting (keeping or losing one's head).
Psychological function:	Keeping one's head while orienting.
Ego function:	COGNITIVE SKILLS, (a) orienting.
Psychological function:	Orienting toward fulfilling one's needs.
Ego function:	MANAGEMENT OF ENERGY, (b) containment of high-level energy.
Psychological function:	Regulating energy by fulfilling a need.
Child's developmental stage/age:	The child lifts its head when lying on the back; holds the head; pulls the head forward (searching toward the breast). The muscle takes part in stabilizing the chest to increase inhalation.

Bodymapping:

Client's position:	On the back.
Tester's position:	By the top of the head.
Activation in test position:	Lift the head slightly with the face turned to the side.
Test location:	Find the area between trapezius, sternocleidomastoid, and the clavicle, and then find the transverse processes of the cervical vertebrae. Scalenus anterior is found just in front of the transverse processes and under the clavicular head of sternocleidomastoid. Note that scalenus anterior runs under the clavicle. Test the muscle belly proximally to the clavicle.
Test direction:	Cranially.

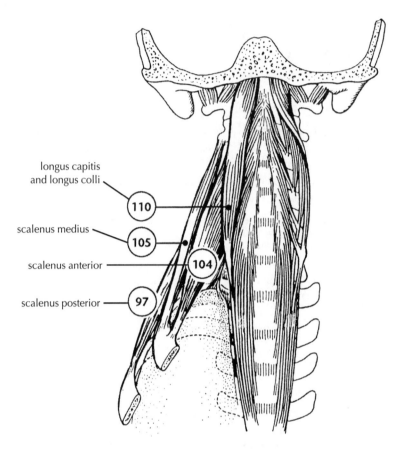

longus capitis
and longus colli

(110)

scalenus medius — (105)

scalenus anterior — (104)

scalenus posterior — (97)

Deep muscles of the neck, ventral view

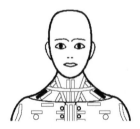

Name:	**Scalenus medius**	**Number: 105**

Origin:	Transverse processes of C2-C7.
Insertion:	Superior surface of 1st rib.
Anatomical function:	Raises 1st rib in inspiration. Acting together, they flex the neck. Acting on one side, it laterally flexes and rotates the neck.
Map:	As a group the scalene muscles are deep but lie more superficially in the lower anterolateral neck between trapezius, sternocleidomastoid, and the clavicle. Scalenus medius is found on the side of the neck, slightly behind the transverse processes.
Is contracted by:	Bending the head to the side and lifting it up again.
Character structure(s):	AUTONOMY
Ego function:	POSITIONING, (e) orienting (keeping or losing one's head).
Psychological function:	Orient oneself in physical space. When entering a new room/house, one looks around curiously to examine everything.
Ego function:	COGNITIVE SKILLS, (a) orienting.
Psychological function:	Curiosity in connecting things (causal thinking).
Ego function:	MANAGEMENT OF ENERGY, (b) containment of high-level energy.
Psychological function:	Containing the energy of curiosity.
Child's developmental stage/age:	The child keeps the head in a upright position; tilts the head so it can see things from different angles. The muscle takes part in stabilizing the chest to increase inhalation.

Bodymapping:

Client's position:	On the back.
Tester's position:	By the top of the head.
Activation in test position:	Lift the head slightly with the face turned to the side.
Test location:	Find the area between trapezius, sternocleidomastoid, and the clavicle. Palpate the transverse processes of the cervical vertebrae. Scalenus medius is found slightly behind the transverse processes. Contract levator scapulae to distinguish scalenus medius.
Test direction:	Cranially.

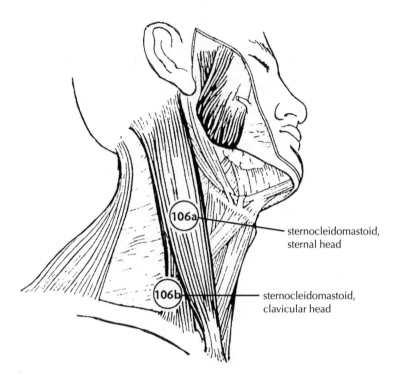

106a ——— sternocleidomastoid,
            sternal head

106b ——— sternocleidomastoid,
            clavicular head

Head and neck, right lateral view

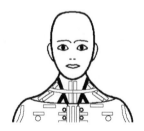

Name:	**Sternocleidomastoid**	Number: 106a, b

Origin:	(a) Sternal head: manubrium of sternum. (b) Clavicular head: medial part of clavicle.
Insertion:	Mastoid process.
Anatomical function:	Acting on one side, it bends the neck laterally and rotates the head. Acting together, they flex the neck, draw the head ventrally and elevate the chin, and draw the sternum superiorly in deep inspiration.
Map:	Is found on the front of the neck (anterolateral) and is seen as full muscle bellies.
Is contracted by:	Moving the head forward, turning it to the side, tilting it to the side.
Character structure(s):	(a) Sternal head, superior part: LOVE/SEXUALITY (a) Sternal head, inferior part: OPINIONS (b) Clavicular head: WILL
Ego function:	POSITIONING, (e) orienting (keeping or losing one's head).
Psychological function:	LOVE/SEX: positioning around alliances (focusing more on one person than another). OPINIONS: positioning around taking a stand. WILL: positioning around choice and consequences.
Ego function:	COGNITIVE SKILLS, (a) orienting.
Psychological function:	LOVE/SEX: orienting oneself in relation to alliances ("Who has an alliance with whom?"). OPINIONS: orienting oneself in relation to own opinions ("Who has which opinion?"). WILL: orienting oneself in relation to choice and consequences ("Who has chosen what, and what are the consequences?").
Ego function:	MANAGEMENT OF ENERGY, (b) containment of high-level energy.
Psychological function:	LOVE/SEX: containing the energy from different alliances at the same time. OPINIONS: containing one's own opinion at the same time as being flexible around seeing other possibilities. WILL: containing one's choice at the same time as seeing the consequences (see what one has to relinquish).
Ego function:	106 (a), sternal head, superior part: GENDER SKILLS, (e) manifestation of sensuality and sexuality.
Psychological function:	LOVE/SEX: flirting with dignity and love.

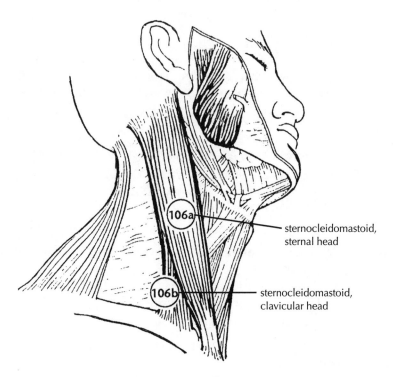

sternocleidomastoid,
sternal head

sternocleidomastoid,
clavicular head

Head and neck, right lateral view

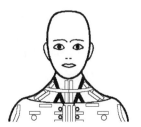

Name:	**Sternocleidomastoid**	Number: 106a, b

Child's developmental stage/age:	The muscle is active in the rotation pattern of walking, allowing a greater awareness while walking toward one's goal. Walking this way, the child actually has a larger view and thereby a larger overview. LOVE/SEX: making constructive alliances with best friends and at the same time being together in a group with others. OPINIONS: the child asks very specifically for the meaning of words (e.g., the word *love*). WILL: the child tries to understand the meaning of choice and the consequence of choice ("There is something I don't get").

Bodymapping:

Client's position:	On the back.
Tester's position:	By the top of the head.
Activation in test position:	Turn the head to the side; the muscle is activated by lifting the head slightly.
Test location:	Turn the head back toward a (symmetrical) neutral position and test the two heads of the muscle. (a) Sternal head: test in two locations, superiorly and inferiorly. (b) Clavicular head: test in one location.
Test direction:	Cranially.

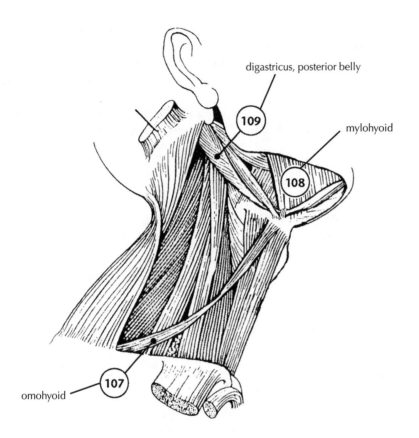

digastricus, posterior belly

mylohyoid

109

108

omohyoid

107

Muscles of hyoid bone, right lateral view

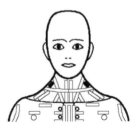

Name:	**Omohyoid**
Origin:	Superior border of scapula.
Insertion:	Inferior belly: bound to the clavicle by a central tendon Superior belly: hyoid bone.
Anatomical function:	Depresses hyoid bone and tightens up the central fascia of the neck.
Map:	A long slim muscle that, in its superficial course, crosses the scalene muscles on the lateral side of neck.
Is contracted by:	Making deep sounds, swallowing, vomiting.
Character structure(s):	SOLIDARITY/PERFORMANCE
Ego function:	GROUNDING AND REALITY TESTING, (c) experience and grounding of extrasensory perceptions.
Psychological function:	Remain in one's dignity when one experiences emotions and instincts.
Ego function:	MANAGEMENT OF ENERGY, (b) containment of high-level energy.
Psychological function:	Preserve one's normal vocal pitch during high-level energy.
Child's developmental stage/age:	The muscle connects the hyoid bone and the neck fascia and takes part in creating a space for containing the voice. The voice becomes more precise and rich because the muscle stabilizes the vocal pitch.

Number: 107

Bodymapping:

Client's position:	On the back.
Tester's position:	By the top of the head.
Activation in test position:	Make a deep sound or swallowing movements.
Test location:	On the muscle belly that lies superficially on the scalene muscles.
Test direction:	Laterally.

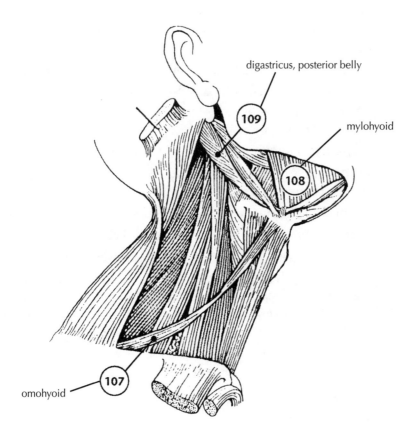

digastricus, posterior belly

mylohyoid

109

108

omohyoid

107

Muscles of hyoid bone, right lateral view

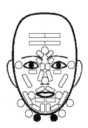

Name:	**Mylohyoid**	Number: 108

Origin:	Inner surface of mandible.
Insertion:	Hyoid bone.
Anatomical function:	Elevates the hyoid bone (forward and upward) and forms the oris diaphragm (floor of the mouth).
Map:	Covers the area under the jaw bone.
Is contracted by:	Opening the mouth, swallowing.
Character structure(s):	NEED
Ego function:	GROUNDING AND REALITY TESTING, (c) experience and grounding of extrasensory perceptions.
Psychological function:	Being able to deeply receive and take in contact, as if "swallowing" it.
Ego function:	MANAGEMENT OF ENERGY, (b) containment of high-level energy.
Psychological function:	Express energy through sounds (crying, laughing).
Ego function:	GENDER SKILLS, (d) containment of sensuality and sexuality.
Psychological function:	Express pleasure/enjoyment/delight.
Child's developmental stage/age:	The muscle is active in the swallowing reflex initiated in the fourth month of the embryonic stage. This reflex remains; if something is placed on the back of the tongue, it will be swallowed. The child develops the ability to swallow actively (consciously), as when breast-feeding and learning to chew and waiting to swallow. The child will drink and explore the ability to swallow.

Bodymapping:

Client's position:	On the back.
Tester's position:	By the top of the head.
Activation in test position:	Press the tongue against the roof of the mouth.
Test location:	On the muscle belly under the jaw bone.
Test direction:	Laterally.

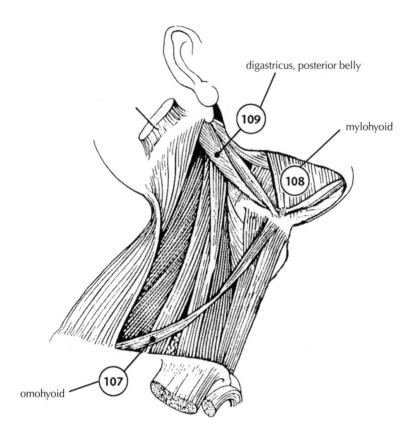

digastricus, posterior belly

mylohyoid

109

108

omohyoid

107

Muscles of hyoid bone, right lateral view

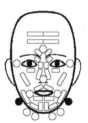

The Bodynamic Psycho-Motor Anatomy

Name:	**Digastricus, posterior belly**	**Number: 109**

Origin:	Mastoid notch of temporal bone.
Insertion:	Intermediate tendon attached to hyoid bone.
Anatomical function:	Raises hyoid bone and opens the mouth.
Map:	Is found superficially behind the jaw.
Is contracted by:	Opening the mouth.
Character structure(s):	EXISTENCE
Ego function:	MANAGEMENT OF ENERGY, (b) containing high-level energy.
Psychological function:	Staying open to taking in information from the physical world.
Ego function:	PATTERNS OF INTERPERSONAL SKILLS, (d) receiving and giving from one's core.
Psychological function:	Staying open to receiving and giving.
Child's developmental stage/age:	IN UTERO: At the end of the embryonic stage, the child can safely open her mouth and swallow the amniotic fluid at the same time as she is sucking her thumb. If there is a problem with the amniotic fluid, the child can use other muscles to close her mouth to stop ingesting the fluid. AFTER BIRTH: The child opens her mouth to be breast-fed and at the same time takes in the current social energy (it is important that the mother breast-feeds in a social atmosphere or context while maintaining her boundaries).

Bodymapping:

Client's position:	On the back.
Tester's position:	By the top of the head.
Activation in test position:	Open the mouth.
Test location:	Where the muscle belly can be palpated between the jaw and sternocleidomastoid muscle.
Test direction:	Cranially, laterally.

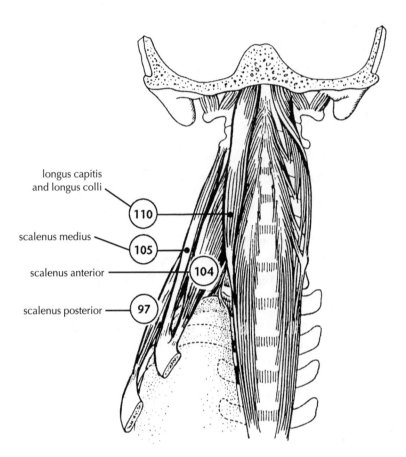

longus capitis
and longus colli — (110)

scalenus medius — (105)

scalenus anterior — (104)

scalenus posterior — (97)

Deep muscles of the neck, ventral view

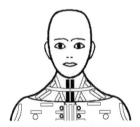

Name:	**Longus capitis and longus colli**	**Number: 110**

Origin:	Longus capitis: anterior tubercle of transverse processes C3–C6. Longus colli: anterior surface of C1–T3 running to 2–3 levels above.
Insertion:	Longus capitis: basal portion of occipital bone. Longus colli: anterior tubercles of transverse processes C1–C6.
Anatomical function:	Flexes the head and neck, side flexes the neck to the same side, and rotates to the opposite side.
Map:	Is found anteriorly (on the front) of the cervical vertebrae.
Is contracted by:	Moving the nose slightly downward while lengthening the back of the neck.
Character structure(s):	EXISTENCE
Ego function:	POSITIONING, (a) stance toward life. (e) orienting (keeping or losing one's head).
Psychological function:	(a) integrate spiritual life into the physical life. (e) orient oneself in the integration of spirituality, thoughts, and the sensation of the body.
Ego function:	GROUNDING AND REALITY TESTING, (c) experience and grounding of extrasensory perceptions.
Psychological function:	Integrate the surroundings through the kinesthetic sense (motor system)
Ego function:	COGNITIVE SKILLS, (a) orienting.
Psychological function:	Preserve the connection between intuition, thoughts, and body.
Ego function:	MANAGEMENT OF ENERGY, (b) containment of high-level energy.
Psychological function:	Accepting the energy of the instincts.
Child's developmental stage/age:	The child is able to maintain the balance of the head on the neck; lengthens the back of the neck.

Bodymapping:

The client's position:	On the back.
Tester's position:	By the top of the head.
Activation in test position:	A slight lift of the head.
Test location:	Find the transverse processes behind sternocleidomastoid; let the fingers slide toward the midline on the cervical vertebrae.
Test direction:	Cranially.

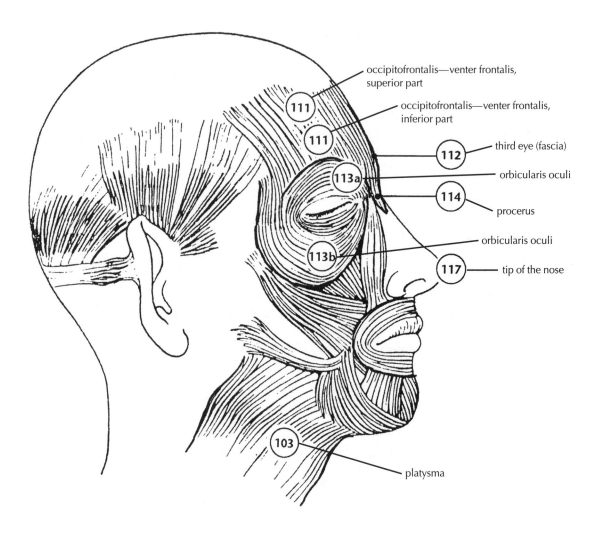

occipitofrontalis—venter frontalis, superior part **111**

occipitofrontalis—venter frontalis, inferior part **111**

third eye (fascia) **112**

orbicularis oculi **113a**

114 procerus

orbicularis oculi **113b**

117 tip of the nose

103 platysma

Superficial muscles of the face, right lateral view

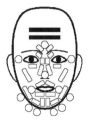

Name:	**Occipitofrontalis—venter frontalis**	**Number: 111**

Origin:	Galea aponeurotica.
Insertion:	Skin above the nose and eyes.
Anatomical function:	Wrinkles the forehead, raises eyebrows.
Map:	Muscle fibers on the forehead that insert in galea aponeurotica.
Is contracted by:	Lifting the eyebrows.
Character structure(s):	Superior part: SOLIDARITY/PERFORMANCE Inferior part: OPINIONS
Ego function:	COGNITIVE SKILLS, (f) contemplation/consideration.
Psychological function:	SOL/PERF: form opinions from ideas. OPINIONS: form opinions from new information.
Child's developmental stage/age:	Facial expression when something is realized/understood.

Bodymapping:

Client's position:	On the back.
Tester's position:	By the top of the head.
Activation in test position:	Lift the eyebrows.
Test location:	Test in two different locations on the muscle cranially to the eyebrows.
Test direction:	Cranially.

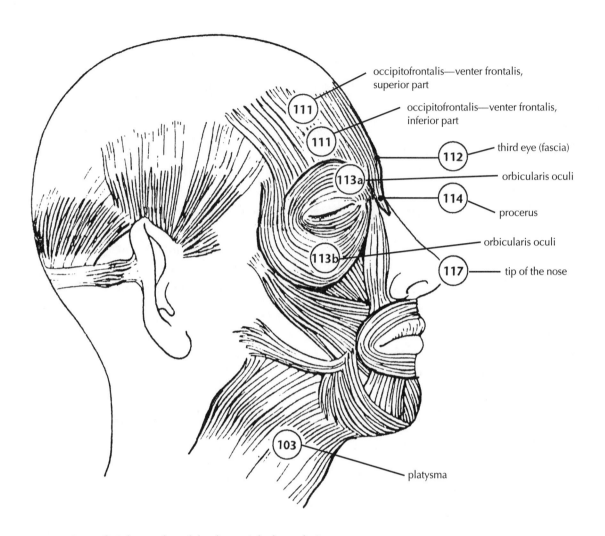

occipitofrontalis—venter frontalis, superior part — 111

occipitofrontalis—venter frontalis, inferior part — 111

third eye (fascia) — 112

orbicularis oculi — 113a

procerus — 114

orbicularis oculi — 113b

tip of the nose — 117

platysma — 103

Superficial muscles of the face, right lateral view

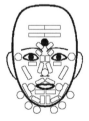

Name:	"Third eye"	Number: 112

Origin:	
Insertion:	
Anatomical function:	
Map:	Connective tissue between the eyebrows.
Is contracted by:	
Character structure(s):	EXISTENCE
Ego function:	GROUNDING AND REALITY TESTING, (c) experience and grounding of extrasensory perceptions.
Psychological function:	Physical and emotional sensation of extrasensory phenomena.
Ego function:	COGNITIVE SKILLS, (f) contemplation/consideration.
Psychological function:	Accepting intuitive knowledge.
Child's developmental stage/age:	The energetic spot for extrasensory perceptions and intuitive knowledge (the pineal gland).

Bodymapping:

Client's position:	On the back.
Tester's position:	By the top of the head.
Activation in test position:	
Test location:	Between the eyebrows.
Test direction:	Cranially.

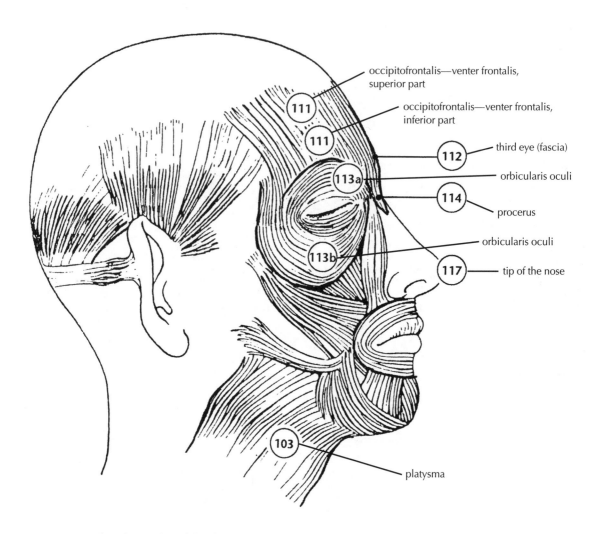

occipitofrontalis—venter frontalis,
superior part

occipitofrontalis—venter frontalis,
inferior part

third eye (fascia)

orbicularis oculi

procerus

orbicularis oculi

tip of the nose

platysma

Superficial muscles of the face, right lateral view

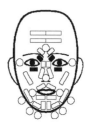

Name:	**Orbicularis oculi**	**Number: 113a, b**

Origin:	Frontal bone and maxilla (medial aspect of orbit).
Insertion:	Continues around orbit and returns to origin.
Anatomical function:	Closing of eyes and scrunching up the eyes.
Map:	Circular-shaped muscle around the eye.
Is contracted by:	Closing the eyes and scrunching up the eyes.
Character structure(s):	NEED
Ego function:	PATTERNS OF INTERPERSONAL SKILLS, (d) receiving and giving from one's core.
Psychological function:	Using eyes as means of making contact. Ask for, receive, give, accept, and reject/close.
Child's developmental stage/age:	Closing the eyes, scrunching up the eyes.

Bodymapping:

Client's position:	On the back.
Tester's position:	By the top of the head.
Activation in test position:	Scrunch up the eyes.
Test location:	(a) In the corner above the eye. (b) Right beneath the eye.
Test direction:	(a) Laterally according to the shape of the corner of the eye. (b) Medially.

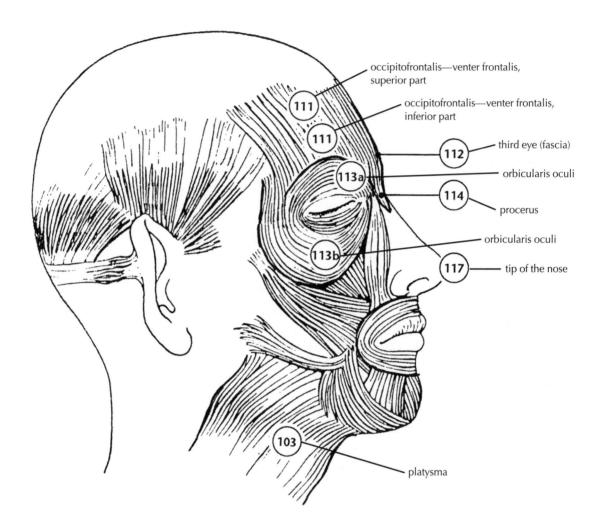

occipitofrontalis—venter frontalis, superior part

occipitofrontalis—venter frontalis, inferior part

third eye (fascia)

orbicularis oculi

procerus

orbicularis oculi

tip of the nose

platysma

Superficial muscles of the face, right lateral view

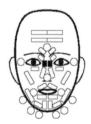

Name:	**Procerus**	**Number: 114**

Origin:	Skin at the bridge of the nose.
Insertion:	Skin of the forehead, between the eyebrows.
Anatomical function:	Pulls the skin of the forehead downward.
Map:	Is found at the top of the bridge of the nose.
Is contracted by:	Wrinkling the nose.
Character structure(s):	NEED AUTONOMY
Ego function:	COGNITIVE SKILLS, (f) contemplation/consideration.
Psychological function:	NEED: alertness, "what is that?" AUT: researching curiosity to people and things; "poking one's nose" into things.
Child's developmental stage/age:	NEED: the child integrates knowledge about things with the sense of smell; wrinkling the nose in alertness as when offered food or something new. AUT: when the child relates to things, he also smells them.

Bodymapping:

Client's position:	On the back.
Tester's position:	By the top of the head.
Activation in test position:	Wrinkle the nose.
Test location:	On the bridge of the nose between the eyes.
Test direction:	Cranially.

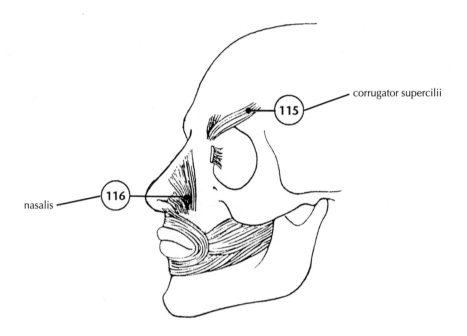

Deep muscles of the face, left lateral view

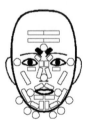

Name:	**Corrugator supercilii**	Number: 115

Origin:	Superciliary arch of frontal bone.
Insertion:	Skin above the eyebrows.
Anatomical function:	Pulls the eyebrows downward, making vertical wrinkles in the forehead.
Map:	Is found between the eyebrows.
Is contracted by:	Wrinkling the eyebrows, e.g., when frowning.
Character structure(s):	WILL
Ego function:	COGNITIVE SKILLS, (f) contemplation/consideration.
Psychological function:	Concentrate and consider things, remember situations.
Child's developmental stage/age:	The child is able to wrinkle the brows, concentrate, put together/distinguish, and thus it helps with grasping what is going on in the world.

Bodymapping:

Client's position:	On the back.
Tester's position:	By the top of the head.
Activation in test position:	Wrinkle the eyebrows; pull them together.
Test location:	On the medial third of the eyebrow.
Test direction:	Obliquely cranially, laterally.

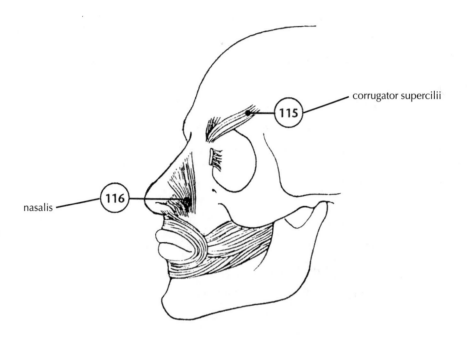

corrugator supercilii

115

116

nasalis

Deep muscles of the face, left lateral view

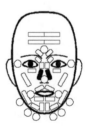

Name:	Nasalis	Number: 116

Origin:	Transverse part: middle of maxilla. Alaris part: greater alar cartilage, skin on nose.
Insertion:	Transverse part: muscle of opposite side over bridge of nose. Alaris part: skin at point of nose.
Anatomical function:	Both parts maintain opening of external nares during forceful inspiration. Transverse part compresses the nostrils/nasal openings. Alaris part dilates the nostrils/nasal openings.
Map:	Is found on the sides of the nose.
Is contracted by:	Compressing the nasal openings. Dilating the nasal openings.
Character structure(s):	OPINIONS
Ego function:	COGNITIVE SKILLS, (f) contemplation/consideration.
Psychological function:	Understanding the coherence or truth of a matter, ambiguity (i.e., "I don't believe this," "I smell a rat.").
Ego function:	SELF-ASSERTION, (b) asserting oneself in one's roles.
Psychological function:	Asserting oneself and creating an image of oneself.
Child's developmental stage/age:	The muscle is used in snorting: "So, that's what you mean." The child uses the sense of smell to understand situations, i.e., that the parents have had an argument; she smells emotions, i.e., "I smell a rat."

Bodymapping:

Client's position:	On the back.
Tester's position:	By the top of the head.
Activation in test position:	Open the nostrils wide.
Test location:	On the side of the nose.
Test direction:	Obliquely cranially, medially.

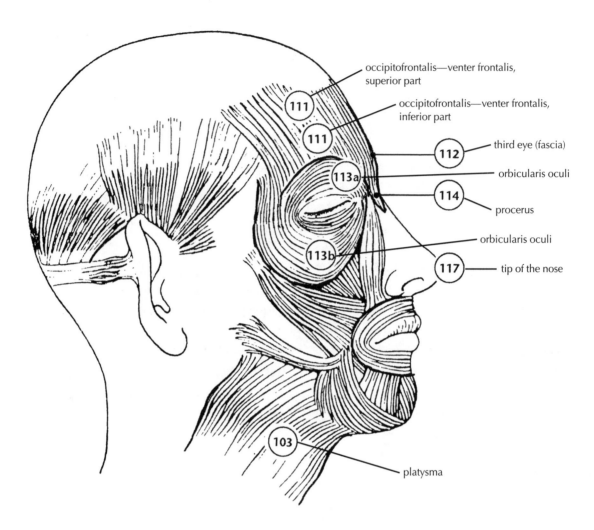

occipitofrontalis—venter frontalis, superior part

occipitofrontalis—venter frontalis, inferior part

third eye (fascia)

orbicularis oculi

procerus

orbicularis oculi

tip of the nose

platysma

Superficial muscles of the face, right lateral view

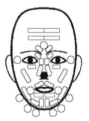

Name:	**Tip of the nose**	**Number: 117**

Origin:	
Insertion:	
Anatomical function:	Fascia on the tip of the nose.
Map:	Is found on the tip of the nose.
Is contracted by:	
Character structure(s):	WILL
Ego function:	SELF-ASSERTION, (a) self-assertion (manifesting one's power).
Psychological function:	Assert one's independence and one's rigid ideas
Child's developmental stage/age:	The child is "poking his nose" into everything. He asserts himself, i.e., by saying "My dad is bigger than yours." A game: "stealing your nose" ("along came a blackbird and pecked off your nose") = "taking the child's independence."

Bodymapping:

Client's position:	On the back.
Tester's position:	By the top of the head.
Activation in test position:	
Test location:	On the tip of the nose.
Test direction:	Cranially.

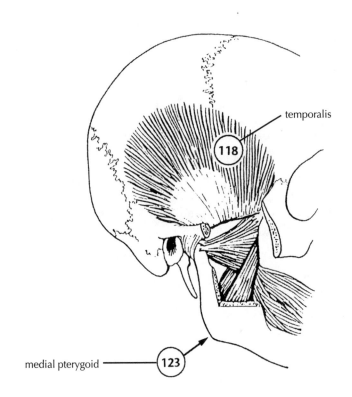

temporalis **118**

medial pterygoid ——**123**

Muscles of mastication, right lateral view

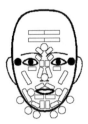

Name:	**Temporalis**	**Number: 118**

Origin:	Lateral surface of temporal bone.
Insertion:	Coronoid process and ramus of mandible.
Anatomical function:	Strong muscle that closes the mouth. The most dorsal fibers pull the mandible backward and have influence on the movements of the jaw.
Map:	Is found on the temples.
Is contracted by:	Biting the teeth together; chewing movements/mastication.
Character structure(s):	Insertion: EXISTENCE (is not tested separately) Muscle: SOLIDARITY/PERFORMANCE-PUBERTY
Ego function:	GROUNDING AND REALITY TESTING, (c) experience and grounding of extrasensory perceptions.
Psychological function:	EX: mixing feelings and emotions with sensations and making sense SOL/PERF-PUB: understanding abstract thoughts, and has the ability to create them both concretely and emotionally.
Ego function:	COGNITIVE SKILLS, (f) contemplation/consideration.
Psychological function:	EX: the same as in grounding and reality testing. SOL/PERF-PUB: understanding the philosophical way of thinking/ideas.
Child's developmental stage/age:	EX: The child senses the gums when it is sucking. SOL/PERF: The child uses the back molars for chewing. PUB: When wisdom teeth appear, the child starts using them for chewing; the action becomes further differentiated to the very back of the mouth.

Bodymapping:

Client's position:	On the back.
Tester's position:	By the top of the head.
Activation in test position:	Bite the teeth together; make chewing movements.
Test location:	Between the ear and the eye above the zygomatic arch where the muscle tenses.
Test direction:	Cranially.

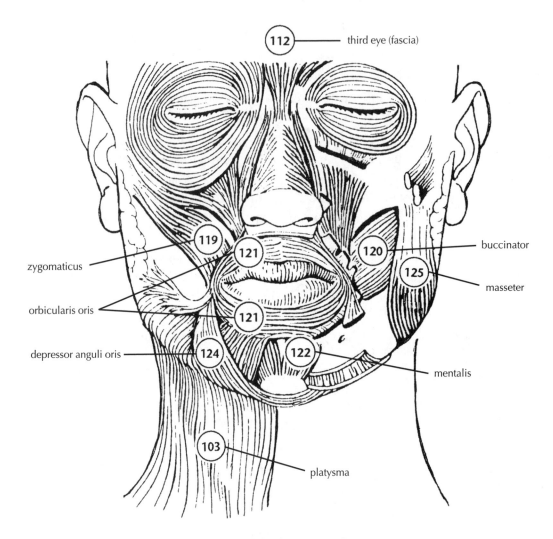

Muscles of the face, ventral view

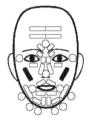

Name:	**Zygomaticus**	Number: 119

Origin:	Zygomatic bone.
Insertion:	Angle of mouth, blending with orbicularis oris.
Anatomical function:	Pulls the corner of the mouth upward and backward.
Map:	Is found between the cheekbone and the mouth.
Is contracted by:	Smiling, moving the corners of the mouth obliquely upward.
Character structure(s):	LOVE/SEXUALITY
Ego function:	MANAGEMENT OF ENERGY, (b) containment of high-level energy.
Psychological function:	Containing high-level energy by smiling, helping to deflect high-level energy in order to manage better.
Child's developmental stage/age:	The child can smile deliberately, giving a facade or image smile. The child can give a smile that means that she likes the contact. She can contain the high energy of both positive and negative contact experiences.

Bodymapping:

Client's position:	On the back.
Tester's position:	By the top of the head.
Activation in test position:	Smile; pull the corners of the mouth obliquely upward.
Test location:	Just beneath the zygomatic arch (the cheekbone).
Test direction:	Obliquely cranially, laterally.

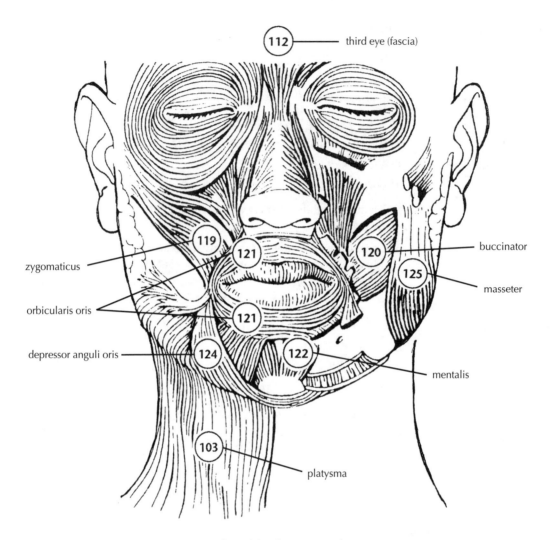

third eye (fascia) — 112

zygomaticus — 119

orbicularis oris — 121, 121

depressor anguli oris — 124

buccinator — 120

masseter — 125

mentalis — 122

platysma — 103

Muscles of the face, ventral view

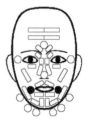

Name:	Buccinator	Number: 120

Origin:	Outer surface of maxilla and mandible.
Insertion:	Deep part of muscles of the lips.
Anatomical function:	Compresses the cheek.
Map:	Is found under the cheekbone, level with the molars.
Is contracted by:	Inflating a balloon, blowing a horn.
Character structure(s):	NEED
Ego function:	SOCIAL BALANCE, (a) balancing own needs/feelings/desires against others' expectations.
Psychological function:	Ability to satisfy the needs one has from others and to "spit out" what you do not want.
Ego function:	GENDER SKILLS, (d) containment of sensuality and sexuality.
Psychological function:	Instinctual and emotional enjoyment of sensation.
Child's developmental stage/age:	The muscle is active in exhaling/puffing out, sucking, and is active around receiving. The child is able to process food/things and spit out what he does not want.

Bodymapping:

Client's position:	On the back.
Tester's position:	By the top of the head.
Activation in test position:	Suck in the cheeks, pretending you are blowing a trumpet.
Test location:	Deeply, level with the corners of the mouth.
Test direction:	Obliquely laterally, cranially.

		Number: *
Name:	**Risorius**	

Origin:	Fascia over masseter.
Insertion:	Skin at angle of mouth.
Anatomical function:	Pulls the corners of the mouth backward.
Map:	Is found lateral to the corners of the mouth.
Is contracted by:	Grinning, showing the teeth, "Mona Lisa" smile.
Character structure(s):	LOVE/SEXUALITY
Ego function:	SOCIAL BALANCE, (c) degree of "facade" and maintaining one's front.
Psychological function:	Ability to be polite without losing oneself.
Child's developmental stage/age:	The child can smile out of politeness/give a polite smile. The child can show her teeth, e.g., when the teeth are brushed.

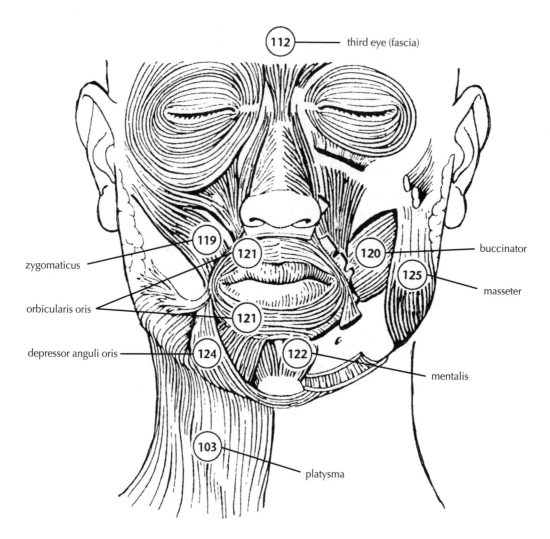

third eye (fascia) — **112**

zygomaticus — **119**

121

120 — buccinator

125 — masseter

orbicularis oris — **121**

depressor anguli oris — **124**

122 — mentalis

103 — platysma

Muscles of the face, ventral view

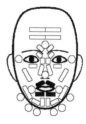

Name:	**Orbicularis oris**	**Number: 121**

Origin:	Muscle fibers surrounding the mouth derived from other facial muscles.
Insertion:	Skin and mucous membrane.
Anatomical function:	Closure and protrusion of lips.
Map:	Circular muscle around the mouth.
Is contracted by:	Closing/"lacing up" the mouth tight, pursing one's lips, whistling.
Character structure(s):	NEED
Ego function:	SELF-ASSERTION, (a) self-assertion (manifesting one's power).
Psychological function:	Self-assertion in both accepting and rejecting ("yes" and "no").
Ego function:	PATTERNS OF INTERPERSONAL SKILLS, (d) receiving and giving from one's core.
Psychological function:	Ability to receive and reject; giving from and receiving into one's core from both the instinctive layer and emotional layer.
Ego function:	GENDER SKILLS, (e) manifestation of sensuality and sexuality.
Psychological function:	Sensual pleasure/enjoyment via the mouth.
Child's developmental stage/age:	The child is exploring sensation with the mouth, i.e., reaching out, spitting out, receiving; one of the primary sense organs for perceiving the world and surviving. Active in the seeking reflex.

Bodymapping:

Client's position:	On the back.
Tester's position:	By the top of the head.
Activation in test position:	Purse the mouth, close the mouth tight.
Test location:	Above the mouth, above the lip edge. Beneath the mouth, below the lip edge.
Test direction:	Laterally.

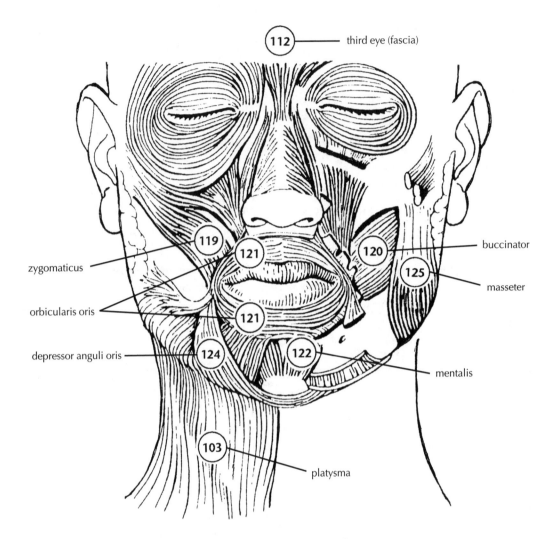

Muscles of the face, ventral view

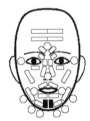

Name:	**Mentalis**	Number: 122

Origin:	Incisive fossa of mandible.
Insertion:	Skin of chin.
Anatomical function:	Raises and protrudes the lower lip; wrinkles skin of the chin.
Map:	Is found on the chin.
Is contracted by:	Pushing out the lower lip (pouting).
Character structure(s):	NEED WILL
Ego function:	SOCIAL BALANCE, (c) degree of "facade" and maintaining one's front.
Psychological function:	NEED and WILL: express dissatisfaction.
Child's developmental stage/age:	NEED: is active just before bursting into tears and crying. WILL: is active in looking moody, sullen, feeling sorry for oneself; part of a "poker face" expression.

Bodymapping:

Client's position:	On the back.
Tester's position:	By the top of the head.
Activation in test position:	Push out the lower lip.
Test location:	On the chin.
Test direction:	Cranially.

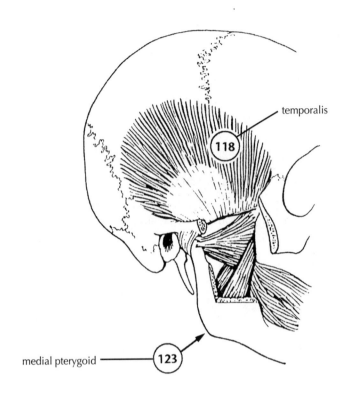

temporalis

118

medial pterygoid ——(123)

Muscles of mastication, right lateral view

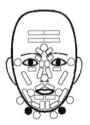

Name:	**Medial pterygoid**	**Number: 123**

Origin:	Tuberosity of maxilla and medial surface of lateral pterygoid plate.
Insertion:	Medial surface of ramus and angle of the mandible.
Anatomical function:	Closes the lower jaw, clenches teeth. Acting together, they help to protrude the mandible. Acting on one side, it protrudes the side of the jaw. Acting alternately, they produce a grinding movement.
Map:	A square muscle that runs obliquely downward and backward, working together with temporalis and masseter.
Is contracted by:	Closing the mouth and protruding the lower jaw.
Character structure(s):	AUTONOMY
Ego function:	MANAGEMENT OF ENERGY, (b) containment of high-level energy.
Psychological function:	Containing the building of emotional energy.
Child's developmental stage/age:	The child is practicing chewing; begins making grinding movements back and forth; pushes the jaw forward and looks angry, protrudes jaw forward and to the side and growls like a dog.

Bodymapping:

Client's position:	On the back.
Tester's position:	By the top of the head.
Activation in test position:	Clench the teeth or push the jaw forward.
Test location:	On the inner side of the jawbone at the corner.
Test direction:	Along the jawbone.

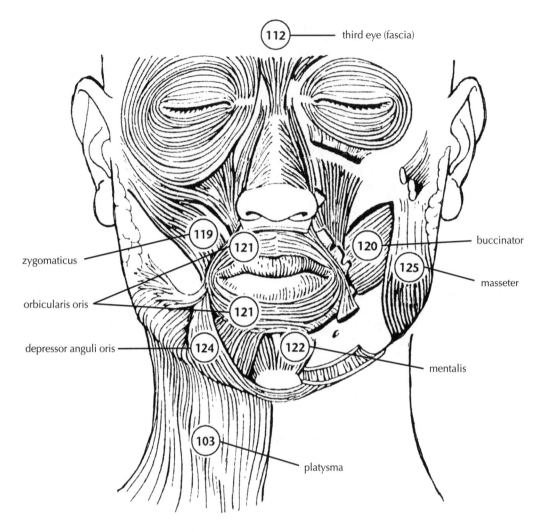

Muscles of the face, ventral view

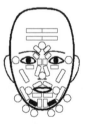

Name:	**Depressor anguli oris**	**Number: 124**

Origin:	Oblique line of the mandible.
Insertion:	Skin at corner of mouth.
Anatomical function:	Lowers the corners of the mouth.
Map:	Is found on the sides of the chin at the corners of the mouth.
Is contracted by:	Pulling the corners of the mouth down.
Character structure(s):	WILL
Ego function:	SOCIAL BALANCE, (c) degree of "facade" and maintaining one's front.
Psychological function:	Showing or holding back the facial expression of discontented feelings.
Ego function:	MANAGEMENT OF ENERGY, (a) containment of emotions.
Psychological function:	Contain emotions.
Ego function:	SELF-ASSERTION, (b) asserting oneself in one's roles.
Psychological function:	Assert one's independence and one's will.
Child's developmental stage/age:	The child can look sulky/sour, huffy, look threatening, ("Look what you have done to me"); is used purposely to punish; "I'm unhappy and I will stay that way," can keep a secret, make a "poker face."

Bodymapping:

Client's position:	On the back.
Tester's position:	By the top of the head.
Activation in test position:	Pull down the corners of the mouth.
Test location:	At the sides of the chin at the corner of the mouth
Test direction:	Toward the ear.

Name:	**Depressor labii**	Number: *

Origin:	Mandible and platysma.
Insertion:	Lower lip.
Anatomical function:	Lowers the lower lip and pulls it laterally.
Map:	Is found on the chin.
Is contracted by:	Pulling the lower lip down; is often activated together with platysma.
Character structure(s):	OPINIONS
Ego function:	SOCIAL BALANCE, (c) degree of "facade" and maintaining one's front.
Psychological function:	Keeping up appearances/facade when one is feeling a total outsider/totally different.
Ego function:	MANAGEMENT OF ENERGY, (b) containment of high-level energy.
Psychological function:	Containment of provocative energy.
Child's developmental stage/age:	The muscle stabilizes platysma; helps to express annoyance or holds it back when the child experiences things that are on the edge of cultural norms; strange tastes, smells, and unexpected behavior.

Name:	**Depressor septi**	**Number: ***
Origin:	Incisive fossa of maxilla.	
Insertion:	Nasal septum and ala.	
Anatomical function:	Pulls the tip of the nose downward, narrowing the nostrils.	
Map:	Is found right under the nose.	
Is contracted by:	Pulling the tip of the nose downward.	
Character structure(s):	OPINIONS	
Ego function:	SELF-ASSERTION, (a) self-assertion (manifesting one's power).	
Psychological function:	Underlining one's opinions with a facial expression.	
Child's developmental stage/age:	The child can snort, close the nostrils (shut out "smell").	

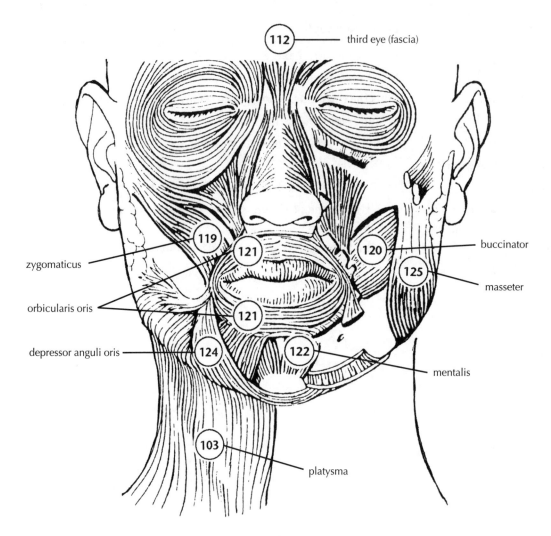

Muscles of the face, ventral view

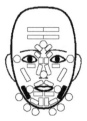

Name:	Masseter	Number: 125

Origin:	Process and arch of zygoma.
Insertion:	Ramus and angle of mandible.
Anatomical function:	Closing the lower jaw; clenching the teeth (biting).
Map:	Is found between the zygomatic arch (cheekbone) and the lower jaw bone.
Is contracted by:	Closing the mouth; biting.
Character structure(s):	WILL
Ego function:	MANAGEMENT OF ENERGY, (b) containment of high-level energy.
Psychological function:	Regulating high-level energy.
Child's developmental stage/age:	The muscle is active in chewing, clenching the teeth, and clenching the jaw to endure something that is unsupportable/exhausting. 2-2½ years of age: grinding chewing movements from side to side (all kinds of teeth have appeared—front teeth, canine teeth, and molars).

Bodymapping:

Client's position:	On the back.
Tester's position:	By the top of the head.
Activation in test position:	Bite the teeth together; chewing movements.
Test location:	Slightly anterior to the joint of the jaw, where the muscle is full.
Test direction:	Toward the ear (across the direction of fibers) or cranially in the direction of the fibers.

Section 3

The Bodynamic Character Structure System

The Character Structures
in the Bodynamic System

The Character Structure table on page 357 presents the Character Structures and their age levels and positions. In order to compare our interpretation of age levels with others, we have placed Freud's, Erik Erikson's, and Alexander Lowen's models of development at the left of the table. We interpreted Freud's model from Jydebjerg and Fonsmark (1970); Erikson's model was interpreted from Erikson (1968); and Lowen's model is from Michael Maley (n.d.), as Lowen himself has not given any precise age graduation in his books.

In this section, a general introduction to the Character Structures is followed by a description of each Character Structure as a whole. For each Character Structure and age level in question, some "Important Themes of Development" are mentioned.

The "Characteristic Body Features" are the body postures that occur when Closed Codings are formed during the different age levels. The muscle responses in the Closed Coding are visible because the muscles and the particular themes that become active at this age level will become either hyporesponsive or hyperresponsive when Closed Codings are formed. A system of muscle tenseness is formed. This Tenseness System makes it possible to "read" and interpret a person's Closed Codings and the positions in the different Character Structures. The Characteristic Features from the Early Position are formed by Closed Codings in an early stage of the age level. If you form Closed Codes later in the developmental stage, the Characteristic Features from the Late Position are formed. Often body features from both the Early and the Late Position are seen, as you may have formed Closed Codings in some themes in the beginning of the age level and in other themes later in the stage of age in question.

"Life Patterns" are the attitudes you have when meeting other people. They are patterns or styles of contact and communication and how you act and react in your life.

"Key Sentences" are the sentences we have heard that people use when they are expressing themselves from this age level.

"Resources" are the resources developed during the different age levels.

"Ideal messages in interaction with the Early and Late Positions" are words and sentences that are useful to establish good contact. It is not always necessary to use the words directly; often holding the intention of the words may be rewarding.

A Bodymap showing all the muscles that are tested in the Character Structure follows.

A review of the muscles and connective tissue in the age level is shown on the opposite page.

On an image of the body, the places of some of the muscles and connective tissue within the Character Structure described are marked, and on the opposite page are their names and "Patterns of Movement."

The Character Structures in the Bodynamic System

Freud	Erikson	Lowen
Gential	Identity vs. role diffusion	
Latency	Industry vs. inferiority	Four variations of rigidity
Phallic	Initiative & responsibility vs. guilty function	
Anal	Autonomy vs. shame and doubt	Masochistic
		Psychopathic
Oral	General trust vs. basic mistrust	Oral
		Schizoid

Age	Structural Issues	Predominant hyporesponse Early position	Predominant hyperresponse Late position	Balanced response Healthy position
The teenager is occupied with decisions about life and how he or she is going to live as a grown-up (choice of direction in life). He/she is establishing an integration of sexuality and social function. At the same time, patterns of all the earlier stages are played out—with the possibility of becoming more closed or integrated in a new way.				
7-12 years	Solidarity/ Performance	Leveling	Competitive	Balancing we/I
5-9 years	Opinion formation	Sullen	Opinionated	Integration of opinions
3-6 years	Love/ Sexuality	Romantic	Seductive	Balancing love and sexuality
2-4 years	Will	Self-sacrificing	Judging	Powerful in actions
8 months-2½ years	Autonomy	Nonverbal activity-changing	Verbal activity-changing	Emotionally autonomous
1 months -1½ years	Need	Despairing	Distrustful	Fulfillment of needs
2nd trimester–3 months	Existence	Mental	Emotional	Secure being
Perinatal	This stage is not a character structure but an imprint of how one manages in stress and shock situations.			

A Theory of Personality Based on Psychomotor Development

We think that the creation of our personality begins before birth and continues throughout life. We also think that there are some sensitive periods of age when the child voluntarily includes new muscles and new patterns of movement at the same time as the child learns new physical and psychological behavioral systems. All this takes place in contact with someone or something and within a social context. As described in the introduction, this forms Code systems that are rooted in the muscles involved.

In every psychomotor stage of development, the child is developing new possibilities in her life and the motor abilities it leads to. These possibilities can be summarized as a developmental theme. This theme is connected to a pattern of muscles that are found in different places in the body. These muscles are used for different aspects of the theme and start working in the specific stage of development attached to it.

Before the individual has reached the age of fourteen, he or she has formed his or her own experiences of acting in relation to the world, and this is connected to the different muscles that belong to each developmental stage. From these experiences the muscles then have adjusted their way of responding. They may become despairing, reluctant, or healthy. This corresponds to a measurable reaction in the elasticity of the muscle: hyporesponsive, hyperresponsive, and neutral. These muscular reactions can be read visually or felt by touch.

These three reactions—hyporesponsive, hyperresponsive, and neutral—are typical for the three Character Positions in each developmental structure. The first is despairing, which corresponds to a Closed Coding system happening early in a specific developmental stage. The second is more reluctant, which corresponds to a Closed Coding system happening late in a specific developmental stage. The third and last is the healthy structure, which corresponds to an undoubted resource.

The different themes and experiences may therefore be observed in the muscular structures. (We do this by visually body-reading or body-testing where the response from the muscles, picked up or assessed through palpation, are marked on a Bodymap; the reading then takes place from this test.) It is rare that a person has problems only in one stage of development. As a rule there are features from many different stages, and maybe from all of them. As a rule, though, there are some stages of development that are clearly closed and others that are clearly filled with resources.

Just as human beings are not static, our body structure is not static either. We change voluntarily through therapy or other kinds of personal development, but our changes also just happen without thinking about them. The reason for this is that in our daily lives we get the challenge, support, and guidance we didn't get when we developed the Closed Codes.

In the same way, we can also change to a more closed position. That happens if, in different challenges, we get the same sort of support and guidance that we got when the Codes were first developed; consequently the Codes will close more firmly. This means that at times, some Character Positions are more obvious than others, and that the impression of the whole may change.

Prenatal and Perinatal

Birth is not a Character Structure as such, though it is an important experience for the child. It is the first time that the baby or fetus produces a rush of adrenaline. A rush of adrenaline is normally only produced in situations with a very high intensity of energy, as in highly dangerous or fatal situations and during high stress (in both what we describe as good and bad stress). Because of this very high level of adrenaline, we say that an imprint is made and not a code. On account of this, later situations with a high level of adrenaline (stress-shock-peak) will have a tendency to activate the behavioral patterns that were imprinted in birth.

Below is a model of the stages of birth, laid out as what happens to the mother, what happens to the child, and what issues are integrated by the child at birth.

Model of the Stages of Birth

	Stage	Mother	Child's bodily reaction	Optimal coding possibility
1.	The time just before birth (1 week before).	She makes herself ready. Puts in order, tidies up, cleans, "makes a nest." May have premonitory pains.	Less room available; bodily anxiety and restlessness; may press toward the pressure.	To experience that one has the time needed.
2.	First-stage labor pains; the stage of expansion.	She lets the labor pains flow through.	Is squeezed; pulls himself together /contracts away from the pressure.	Pulls himself together/contracts; an avoiding reaction.
3.	Stage of transition; transition between first-stage labor pains and second-stage labor pains, which move the uterus in different ways.	Anxiety and restlessness; Sometimes an experience of desperation. What is happening?	Anxiety and restlessness in his whole body.	An experience of confusion; no way out; makes himself ready.
4.	Second-stage labor pains.	In the second-stage labor pains, she presses and she squeezes.	He pushes with all his power.	The experience of using all power and having the right to do so.
5.	Delivery	She presses and lets go.	The stretching reflex from heel to head is released for the first time.	To come out; to come through when applying power.
6.	The time just after delivery and the first days after birth.	She gets a new contact with her child.	Finds mother's breast; sucking; finds mother's and father's eyes; makes contact.	To have the right to make contact in new surroundings; new connection; to have the right to be on earth, in the family, and the right to be met.

In the different stages of birth, complications may arise. This may cause the child to form imprints. In the future, the person will act according to these imprints in stressful situations. The numbers refer to the stages of birth on the opposite page:

1. An experience that there is never time enough.
   Time is something you cannot control.

2. You feel that you have to pull yourself together, i.e., go to bed/fall asleep, wait until the stress has passed.
   It is difficult to start new projects.

3. When you are in a stressful situation, confusion arises, and you don't know what to do.

4. When using your power, something "dangerous," something painful, happens.
   You fall asleep suddenly or you get a fever (e.g., if you were anaesthetized during this stage of birth).
   It feels best to wait until it goes away.

5. When you get through, you'll be left alone/you are on your own (e.g., if the mother's condition is critical and the child is put aside).
   You are cold and freezing (born in a cold room).
   Your eyes and throat hurt in stressful situations because drops were put in your eyes or your throat was suctioned out after birth, etc.

6. If the optimal contact was not available in the sixth stage of birth, in later stressful situations you may feel left alone and unbelonging.
   You may feel unseen, unmet, inexperienced, and not having the right to be here, to be on earth, to be in the family.
   You may have a feeling of being wrong.

The Muscles Marked on a Bodymap

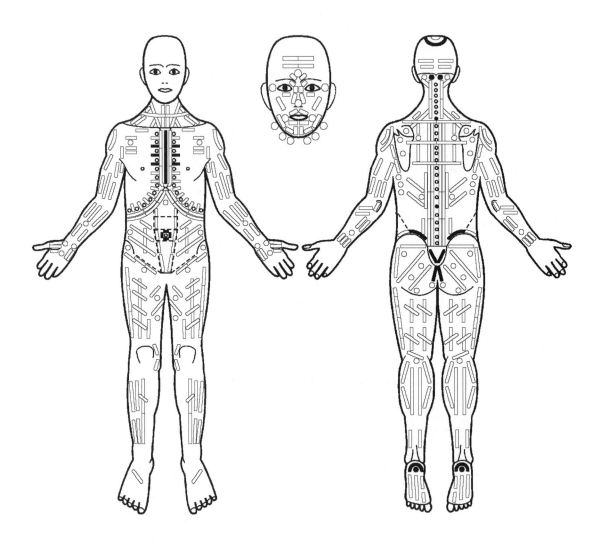

All the Muscles and Connective Tissue in This Age Span

Head and throat:

101b   Galea aponeurotica (half circle around the top of the head)

Back and neck:

100   Suboccipitals, medial part

Shoulders and arms:

*	Connective tissue on top of the shoulder (shoulder plexus)	
*	Connective tissue of medial and lateral rotators of the shoulder joint	(PERINATAL and EX)
*	Connective tissue around elbow and wrist	

Front:

54	Umbilicus	(PERINATAL and EX)
60	Sternal fascia	(PERINATAL and EX)
61	Intercostals, between ribs 2-5	
*	Transversus thoracis, 1st part of 3 (ref. 58)	(PERINATAL and EX)

Hip and legs:

12	Iliac crest, medial part	
13	Sacrum	
21	Sacrotuberous ligament	(PERINATAL and EX)
*	Origin of iliacus (ref. 51a)	
*	Insertion of iliopsoas (ref. 51b)	
33	Plantar aponeurosis	
*	Connective tissue of medial and lateral rotators of the hip joint	(PERINATAL and EX)
*	Connective tissue around knee and ankle	

Some Essential Patterns of Movement in This Age Span

Head and throat:

101b Galea aponeurotica (half circle around the top of the head)

The area of the baby's head that is impacted during second-stage labor contractions. Pressure at this time comes both from the birth canal and from inside the child (the child's own strength/power).
This provides the basic ability to maintain direction and have confidence in the possibility of getting through stressful situations.

Back and neck:

100 Suboccipitals, medial part

The muscles are active in birth when the child squeezes/presses his way out in second-stage labor; active in both the seeking and sucking reflexes.

Shoulders and arms:

* Connective tissue on top of the shoulder (shoulder plexus)

Part of the reflex of pushing out during birth.

* Connective tissue of medial and lateral rotators of the shoulder joint

The connective tissue is part of the reflex system, and during second-stage labor it assists in stabilizing the throat and neck so the power/strength can get through when the child pushes from the heels.

Front:

54 Umbilicus

Affects the flow through the navel cord.

61 Intercostals, between 2–5

Active in breathing.

Hip and legs:

12 Iliac crest, medial part

Reflex contraction in erector spinae begins from the hip bone so the back gains its first curve.

13 Sacrum

Part of the stretch reflex required for pushing oneself through the birth canal during birth.

21 Sacrotuberous ligament

In birth, the sacrotuberous ligament is part of the stretching reflex during second-stage labor, when the child pushes from the heels.

* Insertion of iliopsoas (ref. 51b)

The insertion of iliopsoas is active when the child contracts itself during first-stage labor. When the child is lying alone after birth, he pulls himself into a fetal position.

33 Plantar aponeurosis

Extension reflex in birth. The child contacts the mother's uterus with the heels and then starts extension of the legs; the beginning of the walking reflex.

* Connective tissue of the medial and lateral rotators of the hip joint

In birth, the child initially flexes the whole body, and the limbs rotate inward during first-stage labor. When adrenaline is secreted during second-stage labor, the child starts to rotate the limbs outward and pushes to get through the birth canal with his own power/strength.

The Character Structure EXISTENCE

2nd trimester–3 months

Character Positions

Early position: mental
Late position: emotional
Healthy position: secure being

Important Themes of Development

- Existence
- Spirituality/physical being
- Sensations/emotions
- Contact–physically, emotionally, energetically
- The "Me" (including reflexes)/the "I" (Ego)
- Rhythm and matching
- Experience of contact/experience of oneself without contact
- Mirroring

The Character Structure EXISTENCE

Early position: mental

Late position: emotional

Characteristic Body Features

The energy is drawn into the bones.	Radiates a lot of energy, fills a lot of space in a room.
It may be experienced as if they take up very little room/space.	The energy is located in the bones, muscles, and skin but is missing in some of the connective tissue (fascial layer).
Maladjustments and twists, which derive from the spinal column.	The body seems divided in horizontal layers with more energy in some of the layers than in others.
The head radiates more energy than the body.	The body radiates more energy than the head.
The eyes are unfocused, as if looking toward a distant goal, even in an eye contact situation.	The eyes are focused, fixed on the foreground and the background simultaneously. It may seem as if they hold on to you in eye contact.
Holds on to the energetic and abstract reality.	Holds on to the concrete and emotional reality with the eyes.

Life Patterns

Mental people identify themselves with abstract thinking and imaginings/ideas. This way they lose the consciousness of sensations, emotions, and concrete thinking.	Emotional people identify themselves with emotions and bodily experiences. This way they lose the cognitive comprehension and the understanding of causal relations.
They seek energetic and philosophical contact.	Insist on emotional and physical contact.
Withdraw from emotional and physical contact.	Become desperate when the contact is nonverbal or interrupted.
Compensate by developing fanatical ideologies when they sense a conflict.	Become desperate when they sense a hidden conflict.
Emotions are experienced as threats and are converted into abstract thoughts or mathematical logic.	Abstractions without concretizing are experienced as distance and threats and converted to emotions.
Accumulate energy by abstractions; as it is difficult to contain energy, it is channeled through ideas or projects very often without a plan of action.	Accumulate energy from emotions; as it is hard to contain these, they are often acted out in emotionally intense situations.
Feel connected to others by energy and thoughts.	Feel connected to others by emotions and words (concretizing).
Feel isolated.	Feel lonely.

Early position: mental	Late position: emotional

Key Sentences

I think, therefore I am.	I feel, I experience, therefore I am.
I fall apart or I go to pieces like a jigsaw puzzle.	I go mad when the contact is suddenly gone/disappears.
My head (my thoughts) is too much.	If I show my emotions, the other person withdraws/backs out of contact.
Sometimes . . . it happens . . . OK.	Always . . . never . . . fantastic . . . huge.

Resources

Sensitive to others.	See others and express it.
Creative and full of ideas.	Energetic and emotionally engaged.
Good at giving others permission to be.	Good at catching hold of others if they need contact or something else.
Good at analyzing a hidden conflict.	Good at opening a hidden conflict, though often in an explosive way.
Notice what happens and observe from the sidelines.	Filled with energy, lively, and make things happen.

Ideal Messages in Interaction

I love you.	I love you.
I'm staying here.	I'm here.
You have the right to exist/be.	I sense/feel you, and I'm staying here.
You are wanted here on earth as the human being/person you are.	You have the right to have/get contact.
I'm staying with you even when you withdraw yourself.	I'm staying with you even when you express your emotions/feelings.

The Healthy Position

In the body, they are not locked, as described in the two positions above; they maybe experienced by people with an absence of these body features. They will have life patterns in which they can use the resources from both positions in a flexible way. The developmental themes have been integrated, and they are able to use the themes in a flexible way.

The Muscles Marked on a Bodymap

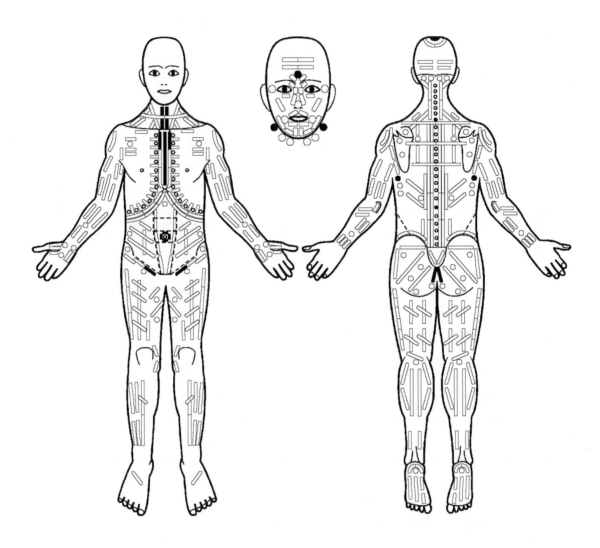

The Bodynamic Character Structure System

All the Muscles and Connective Tissue in This Age Span

The skin

Head and throat:

109	Digastricus, posterior belly
110	Longus capitis and longus colli
101a	Galea aponeurotica (a spot on top of the head)
112	"Third eye" (fascia)
*	Insertion of temporalis (ref. 118)

Back and neck:

*	Connective tissue of the back level with thoracic vertebrae 3-5
*	Origins and insertions of suboccipitals (ref. 100)

Shoulders and arms:

8a	Serratus anterior, superior part	
*	Connective tissue of medial and lateral rotators of the shoulderjoint	(PERINATAL and EX)
*	Insertions of flexors and extensors on the proximal phalanx of the little finger	(EX and NEED)

Front:

54	Umbilicus	(PERINATAL and EX)
59	Origin of pectoralis major, sternal head, superior part	
60	Sternal fascia	(PERINATAL and EX)
*	Transversus thoracis, 1st part of 3 (ref. 58)	(PERINATAL and EX)

Hip and legs:

21	Sacrotuberous ligament	(PERINATAL and EX)
50	Inguinal ligament, medial part	
*	Connective tissue of medial and lateral rotators of the hip joint	(PERINATAL and EX)
*	Insertions of abductor, flexors and extensors on the proximal phalanx of the little toe	(EX and NEED)
*	Iliacus, inferior part (ref. 51a)	

The Location of Some of the Muscles
and Connective Tissue in the Body

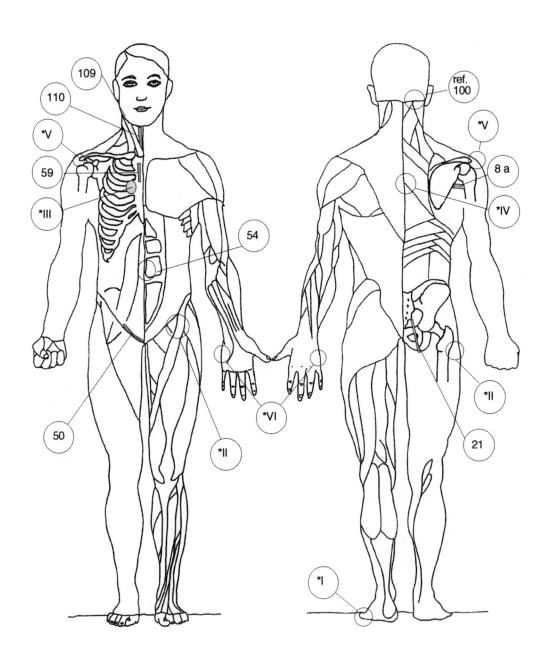

Some Essential Patterns of Movement in This Age Span

Head and throat:

109	Digastricus, posterior belly	Opens the mouth, active in sucking.
110	Longus capitis and longus colli	Lifting the head when lying on the back; lengthens the back of the neck. The child is able to maintain the balance of the head on the neck.

Back and neck:

*IV	Connective tissue of the back level with thoracic vertebrae 3-5	The place on the fetus/child's back where it has contact with the uterus most frequently.
ref. 100	Origins and insertions of suboccipitals	The reflex movements of the head, active in both the seeking and sucking reflexes and active in the falling reflex, holding the head back; are automatically activated if the head is dropping or is unsupported.

Shoulders and arms:

8a	Serratus anterior, superior part	The child reaches out all the way from the inside (the heart) with inhalation/breathing in. The child pulls herself into contact.
*V	Connective tissue of medial and lateral rotators of the shoulder joint	Is part of the reflex system that is active when the child is moving around in utero.
*VI	Insertions of flexors and extensors on the proximal phalanx of the little finger	Grasp reflex; the child pumps the breast. This reflex movement is a remnant from animals' pumping action.

Front:

54	Umbilicus	Affects the flow through the navel cord.
59	Origin of pectoralis major, sternal head, superior part	Is involved in breathing. The child pulls herself into contact by a reflex action.
*III	Transversus thoracis, 1st part of 3	Breathing reflex; the fetus starts to use this muscle in utero; primary respiratory muscle in the first years.

Note: The locations of these muscles and connective tissue are shown on the opposite page. The muscles and connective tissue are marked by number or *. The right half of the front side and the left half of the back side are used for marking superficial musculature and connective tissue; the deeper layers are marked on the left half of the front side and the right half of the back side.

The Location of Some of the Muscles and Connective Tissue in the Body

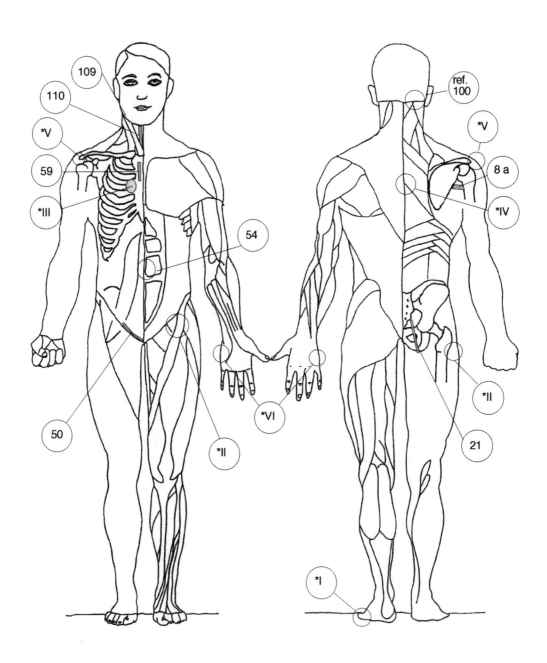

Some Essential Patterns of Movement in This Age Span

Hip and legs:

21	Sacrotuberous ligament	Is involved in the stretch reflex and thus part of the reflex system which keeps the body upright.
50	Inguinal ligament, medial part	Is affected in the stretch reflex; stabilizes the muscles of the stomach area and thus stabilizes emotions.
*II	Connective tissue of medial and lateral rotators of the hip joint	Is part of the reflex system that is active when the child is moving around in utero.
*I	Insertions of abductor, flexors, and extensors on the proximal phalanx of the little toe	A catch/grasp reflex. The child grasps with the little toe reflexively ("pumps") during breast-feeding and bottle-feeding.

Note: The locations of these muscles and connective tissue are shown on the opposite page. The muscles and connective tissue are marked by number or *. The right half of the front side and the left half of the back side are used for marking superficial musculature and connective tissue; the deeper layers are marked on the left half of the front side and the right half of the back side.

The Character Structure NEED

1 month–1½ years

Character Positions

Early position: despairing
Late position: distrustful
Healthy position: fulfillment of needs

Important Themes of Development

- Rhythm, timing, matching
- Saying yes and no
- Feeling oneself seen/met in contact (mirrored, imitated)
- Exploring in contact with others
- Being oneself without contact and exploring one's own movements and different objects around them, e.g., textures and forms
- Concrete thinking
- Connecting words with objects
- Connecting words with emotions and needs
- Claiming the right to have their needs fulfilled
- Having the right to experience a state of being fulfilled
- Balancing between giving and taking

The Character Structure NEED

Early position: despairing

Late position: distrustful

Characteristic Body Features

Weight on the heels.	Weight on the heels.
Hanging in overextended knee joints.	Hanging in overextended knee joints.
Hanging in the hip joint in a bow backward with the stomach pushed forward.	Hanging in the hip joint in a bow with the stomach forward, but slightly straighter than the early position.
Collapse in the thorax in the upper part of the breastbone.	None or just a slight collapse in the thorax by the breastbone.
Head pushed forward like a tortoise (for contact).	Head pushed forward, but much less than in the despairing position.
Full "loose" lips.	Possibly tight mouth (sullen).
The eyes have a yearning/sucking, seeking expression.	The eyes change among a seeking, sucking, and distrustful expression, or often one eye is seeking and the other eye is distrustful.

Life Patterns

Cannot feel own needs, but is good at sensing the need of others.	Can feel own needs, but will not reach out (ask for what they need); snarling and distrustful.
Cannot distinguish between their own and others' needs.	Don't believe they will receive the right thing by asking for what they need; believe that it is only given with "genuine" purpose if you get what you need without asking for it.
Seek merging contact.	Tendency to merging or partly merging contact.
Mirroring a lot and often without interpretation (i.e., precisely).	Mirroring a lot, but also interpretative, so it is less precise than in the despairing position.

The Character Structure NEED

Early position: despairing

Late position: distrustful

Key Sentences

I don't know what I need.

I just need love/All I need is love.

I am always abandoned or left behind.

If you are well, then everything is well. If the family is all right, everything is all right, and then I am happy.

I have no energy. I am depressed, despairing. say.

I always get the wrong thing.

No matter what I ask for (reach out for), I get something else.

Everybody else gets what they need. It is only me that has to do without.

If I have to ask for it, then you are only giving it to me because you have to, not because you want to.

I am irritated, and I don't believe what you

Resources

Loving, caring, good at small-talk (babbling).

Precisely mirroring (very little interpretation).

Giving.

Giving.
Have healthy skepticism.

Persevering.

Good at mirroring.

Ideal Messages in Interaction

You have the right to have your needs. You have the right to be seen and met.

You can say yes or no to what I give you, and I'll respect your answers.

I want to be in contact with you about what you need.

I want to give you ideas as to how you can feel what you like and dislike.

You have the right to demand that your needs are met. I accept your dissatisfaction when I cannot meet/fulfill your needs.

You can say yes or no to what I give you. I accept both answers and stay in contact with you.

I want to be in contact with you about your distrust, your negative world view, and I maintain/take care of my own boundaries.

I'll ask you what you want/need, and I'll stay until I get an answer.

The Healthy Position

In the body, they are not locked, as described in the two positions above. They may be experienced by people with an absence of these body features. They will have life patterns in which they can use the resources from both positions in a flexible way. The developmental themes have been integrated, and they are able to use the themes in a flexible way.

The Muscles Marked on a Bodymap

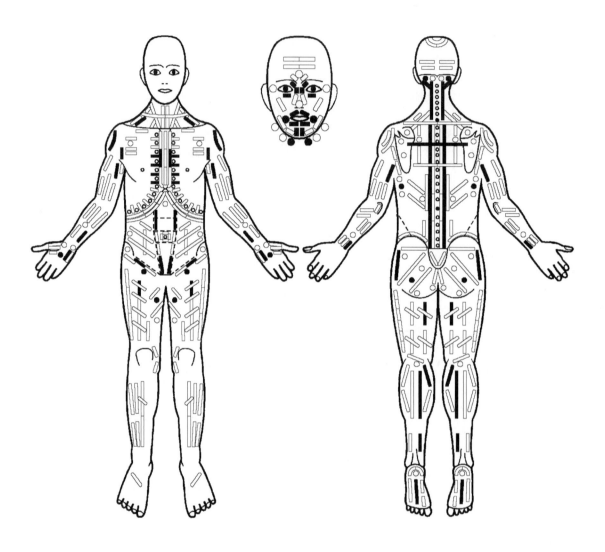

All the Muscles and Connective Tissue in This Age Span

The skin

Head and throat:

104	Scalenus anterior	
108	Mylohyoid	
113a, b	Orbicularis oculi	
114	Procerus	(NEED and AUT)
120	Buccinator	
121	Orbicularis oris	
122	Mentalis	(NEED and WILL)

Back and neck:

1a	Erector spinae
98	Semispinalis capitis
99	Splenius capitis
100	Suboccipitals, lateral part

Shoulders and arms:

2b	Trapezius, middle part	
8b	Serratus anterior, middle part	
*	Pectoralis minor, superior part (ref. 63)	
65	Deltoid, anterior part	
66b	Biceps brachii, short head, proximal part	
69	Subscapularis	
75	Flexor digitorum profundus	
76	Palmar aponeurosis	
82	Flexor digiti minimi brevis	
*	Insertions of flexors and extensors on the proximal phalanx of the little finger	(EX and NEED)
85a	Triceps brachii, long head, proximal part	
92	Extensor digiti minimi	

Front:

53	Rectus abdominis, superior and inferior parts of 4
59	Origin of pectoralis major, sternal head, middle part
*	Transversus thoracis, 2nd part of 3 (ref. 58)
61	Intercostals, between ribs 3-7

The Muscles Marked on a Bodymap

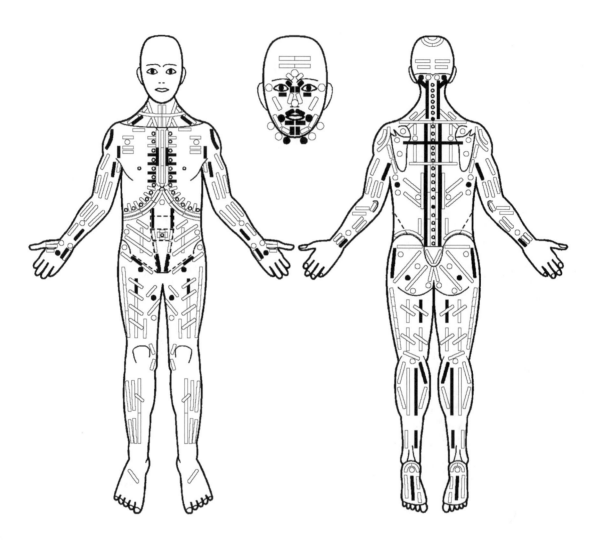

All the Muscles and Connective Tissue in This Age Span

Hip and legs:

18	Gemelli and obturator internus	
*	Pelvic floor: pelvic diaphragm: coccygeus	
22	Tensor fascia lata	
26	Semimembranosus, proximal part	
28b	Gastrocnemius, medial head, proximal part	
30b	Soleus, medial part	
32	Flexor digitorum longus	(NEED and LOVE/SEX)
35	Flexor digitorum brevis	
*	Flexor digiti minimi brevis (is tested together with 34, OPINIONS)	
*	Insertions of abductor, flexors and extensors on the proximal phalanx of the little toe	(EX and NEED)
*	Tibialis posterior	(NEED and LOVE/SEX)
43c	Vastus intermedius, proximal part	
47	Adductor brevis	
50	Inguinal ligament, lateral part	
51b	Iliopsoas	

The Location of Some of the Muscles in the Body

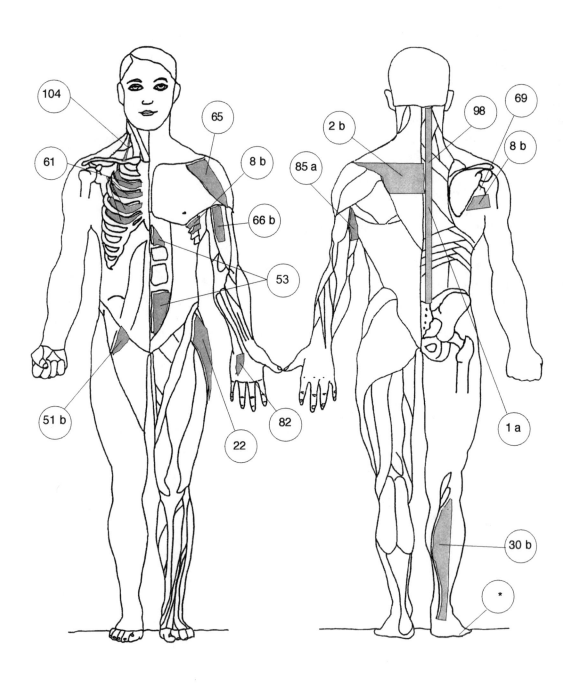

Some Essential Patterns of Movement in This Age Span

Head and throat:

| 104 | Scalenus anterior | It takes part in stabilizing the chest to increase inhalation. The child lifts his head when lying on his back; holds the head; pulls the head forward (searching toward the breast). |

Back and neck:

| 1a | Erector spinae | Postural muscles of the spine; stretches the back. |
| 98 | Semispinalis capitis | The postural muscle of the neck; assists in holding and lifting the head from the position of lying on the stomach. |

Shoulders and arms:

2b	Trapezius, middle part	Draws the shoulder blades together and stabilizes them when the child lifts his head and shoulder up while supporting himself with his arms and when creeping.
8b	Serratus anterior, middle part	Inhalation; stabilizes the shoulder blades when the child lifts himself up from lying on the stomach, in creeping, and when the child reaches out from the inside (the heart).
65	Deltoid, anterior part	It stabilizes the shoulder joint so the arms can be held in a reaching-out gesture. The child lifts the arms forward ("Lift me up"). The muscle is active during play, e.g., when the child is scribbling and when playing with cars.
66b	Biceps brachii, short head, proximal part	Used in pulling in with the arms from the elbow joint, for drawing oneself forward in creeping and drawing oneself up into a standing position.
69	Subscapularis	Rotates inward in the shoulder joint; is active when the child reaches out for something and when rolling from belly to back. It stabilizes when the child pushes himself up from the floor/mat, and it stabilizes the creeping.
82	Flexor digiti minimi brevis	Grips with the little finger. First kind of finger grip/hand grip (ulnar-palmar grip). The child senses what he holds in his hands; pumping while breast-feeding and bottle-feeding.
85a	Triceps brachii, long head, proximal part	Used to push away with the arms from the elbow joint, for pushing oneself up on the arms while lying on the stomach.

Note: The locations of these muscles are shown on the opposite page. The muscles are marked by number or *. The right half of the front side and the left half of the back side are used for marking superficial musculature; the deeper layers are marked on the left half of the front side and the right half of the back side.

The Location of Some of the Muscles in the Body

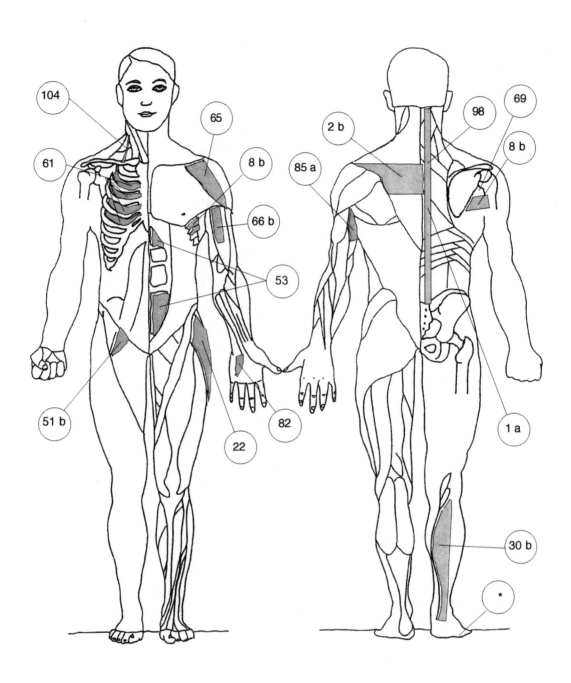

Some Essential Patterns of Movement in This Age Span

Front:

53	Rectus abdominis, superior and inferior parts of 4	Abdominal muscle that gives support in the trunk in cooperation with (1a) erector spinae; active in rolling and creeping, and the child is able to come from a lying to a sitting position.
61	Intercostals, between ribs 3-7	Active in respiration at this age.

Hip and legs:

22	Tensor fascia lata	Pulls the leg outward in the hip joint when the child rolls and creeps.
30b	Soleus, medial part	Pushes forward with the foot; gives stability in calf and ankle joint; takes part in the counter-gravity reflex when the child stands.
*	Flexor digiti minimi brevis (ref. 34)	Grips with little toe.
51b	Iliopsoas	Active in creeping and when the child crosses the leg over the body to initiate rolling; the leg is moved forward in the hip joint; connects trunk and leg.

Note: The locations of these muscles are shown on the opposite page. The muscles are marked by number or *. The right half of the front side and the left half of the back side are used for marking superficial musculature; the deeper layers are marked on the left half of the front side and the right half of the back side.

The Character Structure AUTONOMY

8 months–2½ years

Character Positions

Early position: nonverbal activity changing
Late position: verbal activity changing
Healthy position: emotionally autonomous

Important Themes of Development

- Curiosity/exploring the world
- Learning to distinguish emotions and activities
- Gaining ownership of emotions
- Connecting words and objects
- Needing help to do things themselves
- Awareness of the learning of causal connection
- Being oneself in contact with others
- Mastering one's own activities in interaction with others

The Character Structure AUTONOMY

Early position: nonverbal activity changing   **Late position: verbal activity changing**

Characteristic Body Features

It seems as if the arms are not connected to the body/torso.

It seems as if the legs have a lack of connection to the body/torso.

Energy is in the lower part of the body and in the pelvis.

Energy is in the upper part of the body and in the head.

The kneecaps are locked.

The kneecaps are locked.

Weight is primarily on the middle of the foot; are relatively big distance between the feet (legs).

Weight is mostly on the forefoot and knees extended, feet are rotated outward (from the hip).

Shoulders seem thin (without energy). Pelvis and lower part of body seem/appear broad. Energetically the torso may be described as a triangle with the broad side at the pelvis and pointing upward toward the throat.

Shoulders seem broad and straight (like on a clothes hanger). Pelvis seems thin. Energetically the torso may be described as a triangle with the broad side at the shoulders and pointing downward.

The expression of the eyes changes between an empty look ("They do not see me") and a charming look ("see me").

The expression of the eyes is charismatic, playful, seeking (may seem controlling).

Life Patterns

Walk away from provocative situations without telling, or suddenly change to another activity.

Change provocative situations by sidetracking the conversation or changing the topic of the conversation.

Own impulses, curiosity, and desires disappear in the interaction with others.

Experience a loss of oneself in committing to someone or something.

Become empty.

Are bored.

Wait for initiative from the outside/other people that may give new energy (desire).

Willingly come up with initiatives and try to avoid having others interfere with their activities.

Don't know what help is or what it is to get help.
Help = being swallowed.

Getting help is resigning on one's own impulses or having to do more.

Mirror others and act from the another person's impulses and desires.

Mirror others and come up with new ideas.

Lots of impulses without language.

Lots of impulses that are verbalized.

The Character Structure AUTONOMY

Early position: nonverbal activity changing

Late position: verbal activity changing

Key sentences

Get help—what is that? Then I disappear/vanish.	Get help? Then I just have to do more or give up my own project.
If I tell something about myself, it is taken by the others or used against me. They take away my emotions.	If I really say yes/agree, then I'll lose myself and get bored.
If I do not look at the others, they cannot see me. I disappear. I become empty.	If I fall, I get up again by myself. I keep standing no matter whether I can or cannot.
Something is wrong; it must be me.	I only get love if I can do things on my own.

Resources

Sensitive to control, power, and manipulation.	Dynamic and outgoing.
Helpful.	Charismatic.
Charming in a naive way.	Good at changing situations.
Good at avoiding manipulation.	Good at sensing others' manipulations.
Good at listening and mirroring.	Full of initiative.
	Good at mirroring and coming up with ideas.

Ideal Messages in Interaction

Your emotions belong to you; they are in your body.	Your emotions belong to you; they are in your body.
Help is possible without your activity being taken over.	I want to help you to do it yourself.
I cannot drain you of energy, but you can give more than is good for you.	You can be committed to another and free to be yourself at the same time.
Feel what you want yourself when you are with others, and say this instead of sensing or asking others what they want.	Feel what you want to when others suggest something. Speak and act from this so your desire controls what is going to happen.

The Healthy Position

In the body, they are not locked, as described in the two positions above. They may be experienced by people with an absence of these body features. They will have life patterns in which they can use the resources from both positions in a flexible way. The developmental themes have been integrated, and they are able to use the themes in a flexible way.

The Muscles Marked on a Bodymap

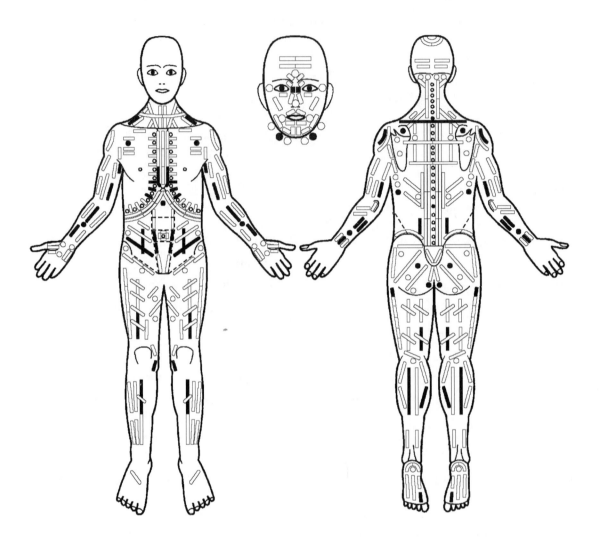

All the Muscles and Connective Tissue in This Age Span

Head and throat:

105	Scalenus medius	
114	Procerus	(NEED and AUT)
123	Medial pterygoid	

Back and neck:

11   Quadratus lumborum

Shoulders and arms:

2a	Trapezius, superior part
8c	Serratus anterior, inferior part
63	Pectoralis minor, inferior/lateral part
66b	Biceps brachii, short head, distal part
67	Coracobrachialis
70	Pronator teres
73	Flexor digitorum superficialis
74	Flexor pollicis longus
84a	Deltoid, middle part
85a	Triceps brachii, long head, distal part
89	Extensor carpi ulnaris
90	Extensor digitorum
91	Supinator
93	Extensor indicis
95	Supraspinatus

Front:

52	Obliquus externus and internus, inferior part
53	Rectus abdominis, two middle parts of 4
58	Transversus thoracis, 3rd part of 3
59	Origin pectoralis major, sternal head, inferior part
61	Intercostals, between ribs 6-9

Hip and legs:

17	Piriformis	37	Flexor hallucis brevis
20	Obturator internus, near pelvic floor	39	Tibialis anterior, proximal part, deep
*	Pelvic floor: pelvic diaphragm: levator ani		
23	Iliotibial tract, 1st part of 6	43c	Vastus intermedius, distal part
26	Semimembranosus, distal part	49	Gracilis
28b	Gastrocnemius, medial head, distal part	55	Psoas major
30a	Soleus, lateral part		

The Location of Some of the Muscles in the Body

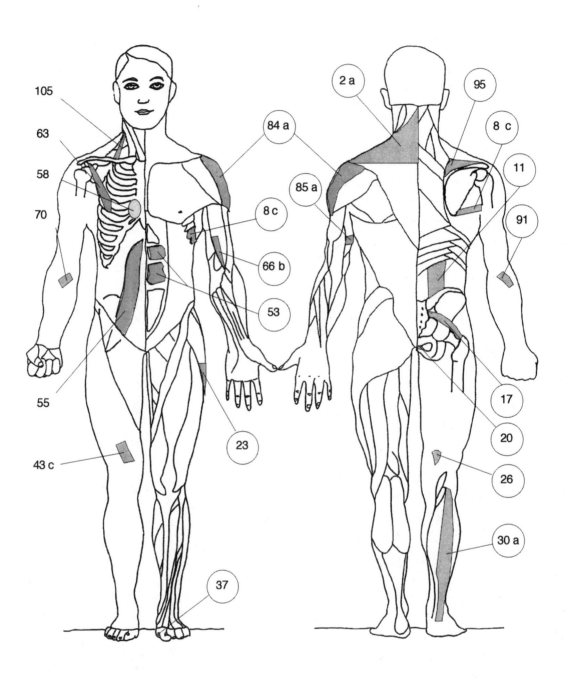

Some Essential Patterns of Movement in This Age Span

Head and throat:

105	Scalenus medius	Inhalation in the upper part of the chest; assists in holding the head.

Back and neck:

11	Quadratus lumborum	Moves the hip forward in crawling; stabilizes the pelvis in the standing position and in walking.

Shoulders and arms:

2a	Trapezius, superior part	Lifts the shoulders; moves the shoulders forward in crawling and stabilizes the shoulder blades.
8c	Serratus anterior, inferior part	Active in respiration; stabilizes the shoulder blades and the chest, when the child stands on all fours; both stabilizing and active in crawling and pulling oneself up into a standing position, and when reaching out from the inside (the heart).
63	Pectoralis minor, inferior/lateral part	Draws the shoulder blades forward/downward; gives stability to the shoulder girdle so the arms can reach out. The child is pointing and saying "What is that?" Both stabilizing and active when the child pulls herself forward in creeping and crawling and when she pulls herself to a standing position.
66b	Biceps brachii, short head, distal part	Bends the arm in the elbow joint; is used in crawling and in pulling oneself up to a standing position; pulls people and objects toward oneself.
70	Pronator teres	Rotates the forearm, so the palm points backward/downward; is used in the movement of giving and taking.
84a	Deltoid, middle part	The child lifts the arms up and out so others have to move away. She lifts the arm when pointing at things; throws a ball without precision.
85a	Triceps brachii, long head, distal part	Stretches the arm in the elbow joint; is used in crawling and in pushing away in contact.
91	Supinator	Rotates the forearm, so the palm points forward/upward; is used in the movement of giving and taking.
95	Supraspinatus	Makes the first part of the movement of the arm out from the body in the shoulder joint; stabilizes the shoulder joint so the arm can be lifted and moved to all positions. The child is doing "flying" movements.

Note: The locations of these muscles are shown on the opposite page. The muscles are marked by number or *. The right half of the front side and the left half of the back side are used for marking superficial musculature; the deeper layers are marked on the left half of the front side and the right half of the back side.

The Location of Some of the Muscles in the Body

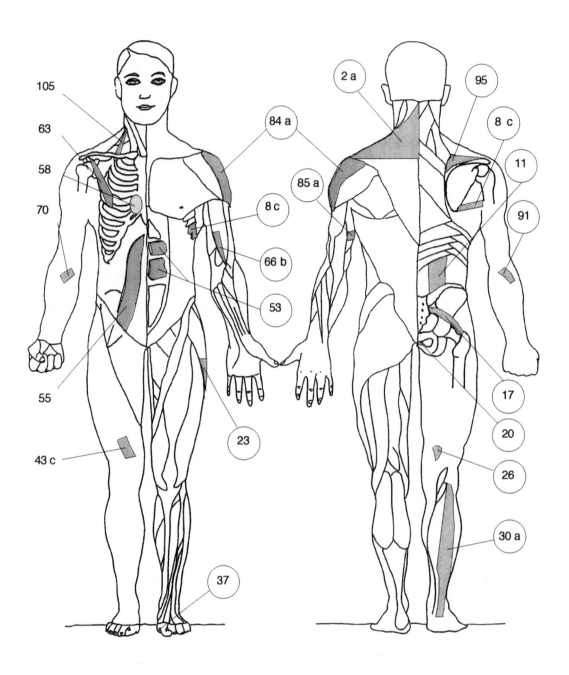

Some Essential Patterns of Movement in This Age Span

Front:

53	Rectus abdominis, two middle parts of 4	Abdominal muscle that bends the trunk; gives support in the abdominal wall; active in rolling and crawling.
58	Transversus thoracis, 3rd part of 3	Is part of the respiration reflex.

Hip and legs:

17	Piriformis	Rotates the leg outward in the hip joint; is used in crawling and later in standing and walking.
20	Obturator internus, near pelvic floor	Rotates the leg outward in the hip joint; activates tension in the pelvis floor, especially around the anus.
23	Iliotibial tract, 1st part of 6	The tract helps keep the muscles of the leg together. It assists in tightening the big fasciae system around the leg as a "stocking"; works together with the postural muscles; affects the mobility in the hip joint. The movements of the leg/knee get stronger and more precise as the child gets older.
26	Semimembranosus, distal part	Bends the knee; gives stability and flexibility in the standing position.
30a	Soleus, lateral part	Postural muscle in the calf; active in the standing position.
37	Flexor hallucis brevis	Pushes against the floor with the big toe. Used in walking, especially when the child begins to walk quickly and "run," and when walking on the toes.
43c	Vastus intermedius, distal part	Stretches the knee and locks the kneecap; gives stability and flexibility in the standing position.
55	Psoas major	Sways the back and bends the hip; lifts the leg when taking a step forward; is active in crawling and walking; stabilizes the spinal column.

Note: The locations of these muscles are shown on the opposite page. The muscles are marked by number or *. The right half of the front side and the left half of the back side are used for marking superficial musculature; the deeper layers are marked on the left half of the front side and the right half of the back side.

The Character Structure WILL

2–4 years

Character Positions

Early position: self-sacrificing
Late position: judging
Healthy position: powerful in actions

Important Themes of Development

- Will—choice and consequences
- Experimenting with coping with things, including body functions (managing, power/being without power)
- Balancing between acting from myself or out of altruism
- Distinguishing between intention and action
- Distinguishing between physical/material reality versus imagination and extrasensory experience
- Guilt, punishment, self punishment
- Expression of all emotions at full blast; containing one's own power
- Experiencing two emotions simultaneously
- Experimenting with roles and humor
- Operative thinking, understanding of dualities and generalized thoughts
- Short-term planning, consciousness of time: being able to act as planned on purpose (can wait)

The Character Structure WILL

Early position: self-sacrificing   **Late position:** judging

Characteristic Body Features

A lot of energy is restrained and bound just beneath the skin (therefore skin is often reddish).

A lot of restrained bound energy. A sensation that they retain/hold back their energy.

The torso looks like it is held in an invisible vice from the neck to the coccyx.

Like the early position, although straighter from solar plexus (diaphragm) and up through the chest.

Weighed-down shoulders, bent as if ready to carry a yoke

The shoulders are less bent forward, appear more restrained.

The "tail" is drawn between the legs (quadratus femoris).

Neck is reminiscent of a bull's neck. Flat bottom (tightness in gluteus minimus) Tightness in semitendinosus.

It often looks as if their pants are sliding down.

It often looks as if their pants are sliding down.

Eye expression: "It is hard on me, but I am proud of being able to cope."

Eye expression: appraising and judging.

Life Patterns

Hold back the power in emotions because they think/experience that others cannot cope with them (grow sullen).

Do things on their own at full blast/with the utmost power. In interaction they restrain their power in order not to overwhelm the others (in their own imagination). Become angry and push away e.g., by being sarcastic.

Sacrifice themselves in order to please others; become martyrs when their actions are not seen or if they are not appreciated for what they do.

Resists everyone's suggestions in order to experience that they get time for themselves to make their choice/decision.

See themselves as helpful (and they are!) and flexible when they do what they imagine that other people want them to do.

Believe that they have a monopoly on what is right and wrong. Forget to ask what the others want (they think they know).

Easily experience themselves as guilty ("It is not right/good enough no matter what I do").

Experience that "It is the others' fault."

Cannot foresee consequences or time framework and therefore they have difficulties making choices and planning.

Act on unverbalized (for themselves natural/ obvious) rituals, rules, and plans.

Experience themselves as inadequate because they think they should know everything without asking or learning.

When making a choice in a group process, they hold on to their own opinions and choice in a rigid way; if not they easily experience chaos.

Often live according to altruistic or self-punishing decisions.

Altruistic, as long as they do not feel threatened.

The Character Structure WILL

Early position: self-sacrificing

Confuse reality, imagination with extrasensory experiences.

Afraid of their own negative thoughts (magical thinking).

Late position: judging

When they feel threatened, they become angry. The anger is expressed through humor but instead of humorous they become sarcastic or humiliate others.

Avenge themselves to bear their own pain.

Key sentences

What I do is me (no distinction between intention and action).

When I follow my own will or speed, I'll be alone.

If I choose to let go of my power, then I'll be crushed, or others cannot contain me/take it.

When I act with my power, I'll crush or overwhelm others.

It is my own fault.

They are all stupid.

I feel like I get sucked down into a swamp.

I feel like I have a bomb inside.

No matter what I do, it will be wrong.

Do not tell me what to do.

If I release/lose control, everything will be chaos.

Do not push me to do something I do not want to.

Resources

Enduring, self-sacrificing, patient.
Self-critical.
Altruistic, active.
Good dramatists and party people.

Enduring, humorous.
Critical.
Helpful, promoters/starters.
Good dramatists and party people.

Ideal Messages in Interaction

You can be furious with a person even though you love him/her (two emotions simultaneously).

I can contain your power no matter what emotion you express.

I like you and I respect your intention, though I do not like what you do (your action).

It is your actions that I do not like (i.e., sarcasm), not your emotions or intentions.

If you choose to do this, it has the following consequences ...

I like your power, although I want you to keep it to yourself right now. (I like your questions, although I do not have an answer right now).

I believe that you hear and see something, even though it may not belong to physical /material reality.

I believe that you know or experience something even though I cannot follow you right away.

I like you for who you are not for what you do.

You may be bigger/more than me, like me, or smaller/less than me, and I'll still like you.

The Healthy Position

In the body, they are not locked, as described in the two positions above. They may be experienced as people with an absence of these body features. They will have life patterns in which they can use the resources from both positions in a flexible way. The developmental themes have been integrated, and they are able to use the themes in a flexible way.

The Muscles Marked on a Bodymap

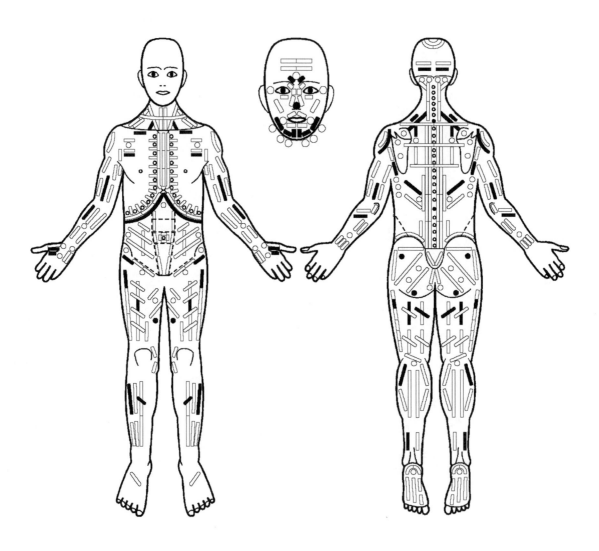

All the Muscles and Connective Tissue in This Age Period

Head and throat:

102	Occipitofrontalis-venter occipitalis	
106b	Sternocleidomastoid, clavicular head	
115	Corrugator supercilii	
117	Tip of the nose	
122	Mentalis	(NEED and WILL)
124	Depressor anguli oris	
125	Masseter	

Back and neck:

*	Serratus posterior superior, cranial part (ref. 4)
9a	Latissimus dorsi, superior part
97	Scalenus posterior

Shoulders and arms:

3a	Rhomboid minor	79	Adductor pollicis
5	Teres major	84b	Deltoid, posterior part
62c	Pectoralis major, abdominal part	85c	Triceps brachii, medial head
68	Brachialis	88	Extensor carpi radialis longus and brevis
71	Flexor carpi radialis		
78	Flexor pollicis brevis	96	Levator scapulae

Front:

57	Diaphragm	64	Subclavius

Hip and legs:

16	Gluteus minimus	
19	Quadratus femoris	
*	Pelvic floor: sphincter ani externus	
23	Iliotibial tract, 2nd part of 6	
24b	Biceps femoris, long head, proximal part, deep	
25	Semitendinosus, proximal part	
28a	Gastrocnemius, lateral head, proximal part	
31	Flexor hallucis longus	(WILL and SOL/PERF)
39	Tibialis anterior, proximal part, superficial	
42a	Peroneus longus	
43b	Vastus lateralis, proximal part	
43c	Vastus intermedius, middle part	
44a	Sartorius, proximal part	
48	Adductor magnus	

The Location of Some of the Muscles in the Body

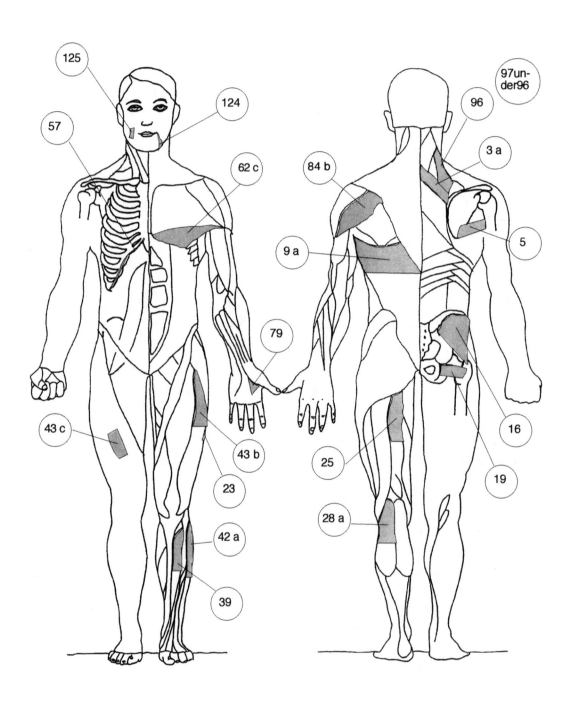

Some Essential Patterns of Movement in This Age Period

Head and throat:

124	Depressor anguli oris	Draws the angles of the mouth downward. The child can look sulky/sour, huffy, and look threatening ("Look what you have done to me"). Is used purposely to punish; "I'm unhappy and I will stay that way!" Can keep a secret, make a "poker face."
125	Masseter	The muscle is active in chewing, clenching the teeth, clenching one's jaw to endure something that is unsupportable/exhausting.

Back and neck:

9a	Latissimus dorsi, superior part	Rotates the arm inward in the shoulder joint and moves the arm backward; supportive muscle in the lower back. The child throws a small ball with both an underhand and overhand motion.
97	Scalenus posterior	Rotates the lower part of the neck on the spinal column; makes the neck short and turns the head backward. The muscle takes part in creating a "bull neck" and thus the "shoulder yoke" together with levator scapulae. The muscle is active in walking, maintaining the face in a forward position during the four phases of rotation.

Shoulders and arms:

3a	Rhomboid minor	Pulls the upper part of the shoulder blades together; stabilizes the shoulder blades when the child throws a ball overhand.
5	Teres major	Rotates the arm inward and stabilizes the shoulder joint; works together with (9a) latissimi dorsi, superior part. The child is able to catch a big ball with his arms; the muscle stabilizes the shoulder joint when lifting heavy things; gives power to an underhand throw, and ability to throw with an overhand motion.
62c	Pectoralis major, abdominal part	Moves the arm forward in the shoulder joint; together with (9a) latissimus dorsi, superior part, and (3a) rhomboid minor is a prerequisite for the ability to use greater strength in the arms, e.g., when lifting heavy objects and walking with them; active when you throw and catch a ball; active in hugging.
79	Adductor pollicis	Pulls the thumb to the palm; gives power to the grip of the hand.
84b	Deltoid, posterior part	Moves the arm backward in the shoulder joint and rotates it outward; is used when making movements to take space with the arms; is used when swinging the arms during walking. The child carries things on his back, e.g., little sisters or brothers, backpacks (forms the "shoulder yoke"), throws a ball with more power and more precision.
96	Levator scapulae	Lifts the shoulder blade; gives strength in carrying.

Note: The locations of these muscles are shown on the opposite page. The muscles are marked by number or *. The right half of the front side and the left half of the back side are used for marking superficial musculature; the deeper layers are marked on the left half of the front side and the right half of the back side.

The Location of Some of the Muscles in the Body

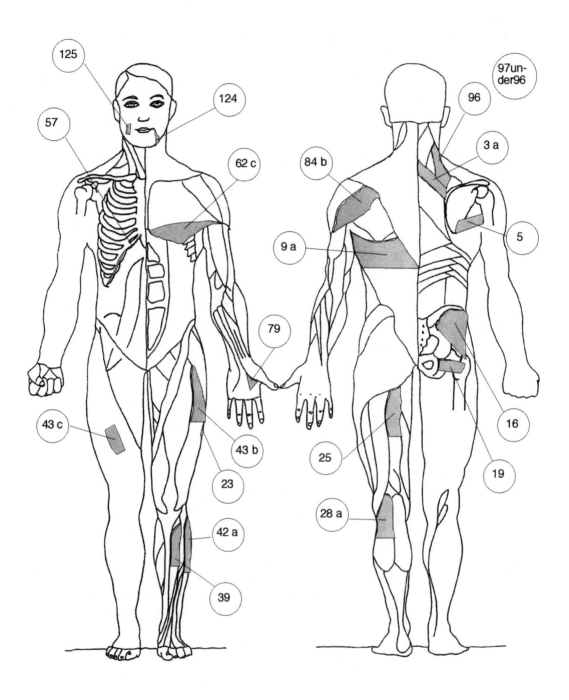

Some Essential Patterns of Movement in This Age Span

Front:

57	Diaphragm	Large respiratory muscle, both reflex and voluntary movement; allows control over the abdominal press and possibility for forceful abdominal respiration.
		The muscle becomes active when the child's body has grown relatively large, so there is more room for the intestines. This happens at the age of 2-4, and the child is now capable of using the diaphragm to the fullest.

Hip and legs:

16	Gluteus minimus	Rotates in the hip joint and moves the leg out to the side
		The child brings foot position to parallel from being turned out during the Autonomy stage. The ability to push off through the foot begins at this age.
		Takes part in rotation of the hip joint while walking, while standing on one leg and lifting the other leg outward, while walking on a broad tree trunk, and when changing direction.
19	Quadratus femoris	Tucks the tailbone between the legs; rotates outward in the hip joint and stabilizes it.
		The muscle enables the child to change direction while walking. Pelvis is free, "tail is lifted."
23	Iliotibial tract, 2nd part of 6	The tract helps keep the muscles of the leg together. It assists in tightening the big fasciae system around the leg as a "stocking"; works together with the postural muscles; affects the mobility in the hip joint.
		The movements of the leg/knee get stronger and more precise as the child gets older.
25	Semitendinosus, proximal part	Moves the thigh backward; adds power in moving forward when walking.
		The child pushes off in walking and jumping up.
28a	Gastrocnemius, lateral head, proximal part	Used in the take-off in walking; moves the ankle joint; stabilizes the ankle joint together with (39) tibialis anterior, so it is possible to stamp and tramp.
39	Tibialis anterior, proximal part, superficial	Involved in the beginning of being able to have a springiness in the ankle joint when landing after having made a jump; lifts the forefoot so it is possible to roll on the foot in walking.

Note: The locations of these muscles are shown on the opposite page. The muscles are marked by number or *. The right half of the front side and the left half of the back side are used for marking superficial musculature; the deeper layers are marked on the left half of the front side and the right half of the back side.

The Location of Some of the Muscles in the Body

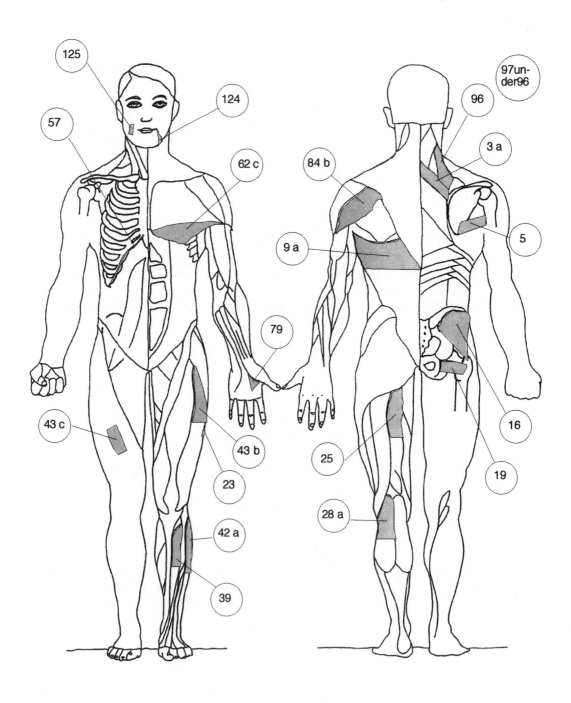

Some Essential Patterns of Movement in This Age Span

42a	Peroneus longus	Tilts the foot outward; gives stability in the ankle joint; is active in balancing, e.g., when balancing on one foot and when balancing on tree trunks.
43b	Vastus lateralis, proximal part	Stretches the knee; gives power in standing, walking, kicking, and stamping the floor.
43c	Vastus intermedius, middle part	Stretches the knee; gives more stability in the standing position and in upright movements. The child stands with good posture, with slightly bent knees and hips (as if ready to carry/lift something); stands on one leg and kicks with the other leg.

Note: The locations of these muscles are shown on the opposite page. The muscles are marked by number or *. The right half of the front side and the left half of the back side are used for marking superficial musculature; the deeper layers are marked on the left half of the front side and the right half of the back side.

The Character Structure
LOVE/SEXUALITY

3–6 years

Character Positions

Early position: romantic
Late position: seductive
Healthy position: balancing love and sexuality

Important Themes of Development

- Becoming conscious/aware of one's gender
- Developing and integrating love and sexuality/sensuality (heart and sex)
- Being in love with (1) the parent of the opposite sex (homosexuals often of the same sex), (2) with other grown-ups, and (3) with peers/children of the same age
- Practicing the creation of constructive alliances
- Becoming aware of gender roles and different aspects of the gender roles in the family, in groups, and in other families
- Becoming aware of muscular tension and relaxation
- Gaining ability to speak in long sentences and ability to reason and participate in talking (from concrete to abstract thinking)
- Gaining ability to change focus from the imagination/fantasy world to concrete reality, from romantic fantasies to hard-core reality
- Learning to balance one's loving, intimate, and sexual emotions and actions in the social context

The Character Structure LOVE/SEXUALITY

Early position: romantic   **Late position: seductive**

Characteristic Body Features

Weighted on the outer edge, the feet are slightly inwardly rotated (a little shy).

The feet rest on the surface of the foot; while walking the foot rolls from the heel to the toes.

The private parts are "hidden" (drawn back) as the pelvis is tilted forward.

The private parts are "shown" as the pelvis is tilted backward.

Tight uplifted buttocks that may be experienced as chaste and snooty.

Tight uplifted buttocks that may be experienced as sexually aggressive or snooty.

Wasp waist.

The waist is not particularly visible.

The posture of the neck is held high, the head slightly tilted downward (wounded pride).

The posture of the neck is straight (pride).

The little finger is often slightly extended from the others.

All fingers are slightly spread.

Their eyes flirt unconsciously and also express longing or wounded pride, shyness.

The expression of the eyes is consciously direct and sexually aggressive (undress others with the eyes).

Life Patterns

Identify with their love and repress their sexuality.

Identify with their sexuality and repress their love.

Romanticize contact.

Sexualize contact.

Leave the initiative for the contact to others while they are playing up to it in a romantic way.

Active in establishing sexual contact; may often act promiscuously.

Unconsciously give flirting sexualized contact to get love.

Consciously show love in order to get sex (good at seducing/"scoring").

The Character Structure LOVE/SEXUALITY

Early position: romantic

Late position: seductive

Key Sentences

If you marry me, I'll love you forever.	In reality, love is a sexual need.
I love him/her, but he/she only wants sex.	I want sex before I open to talking.
My love is pure.	"Sex makes the world go round."
If we only love each other enough, everything will be fine.	If sexuality disappears, there is no love.
Some day Mr. Right/the right prince will turn up on a white horse to fetch me.	You can always find another man/woman; "There are plenty of fish in the sea."
Some day I'll meet the right woman/man who can see the purity of my heart. I'll give my heart to her/him.	It is the seduction/"score" that gives the "kick."

Resources

Romantic, attractive.	Sexually self-assured, active.
Idealistic about love relations.	Charming.
Good at flirting.	Seductive.

Ideal Messages in Interaction

I accept your sexuality. You can never marry your Mom/your Dad.	I have my sexuality, and I enjoy it with my partner.
I value and respect the sexuality you feel toward another person.	I value and respect the love you feel toward another person.
It is OK that you sense both love and your sexuality when you are together with people other than your partner. It is you who decides how to act on your feelings of love and sexuality.	It is OK that you sense and fill yourself up with your love and sexuality when you are with others. It is your responsibility how you act with the feelings of love and sexuality.
You cannot give your heart away. You can give from your heart and take into your heart.	Your heart cannot be broken or break into pieces. It might feel like it because it hurts to lose someone you love.
Justice does not exist.	Justice does not exist.

The Healthy Position

In the body, they are not locked, as described in the two positions above. They may be experienced by people with an absence of these body features. They will have life patterns in which they can use the resources from both positions in a flexible way. The developmental themes have been integrated, and they are able to use the themes in a flexible way.

The Muscles Marked on a Bodymap

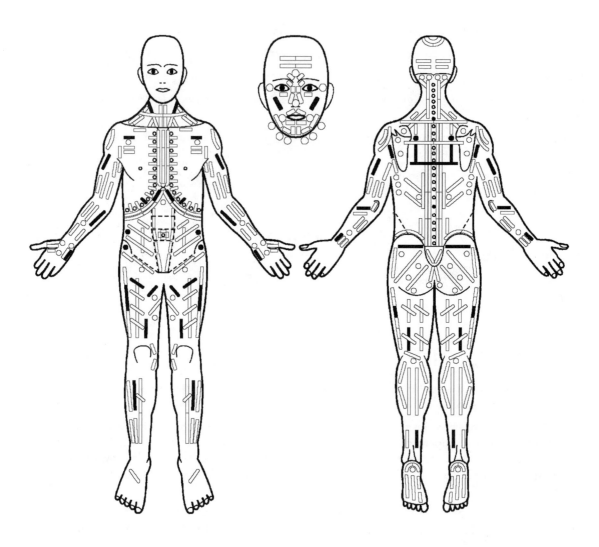

All the Muscles and Connective Tissue in This Age Span

Head and throat:
106a	Sternocleidomastoid, sternal head, superior part
119	Zygomaticus
*	Risorius

Back and neck:
4	Serratus posterior superior, caudal part
*	Splenius cervicis

Shoulders and arms:
2c	Trapezius, inferior part
3b	Rhomboid major
6	Teres minor
62a	Pectoralis major, clavicular part
66a	Biceps brachii, long head, proximal part
72	Flexor carpi ulnaris
81	Abductor digiti minimi
85b	Triceps brachii, lateral head, proximal part
87	Brachioradialis
94	Extensor pollicis brevis and abductor pollicis longus

Front:
56	Costal curve, medial one-third
51c	Transversus abdominis
61	Intercostals, between ribs 9-10

Hip and legs:
15	Gluteus medius	
*	Pelvic floor, urogenital diaphragm	
23	Iliotibial tract, 3rd part of 6	
24d	Biceps femoris, short head	
*	Tibialis posterior	(NEED and LOVE/SEX)
32	Flexor digitorum longus	(NEED and LOVE/SEX)
*	Quadratus plantae	
40	Extensor digitorum longus	
43a	Rectus femoris, 1st part of 4	
43b	Vastus lateralis, middle part	
43d	Vastus medialis	(LOVE/SEX and PUB)
45	Pectineus	
51a	Iliacus, superior part	

The Location of Some of the Muscles in the Body

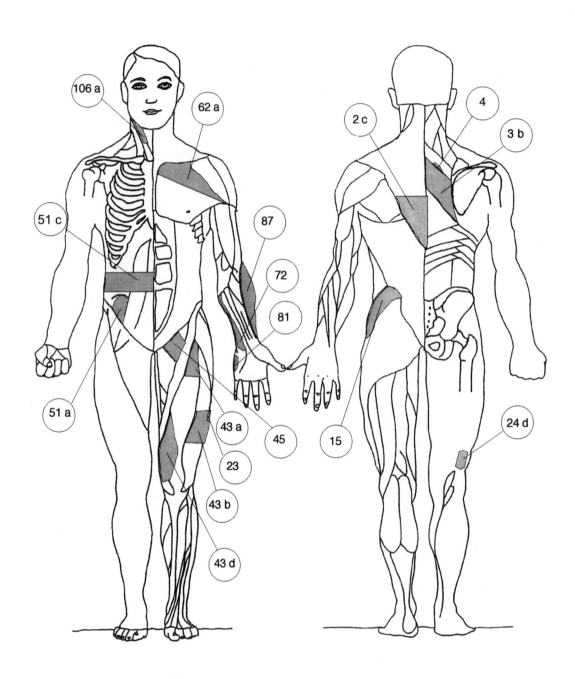

Some Essential Patterns of Movement in This Age Span

Head and throat:

106a	Sternocleidomastoid, sternal head, superior part	Big muscle on the front of the neck; holds and rotates the head, tilts it to the same side.

Back and neck:

4	Serratus posterior superior, caudal part	Respiratory muscle located on the back side of the trunk between the shoulder blades.

Shoulders and arms:

2c	Trapezius, inferior part	Draws the shoulder blades together and downward; gives support in the middle of the back; activation of this muscle together with (3b) rhomboid major and (4) serratus posterior superior produces a straightness in the upper part of the back, pushing the chest forward. Takes part in flirting with the shoulder together with (62a) pectoralis major, clavicular head.
3b	Rhomboid major	Draws the lower part of the shoulder blades together; adds power and precision in the overhand throw.
62a	Pectoralis major, clavicular part	Pulls the arm forward in the shoulder joint; the movement occurs in the area of the collar bone; active in hugging and flirting with the shoulder together with (2c) trapezius, inferior part.
72	Flexor carpi ulnaris	Bends the wrist on the little finger side. The child is able to tilt the hand when drinking, wave like royalty, and catch and throw a ball with one hand.
81	Abductor digiti minimi	Draws the little finger to the side; gives more range to the grip of the hand, e.g., catching a ball.
87	Brachioradialis	Bends the elbow joint. Is active when the child is playing ball-games, throwing, skipping rope, carrying dolls, carrying heavy things, holding handlebars (of a bicycle), pulling on the handlebars when pedaling up hills.

Front:

51c	Transversus abdominis	Pulls the stomach inward; gives a slender waist when contracted, and keeps the stomach together. The fascial layer connected to the muscle inserts on the front of the spine and is involved in the reflex system that keeps the spine straight. The muscle connects the upper and lower parts of the body, stabilizes the trunk, e.g., maintaining balance while kicking a ball. Bracing the belly to receive a punch in "boy's play"; to shut one's mind to emotions. The child is able to practice and master a hula hoop.

Note: The locations of these muscles are shown on the opposite page. The muscles are marked by number or *. The right half of the front side and the left half of the back side are used for marking superficial musculature; the deeper layers are marked on the left half of the front side and the right half of the back side.

The Location of Some of the Muscles in the Body

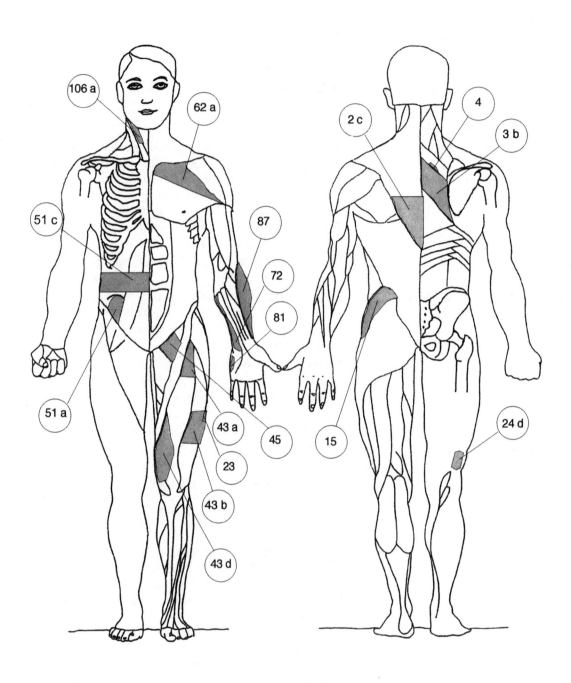

Some Essential Patterns of Movement in This Age Span

Hip and legs:

15	Gluteus medius	Lifts the leg to the side of the trunk; moves the pelvis from side to side in walking; keeps the pelvis in balance when standing on one leg and when moving the other in all directions and rotating more with the pelvis while walking. At the end of this stage, the child is able to use a hula hoop.
23	Iliotibial tract, 3rd part of 6	The tract helps keep the muscles of the leg together. It assists in tightening the big fasciae system around the leg as a "stocking"; works together with the postural muscles; affects mobility in the hip joint; and stabilizes the stretched knee. The movements of the leg/knee get stronger and more precise as the child gets older.
24d	Biceps femoris, short head	Bends the knee; is active in jumping over something and hopping on one leg.
32	Flexor digitorum longus	Bends the four smaller toes. Pushes off with the toes while walking; curls the toes when being shy. The child is fascinated by his toes and feet.
43a	Rectus femoris, 1st part of 4	Bends the hip joint; active in kicking movements. Contracting the muscle from the knee up allows a more powerful kick. The following actions apply to quadriceps femoris as a whole: jumping/hopping (away-toward); maintaining balance; running; riding a bicycle.
43b	Vastus lateralis, middle part	Stretches the knee from the outer side of the thigh; gives the first access to more power in standing, walking, kicking, jumping, and stamping the floor.
43d	Vastus medialis	Stretches the knee from the inner side of the thigh; gives balance between the outer and inner side of the thigh; gives better balance and possibility for refinement of the movements of the knee. More power and accuracy in kicking; able to tackle for a ball; kick away.
45	Pectineus	Pulls the legs together close to the genitals. The child pulls the leg medially in flirting, shyness, "hold on with the legs," playing "doctor," desire to examine one's body and others' bodies, and ability to stop when it feels wrong.
51a	Iliacus, superior part	Important muscle involved in the tilting of the pelvis. The muscle tilts the pelvis back and forth, e.g., when the child swings/rocks, stands on one foot and maintains his balance at the same time.

Note: The locations of these muscles are shown on the opposite page. The muscles are marked by number or *. The right half of the front side and the left half of the back side are used for marking superficial musculature; the deeper layers are marked on the left half of the front side and the right half of the back side.

The Character Structure OPINIONS

5–9 years

Character Positions

Early position: sullen
Late position: opinionated
Healthy position: integration of opinions

Important Themes of Development

- Knowing the difference between right and left side of oneself, east/west
- Understanding the meanings of words and why things are as they are
- Reality testing
- Understanding unified wholes and grasping the differences in opinions and ways of life in one's own family, school, age group, neighbors, other families, etc.
- Forming one's own opinions and rules and fighting for them by arguing
- Using arguments in a confronting contact manner

The Character Structure OPINIONS

Early position: sullen

Late position: opinionated

Characteristic Body Features

They are energetically filled out to the surface of the muscles.	Tensions in the surface of the muscles (just beneath the skin).
The shoulder is filled out but the chest muscle (in the middle) and the surface muscle on the back are not quite filled out.	Tension in the big chest muscle in the middle and the big surface muscle (latissimus dorsi) on the back.
When they look back they have a tendency to swing around in stead of rotating the spinal column.	Turn the whole torso from the lower back to look backward.
Rotate the torso/body in a loose swinging manner/gangling.	Have a tendency to take a step forward on one leg when they express their opinions.
Difficulties in making the opposed position with the thumb and the little finger.	The thumb is often locked in the opposed position (thumb against little finger).
Slightly raised eyebrows with a passive given-up and a know-all expression in the eyes; at the same time a silent snuffle with the nostrils saying, "Oh, that's what you think."	The eyes are insisting, and the expression is "ready to fight."

Life Patterns

Lack of skills to form their own opinions or let go of them easily.	Actively seek to confront others with their own opinions.
Give up expressing their points of view.	Stick to own opinions regardless of logic or obvious arguments.
Passively oppose others' opinions and nonverbally indicate that what is going on is ridiculous.	Difficulties in listening to and accepting that others may have different opinions, therefore they argue to convince others that their opinions are right/correct.
Declare that discussions are unimportant.	In a discussion they are often not able to relate to new information in order to examine it.

Early position: sullen

Late position: opinionated

Key sentences

I do not have an opinion—what do you think?

If I do not prove myself right, none of my points of view are worth anything.

If I express an opinion/say what I think, everything goes wrong.

I am right!/I know what is right.

It is stupid/ridiculous (often they don't say so, but "look" that way).

If I do not fight for my point of view, they will take me over.

It doesn't matter.

There you are! I was right.

That was what I thought/expected.

If they had done what I said . . .

Resources

Good at getting others to express their opinions.

Stubborn and persevering in negotiations.

Adaptive to others' opinions.

Active and enthusiastic about things they believe in.

Good at disclaiming responsibility.

Start discussions.

Ideal Messages in Interaction

I would like to hear what you think.

I would like to hear your opinions and your reasons.

No matter what you think and how you express it, it is important for the situation.

I would like to discuss opinions with you so we can test them in reality.

I would like you to repeat what you said earlier, so I have the possibility to relate/ respond to it while we are in contact.

I like it when you argue for your opinions and insist on your point of view.

I appreciate that you have an opinion and that you express it.

It is okay that we disagree (have different opinions).

The Healthy Position

In the body, they are not locked, as described in the two positions above. They may be experienced by people with an absence of these body features. They will have life patterns in which they can use the resources from both positions in a flexible way. The developmental themes have been integrated, and they are able to use the themes in a flexible way.

The Muscles Marked on a Bodymap

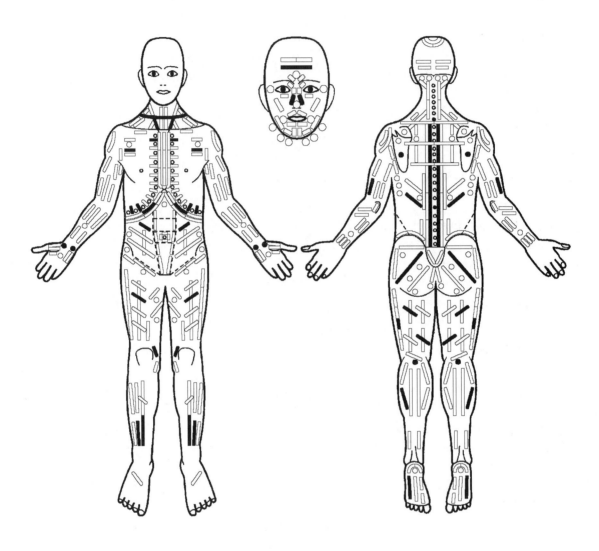

All the Muscles and Connective Tissue in This Age Span

Head and throat:

103	Platysma
106a	Sternocleidomastoid, sternal head, inferior part
111	Occipitofrontalis-venter frontalis, inferior part
116	Nasalis
*	Depressor labii
*	Depressor septi

Back and neck:

1b	Erector spinae at spinous processes-rotators	(OPINIONS and SOL/PERF)
9b	Latissimus dorsi, inferior part	(OPINIONS and SOL/PERF)
*	Serratus posterior inferior, cranial one-quarter (ref. 10)	

Shoulders and arms:

7b	Infraspinatus, inferior part	
62b	Pectoralis major, sternal part	(OPINIONS and SOL/PERF)
80	Opponens pollicis	
83	Opponens digiti minimi	
85b	Triceps brachii, lateral head, distal part	

Front:

52	Obliquus externus and internus, superior part	
56	Costal curve, middle one-third	
61	Intercostals, between ribs 1-2 and 10-12	(OPINIONS and SOL/PERF)

Hip and legs:

14	Gluteus maximus, superior part
23	Iliotibial tract, 4th part of 6
24a	Biceps femoris, long head, proximal part, superficial
25	Semitendinosus, distal part
28a	Gastrocnemius, lateral head, distal part
29	Popliteus
34	Abductor digiti minimi
39	Tibialis anterior, distal part
41	Extensor hallucis longus
43a	Rectus femoris, 2nd part of 4
44b	Sartorius, distal part

The Location of Some of the Muscles in the Body

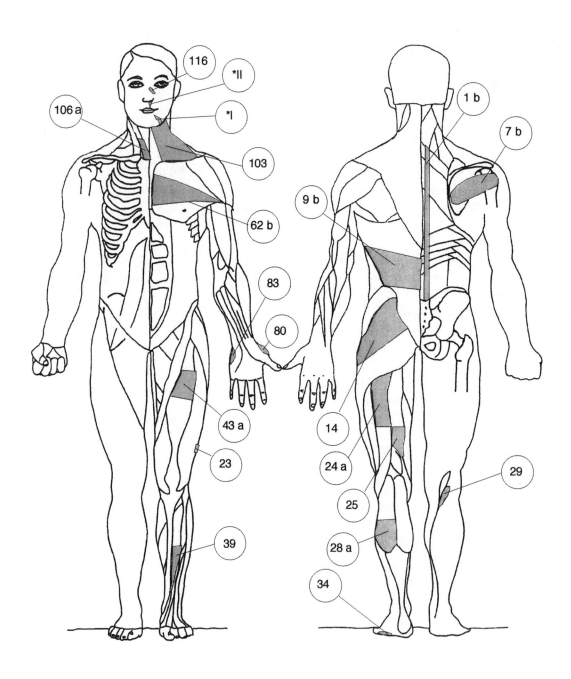

Some Essential Patterns of Movement in This Age Span

Head and throat:

103	Platysma	Muscle of the skin; lies in the skin on the upper part of the chest, neck, and jaw; when it is active together with (*I) depressor labii, the corners of the mouth are drawn downward, giving the mouth a "sullen" expression.
106a	Sternocleidomastoid, sternal head, inferior part	Big muscle on the front of the neck; holds and turns the head. The muscle is active in the rotation patterns of walking, allowing a greater awareness while walking toward one's goal. Walking this way, the child actually has a larger view and thereby a larger overview.
116	Nasalis	Opens the nostrils. The muscle is used in snorting: "So, that's what you mean."
*I	Depressor labii	Draws the corners of the mouth downward; see also under (103) platysma.
*II	Depressor septi	Draws the nose downward; activation of/tension in both (116) nasalis and (*II) depressor septi makes a typical expression from this structure (contempt, distance, disgust, arrogance).

Back and neck:

1b	Erector spinae at spinous processes-rotators	Rotate the spine near the thoracic vertebrae; give flexibility and elasticity in the movements of the spine. Stabilize the back so the child is able to use arms and legs with more strength/power.
9b	Latissimus dorsi, inferior part	Rotates the arm inward in the shoulder joint and moves the arm backward; adds power to pulling movements with the arms; support the lower back area of the trunk; is involved in straightening the back and widening it simultaneously. The child throws a large ball with an underhand and overhand motion.

Shoulders and arms:

7b	Infraspinatus, inferior part	Rotates outward in the shoulder joint; stabilizes the shoulder joint. The child is able to throw a rather heavy ball (a small ball) with an overhand motion.
62	Pectoralis major, sternal part	Adds power and gives precision in movements where the arm is moved forward in the shoulder joint; e.g., pole vault, shot put, discus throwing; beating on one's breast like Tarzan.
80	Opponens pollicis	Opposes thumb to other fingers; enables a form of grip that is used in writing and in fine motor activity.
83	Opponens digiti minimi	Opposes the little finger to the thumb; enables a form of grip that is used in fine motor activity.

Note: The locations of these muscles are shown on the opposite page. The muscles are marked by number or *. The right half of the front side and the left half of the back side are used for marking superficial musculature; the deeper layers are marked on the left half of the front side and the right half of the back side.

The Location of Some of the Muscles in the Body

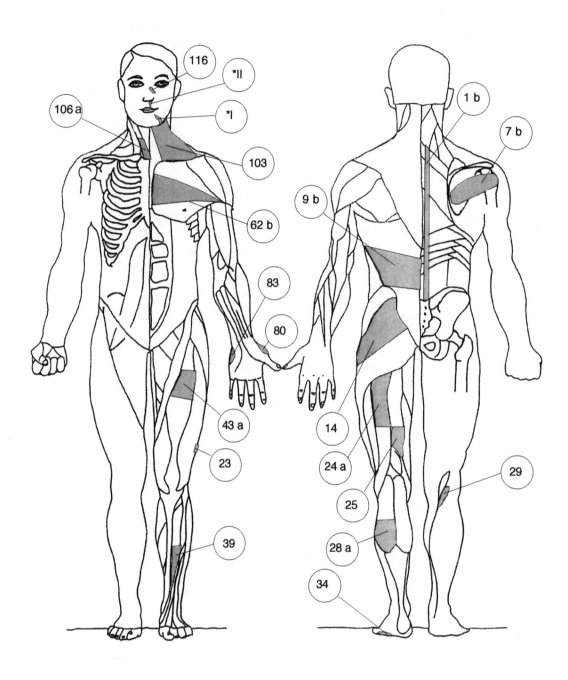

Some Essential Patterns of Movement in This Age Span

Front

Hip and legs:

14	Gluteus maximus, superior part	Extension of the hip joint. The child is able to stand on one leg and extend the other leg. Adds power in push-off and in moving forward; adds strength in running and jumping. It is also used when moving from a sitting position to a standing position.
23	Iliotibial tract, 4th part of 6	The tract helps keep the muscles of the leg together. It assists in tightening the big fasciae system around the leg as a "stocking"; works together with the postural muscles; affects mobility in the hip joint, and stabilizes the stretched knee. The movements of the leg/knee get stronger and more precise as the child gets older.
24a	Biceps femoris, long head, proximal part, superficial	Moves the leg backward in the hip joint; is active in the take-off in walking, running, and jumping; adds power to make long jumps.
25	Semitendinosus, distal part	Bends the knee; is active in take-off, especially in jumping over something.
28a	Gastrocnemius, lateral head, distal part	Moves the ankle joint; is involved in the take-off in walking, running, and jumping. Works together with (39) tibialis anterior, distal part, in doing a karate kick with precision.
29	Popliteus	Bends the knee from a stretched position; unlocks the knee; gives springiness and stability in the knee, e.g., when landing after a jump.
34	Abductor digiti minimi	Moves the little toe away from the other toes, and this way provides the possibility of a better grounding.
39	Tibialis anterior, distal part	Adds more power and better coordination to the springiness movement in the ankle joint, e.g., when landing after a jump; lifts the forefoot so it is possible to roll over the sole in walking.
43a	Rectus femoris, 2nd part of 4	Flexing/bending the hip joint by lifting the leg forward, e.g., in kicking, jumping, balancing, running, bicycling.

Note: The locations of these muscles are shown on the opposite page. The muscles are marked by number or *. The right half of the front side and the left half of the back side are used for marking superficial musculature; the deeper layers are marked on the left half of the front side and the right half of the back side.

The Character Structure
SOLIDARITY/PERFORMANCE

7–12 years

Character Positions

Early position: leveling
Late position: competitive
Healthy position: balancing we/I

Important Themes of Development

- Being engaged in functioning in groups: in/out, up/down (hierarchy/position), close/distant (friends—balancing between best friend and other friends)
- Being engaged in contact between groups: we/they
- Often moving about in groups of the same sex
- Developing solidarity at the time one's own individuality is developed
- Practicing being a leader, a mediator, and a rank-and-file member of different groups
- Competing with oneself and others
- Developing a specialty—wish to be able to do something special and therefore practice physically, psychologically, and cognitively
- Seeking knowledge, education, interests-hobbies
- Developing a sense of responsibility concerning duties
- Developing an understanding of the value of money

Early position: leveling	Late position: competitive

Characteristic Body Features

Motor flexibility, constantly moving the body (arm/hand/foot/leg). Muscle armoring as chain mail.	Rigid/stiff posture (like a guardsman); stable muscle armoring.
Alternate between fine-tuned coordination and loose jointedness. They "hang" to one side in the hip joint and often have a hand on the hip.	Good muscular coordination alternates with stiffness/rigidity.
Slouched in the upper part of the back (from the upper part of the lower back to the neck).	The back is straight (spinal column like a broomstick). Pelvis is kept in a middle position.
Shoulder blades are slightly apart; shoulders fall slightly forward.	The shoulders are held in the middle position or drawn slightly backward.
Expression of the eyes: focused with an examining look on the group ("scanning" look). The expression seems soft.	Expression of the eyes: focused with an expression of goal-directedness and performance; may be seen as a hard expression.

Life Patterns

Can compete with oneself, but do not want to stand forward and perform/be the best at something.	Insist on being capable and the best at doing things.
In groups/teamwork they will insist on having equality and use energy to insure that nobody comes forward in a special way (saying: you are good at . . . the others are good at . . .).	Try to get recognition by coming forward in the world, performing, and competing with others. Have difficulties conforming to groups/being a rank-and-file member of groups.
Maintain solidarity by letting go of own competence.	Insist on having their own special value/ performance by letting go of solidarity.
Always try to take care of the group (secret leader).	Always try to become the leader.

The Character Structure SOLIDARITY/PERFORMANCE

Early position: leveling   **Late position: competitive**

Key Sentences

I cannot do anything that others cannot do also.	I am the architect of my own fortune.
There has to be room/a place for everybody.	I must live up to what is expected here.
Yes, I am good at . . . , but you are good at . . .	If I am not the best, everything is lost.
If I do not show solidarity, I am not equal.	If I am not the best, I am worth nothing.

Resources

Group solidarity.	Good at performing and competing.
Back up others' projects.	Do their best.
Good mediator.	Capable/good leader, but authoritarian.

Ideal Messages in Interaction

You may come forward and be the best.	I like you, also when you fail.
I see your potential and respect when you use it to the utmost so others can see it.	You may be more or less than me or like me; it is OK.
There is always something that you are best at and which you can develop and specialize in.	I want to be with you both when you are good at something and when you are bad at something. I am interested in what you do and how you feel about it.

The Healthy Position

In the body, they are not locked, as described in the two positions above. They may be experienced by people with an absence of these body features. They will have life patterns in which they can use the resources from both positions in a flexible way. The developmental themes have been integrated, and they are able to use the themes in a flexible way.

The Muscles Marked on a Bodymap

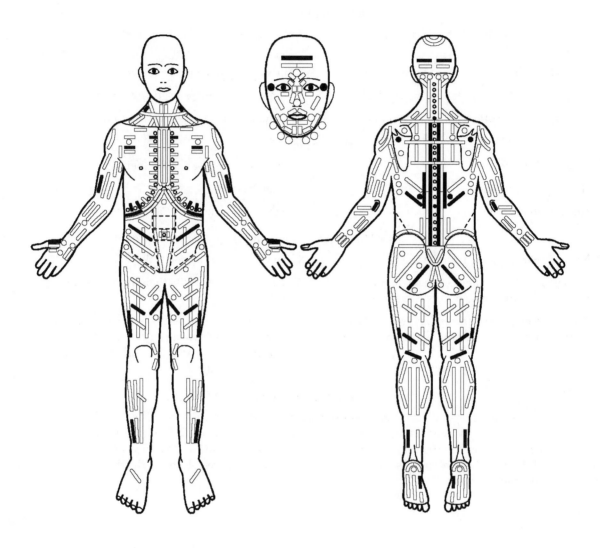

All the Muscles and Connective Tissue in This Age Span

Head and throat:

101c	Galea aponeurotica	
107	Omohyoid	
111	Occipitofrontalis–venter frontalis, superior part	
118	Temporalis	(SOL/PERF and PUB)

Back and neck:

1a*	Erector spinae, lateral fibers level with thoracic vertebrae 8-12	(SOL/PERF and PUB)
1b	Erector spinae at spinous processes-rotators	(OPINIONS and SOL/PERF)
9b	Latissimus dorsi, inferior part	(OPINIONS and SOL/PERF)
10	Serratus posterior inferior, caudal three-quarters	

Shoulders and arms:

7a	Infraspinatus, superior part	
62b	Pectoralis major, sternal part	(OPINIONS and SOL/PERF)
66a	Biceps brachii, long head, distal part	
77	Abductor pollicis brevis	
*	Lumbricals	
86	Anconeus	

Front:

52	Obliquus externus and internus, middle part	
56	Costal curve, lateral one-third	
61	Intercostals between 1-2 and 10-12	(OPINIONS and SOL/PERF)

Hip and legs:

14	Gluteus maximus, inferior part	
23	Iliotibial tract, 5th part of 6	
24c	Biceps femoris, long head, distal part, superficial	
27	Plantaris	
31	Flexor hallucis longus	(WILL and SOL/PERF)
*	Lumbricals	
36	Abductor hallucis	
42b	Peroneus brevis	
43a	Rectus femoris, 3rd part of 4	
43b	Vastus lateralis, distal part	
46	Adductor longus	

The Location of Some of the Muscles in the Body

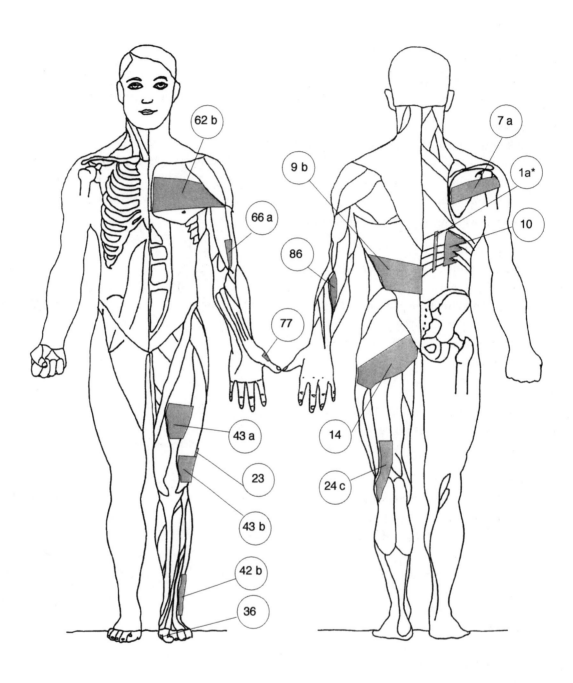

Some Essential Patterns of Movement in This Age Span

Head and throat

Back and neck:

1a*	Erector spinae, lateral fibers level with thoracic vertebrae 8-12	Part of the erectors in the middle of the back; gives a straight back in the standing position.
9b	Latissimus dorsi, inferior part	Rotates the arm inward in the shoulder joint and moves the arm backward; supports the lower back area of the back; is involved in straightening the back and widening it simultaneously. The child throws a large ball with precision with both an underhand and overhand motion.
10	Serratus posterior inferior, caudal three-quarters	Respiratory muscle located on the back side and lower part of the rib cage. Strength in exhalation—the child is able to puff out air in physical training, e.g., karate.

Shoulders and arms:

7a	Infraspinatus, superior part	Rotates outward in the shoulder joint; stabilizes the shoulder joint. Active in playing games where one has to throw a ball and hit others.
62b	Pectoralis major, sternal part	Adds power and precision in movements where the arm is moved forward in the shoulder joint; in many games and sports, e.g., pole vault, shot put, discus throwing; beating on one's breast like Tarzan; is active in greeting good friends (e.g., "give me five").
66a	Biceps brachii, long head, distal part	Bends the elbow joint; provides possibility for using full power in pulling movements. Drawing things toward oneself, reaching out for things and people, doing pull-ups.
77	Abductor pollicis brevis	Moves thumb out from the palm, making the hand broader; gives more power and better fine motoric ability in the grip of the hand.
86	Anconeus	Stretches the elbow joint to the uttermost; gives full power in stretching movements (push/throw). Precision and fine adjustment in activities of throwing, badminton, discus, tennis, etc.

Note: The locations of these muscles are shown on the opposite page. The muscles are marked by number or *. The right half of the front side and the left half of the back side are used for marking superficial musculature; the deeper layers are marked on the left half of the front side and the right half of the back side.

The Location of Some of the Muscles in the Body

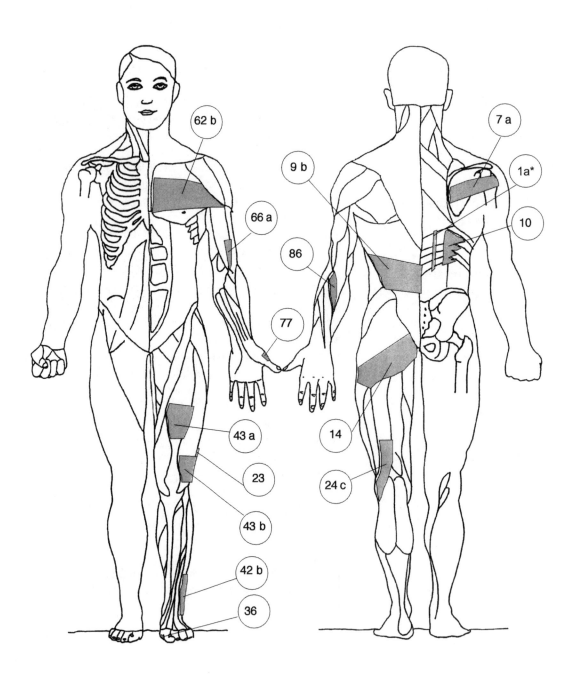

Some Essential Patterns of Movement in This Age Span

Front:

Hip and legs:

14	Gluteus maximus, inferior part	Stretches in the hip joint; adds power to take-off and in moving forward. The child is able to stand on one leg and extend the other leg. Long jumps/triple jumps. In walking with a push-off movement and with strength in running and jumping; it is also used when moving from a sitting position to a standing position.
23	Iliotibial tract, 5th part of 6	The tract helps keep the muscles of the leg together. It assists in tightening the big fasciae system around the leg as a "stocking"; works together with the postural muscles; stabilizes the stretched knee. The movements of the leg/knee get stronger and more precise as the child gets older.
24c	Biceps femoris, long head, distal part, superficial	Bends the knee; is active in the take-off in walking, running, and jumping; adds power to make long jumps and triple jumps.
36	Abductor hallucis	Moves the big toe apart from the other toes; the final push off with the big toe in walking; stabilizing the big toe when changing direction.
42b	Peroneus brevis	Tilts the foot outward; gives stability in the ankle joint; is active in balancing, e.g., when walking on a rail.
43a	Rectus femoris, 3rd part of 4	Stretches the knee, e.g., in kicking, jumping, maintaining balance, running, bicycling.
43b	Vastus lateralis, distal part	Stretches the knee, active in all powerful use of the legs—jumping, kicking, running, bicycling.

Note: The locations of these muscles are shown on the opposite page. The muscles are marked by number or *. The right half of the front side and the left half of the back side are used for marking superficial musculature; the deeper layers are marked on the left half of the front side and the right half of the back side.

PUBERTY

11–19 years

Puberty is a very important developmental stage, even though special structures or positions are not formed as they are in the other stages of age. It is tempting to say that all muscles and themes are "preoccupied." We observe that teenagers activate all the stages and themes again, but this time at random. This is why a person in Puberty can form a new, unique integration of the Ego so that the process of socialization is reenergized at a higher level—in the brain, intellectually, consciously, and in the line of action. The individual develops from a child to a grown-up person or adult.

In a relatively short time—hours to days—a teenager is able to react from all Character Structure Positions, and this gives the person the possibility of changing his or her Closed Codes. This will happen if the person is now met in the way that he or she needed when the Code was first formed so that this change might be constructive. The earlier Closed Code may now be dissolved and healed and become an Open Code, reflected in the Character Structure, where both Life Patterns and the Characteristics of the Body will change toward a more healthy position. The other possibility is that if the individual is met by the same or even more destructive patterns of interaction, the Codes in the different Character Structures will close further, and the Characteristics of the Position will become more obvious both physically and psychologically. It could be said that the Code is formed with more power, so it is pushed deeper into the material from which it is made.

A third possibility is that the individual in puberty carries a certain theme in which more than one Character Structure is "open" at the same time. In this situation, these themes tend to merge and form a new kind of structure. The pubescent person might give this merged combination structure an even deeper imprint by consciously choosing it and practicing the characteristics and features as well as its look. The merged combination structure changes, as the other structures do, from preconscious to unconscious, and as an adult, the person acts unconsciously with the acquired behavioral and muscular patterns from Puberty.

When looking at the body, it will show the underlying Character Structures, but the person's behaviors will not fit, and this confusion may tell the therapist that the problems were probably formed in the teenage years. It is also visible in special characteristics in the Bodymap.

Although we work a lot with this stage of age, the knowledge we have about this age has not yet been precisely described, and Puberty will therefore not be described further in this book. There are some connective tissues and fasciae that we know belong to this stage of age, and therefore they are mentioned.

The Muscles Marked on a Bodymap

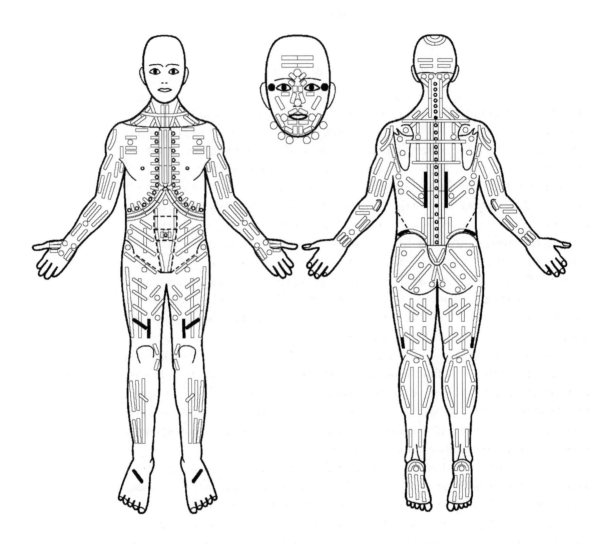

The Bodynamic Character Structure System

All the Muscles and Connective Tissue in This Age Span

Head and throat:

118	Temporalis	(SOL/PERF and PUB)

Back and neck:

1a*	Erector spinae, lateral fibers level with thoracic vertebrae 8-12	(SOL/PERF and PUB)

Shoulders and arms:

Front:

*	Pyramidalis

Hip and legs:

12	Iliac crest, lateral part	
23	Iliotibial tract, at the knee, 6th part of 6	
38	Extensor digitorum brevis and extensor hallucis brevis	
43a	Rectus femoris, 4th part of 4	
43d	Vastus medialis	(LOVE/SEX and PUB)

Some Essential Patterns of Movement in This Age Span

Head and throat:

118	Temporalis	When wisdom teeth appear, the child starts using them for chewing; the action becomes further differentiated to the very back of the mouth.

Back and neck:

1a*	Erector spinae, lateral fibers level with thoracic vertebrae 8-12	Adjusting and balancing the upright position of the spinal column.

Shoulders and arms

Front:

*	Pyramidalis	Active in lifting pubis toward sternum. The muscle is active in sexual contact.

Hip and legs:

12	Iliac crest, lateral part	Full rotation in rapid movements—ability to contract diagonally, e.g., in football/soccer tackling.
23	Iliotibial tract, at the knee, 6th part of 6	The tract helps keep the muscles of the leg together. It assists in tightening the big fasciae system around the leg as a "stocking"; works together with the postural muscles; stabilizes the stretched knee. The movements of the leg/knee get stronger and more precise as the child gets older.
38	Extensor digitorum brevis and extensor hallucis brevis	The child lifts up the toes; the rest of the foot can stay on the ground. Fine adjustment of the different movements of the foot.
43a	Rectus femoris, 4th part of 4	Contracting the muscle from the knee up allows a more powerful kick. The following actions apply to quadriceps femoris as a whole: jumping/hopping (away-toward); maintaining balance; running; riding a bicycle.
43d	Vastus medialis	More power and accuracy in kicking—able to tackle for a ball; kick away.

Section 4

The Bodynamic Ego Function System

The Ego Functions in the Bodynamic System

An overview of the eleven Ego Functions and subfunctions is followed by a general introduction. Each Ego Function is described in the following way:

- An image of the body illustrates the position of the muscles in the body.
- The different graphic patterns in the image show which Character Structure the muscle is a part of.
- On the facing page is a list of all the muscles and connective tissue within the Ego Function, divided into subfunctions.
- A Bodymap shows where the muscles within the Ego Function are marked. The subfunctions are shown in different colors; these colors are not the same as those used for Bodymapping.
- A short description of each Ego Function follows, with examples of its use. If you need more ideas for experiments and experiences with the Ego Functions, we recommend Brantbjerg and Ollars (2005).

In the subsequent section, the muscles that in our experience are impacted by shock are listed. We know that if these muscles are more hyporesponsive or hyperresponsive than the other muscles on the Bodymap, it indicates that the person has some post-traumatic stress disorder from shock trauma that has not been resolved. The muscles involved in PTSD are marked on a Bodymap, and we provide brief information about issues that are worth watching for with clients in therapy.

Overview of the Ego Functions and Their Subfunctions

I. Connectedness
(a) Bonding
(b) Heart contact/opening
(c) Feeling support and self-support

II. Positioning
(a) Stance toward life
(b) Staying power
(c) Standing on one's own
(d) Stance toward values and norms
(e) Orienting (keeping or losing one's head)

III. Centering
(a) Awareness of one's own center
(b) Filling out from the inside
(c) Being oneself in one's different roles
(d) Feelings of self-esteem

IV. Boundaries
(a) The physical boundary
(b) Boundaries of personal space (energetic boundaries)
(c) Boundaries of territorial space
(d) Boundaries of social space
(e) Making space for oneself in social contact

V. Grounding and Reality Testing
(a) Ability to stand one's ground, feel rooted and supported by it
(b) Relationship between reality and fantasy/imagination
(c) Experience and grounding of extrasensory perceptions

VI. Social Balance
(a) Balancing one's own needs/feelings/desires against others' expectations
(b) Degree of pulling oneself together/letting go
(c) Degree of "facade" and maintaining one's front
(d) Balancing a sense of personal identity against being a group member
(e) Balance of managing stress and resolving it

VII. Cognitive Skills
(a) Orienting
(b) Cognitive grasp
(c) Understanding (getting something well enough to go forward with it)
(d) Grasp of reality (ability to apply cognitive understanding to different situations)
(e) Planning
(f) Contemplation/consideration

VIII. Management of Energy
(a) Containment of emotions
(b) Containment of high-level energy
(c) Self-containment
(d) Self-containment—feeling "backed"
(e) Containment of sensuality

IX. Self-Assertion
(a) Self-assertion (manifesting one's power)
(b) Asserting oneself in one's roles
(c) Forward momentum and sense of direction

X. Patterns of Interpersonal Skills
(a) Reaching out
(b) Gripping and holding on
(c) Drawing toward oneself and holding on closely
(d) Receiving and giving from one's core
(e) Pushing away and holding at a distance
(f) Releasing, letting go
(g) Taking on chores (assignments)

XI. Gender Skills
(a) Awareness of gender
(b) Experience of gender
(c) Experience of gender role
(d) Containment of sensuality and sexuality
(e) Manifestation of sensuality and sexuality

The Eleven Ego Functions and Their Embodiment

This section of the book introduces the Ego Functions in the Bodynamic System. The body areas and the groups of muscles that are connected to specific and different functions of the Ego are discussed according to our experience.

The collection of this material has been ongoing since the 1970s, when we focused on the mapping of parallels and coherence between the patterns of motion and the tonus of a particular muscle on the one hand and the character and the psychological themes on the other. These themes later resulted in our understanding of "functions of the Ego." At the same time, further material has been collected as described in the Preface.

The Ego Functions are formed and developed throughout life. They are like paths that run through the stages of age (Character Structures), and the different stages of age give a certain Code in the Ego Functions. The Bodynamic System includes and operates with eleven Ego-functions: I. Connectedness, II. Positioning, III. Centering, IV. Boundaries, V. Grounding and Reality Testing, VI. Social Balance, VII. Cognitive Skills, VIII. Management of Energy, IX. Self-Assertion, X. Patterns of Interpersonal Skills, XI. Gender Skills.

The idea of the model is that all muscles that are mentioned under a certain function are connected with this Ego Function, and therefore these muscles are an ideal starting point when working with a client on the Ego Function in question. It is important to be aware, however, that two or three Ego Functions may be linked or knotted together, and therefore some muscles from other Ego Functions may become visible in the client's body and consciousness during the body work. It is possible to stay focused on the first problem chosen if you ask the client to focus on the muscles that are related to the Ego Function in question.

Here is an example connected to "asserting oneself in one's roles," a subfunction of the Self-Assertion Ego Function: A client explains that even though he knows he is able to do a certain job, he experiences a feeling of insufficiency within himself. In this case, you may help the client to sense, feel, and activate the smaller muscle in the chest, pectoralis minor—subfunction: (b), "asserting oneself in one's roles." When he can sense or feel pectoralis minor, you can ask him to think of the job-situation at the same time as activating the muscle by pulling the shoulder slightly forward and downward. The client often then becomes more aware of the problem or Code that stands in the way of experiencing his self-esteem. Possibly he will remember or experience how the Code was formed, and from this he can move on in the process.

It is also possible to go the opposite way. A client experiences himself "dead" or immobile underneath the big muscle in the chest. On closer examination, the client discovers, with the help of the therapist, that it has to do with pectoralis minor. The therapist can then assume from the Ego Function model that it has to do with Self-Assertion. The client may have specific information on this connection, or the therapist may start questioning him in a certain direction.

The Ego Function model has been taught in Skolen for Kropsdynamik (The School of Body Dynamic Education) since 1975, being developed continuously and becoming more precise over time. In 1975, and at the beginning of the Bodynamic Institute, it was provided as a handout to students, and in 1997 it was published in a manual (Fich 1997a). This manual was a brief but very accurate description of the muscles that are connected to the different Ego Functions according to the Bodynamic System. In this manual, the different subfunctions are also mentioned under each of the Ego Functions.

The model was primarily intended for students and educated therapists within the Bodynamic System, as these people had already been taught the connection between the physical and the psychological. The model was described mostly in an anatomical, technical language without an introduction or explanation.

I. The Ego Function CONNECTEDNESS

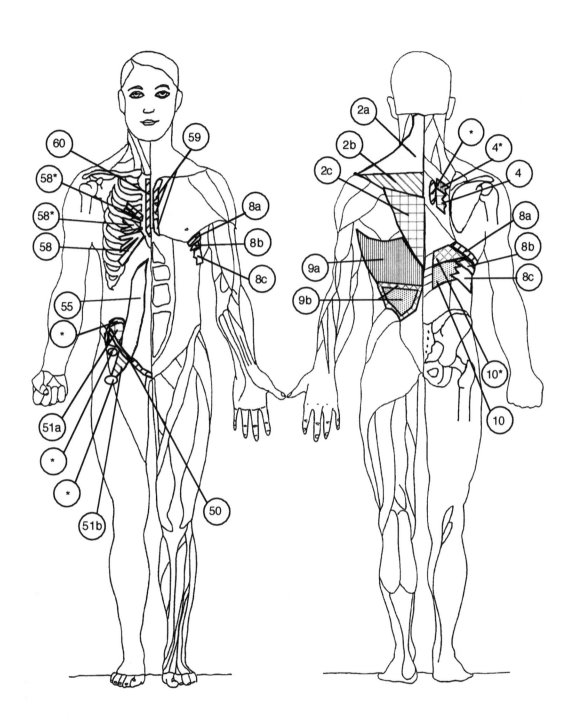

457

The Location of Some of the Muscles and Connective Tissue in the Body

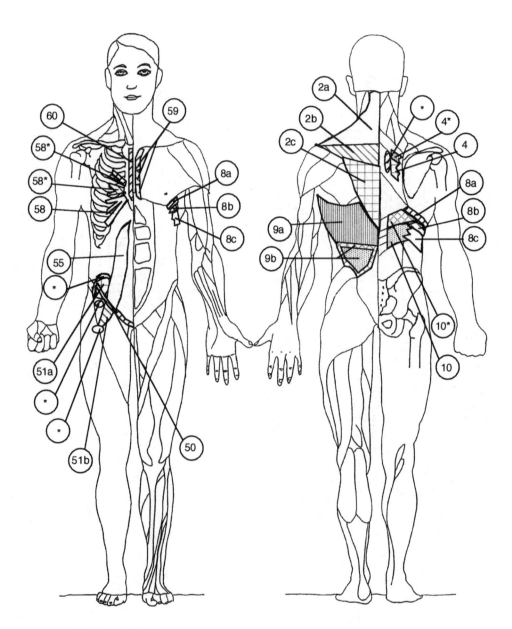

Each graphic pattern represents a Character Structure.

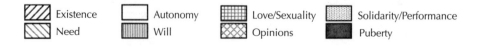

Existence   Autonomy   Love/Sexuality   Solidarity/Performance
Need   Will   Opinions   Puberty

All the Muscles and Connective Tissue in Each Subfunction

(a)   Bonding

*	Connective tissue of the back level with thoracic vertebrae 3-5		EX
50	Inguinal ligament,	medial part	EX
		lateral part	NEED
*	Origin of iliacus (ref. 51a)		PERINATAL
*	Insertion of iliopsoas (ref. 51b)		PERINATAL
*	Iliacus, inferior part (ref. 51a)		EX
51b	Iliopsoas		NEED
55	Psoas major		AUT
51a	Iliacus, superior part		LOVE/SEX
58	Transversus thoracis,	* 1st part	PERINATAL and EX
		* 2nd part	NEED
		3rd part	AUT
59	Origin of pectoralis major, sternal head,	superior part	EX
		middle part	NEED
		inferior part	AUT
60	Sternal fascia		PERINATAL and EX

(b)   Heart contact/opening

8a	Serratus anterior, superior part		EX
8b	Serratus anterior, middle part		NEED
8c	Serratus anterior, inferior part		AUT
4	Serratus posterior superior,	* cranial part	WILL
		caudal part	LOVE/SEX
10	Serratus posterior inferior,	* cranial one-quarter	OPINIONS
		caudal three-quarters	SOL/PERF

(c)   Feeling support and self-support

*	Connective tissue of the back level with thoracic vertebrae 3-5	EX
2b	Trapezius, middle part	NEED
2a	Trapezius, superior part	AUT
9a	Latissimus dorsi, superior part	WILL
2c	Trapezius, inferior part	LOVE/SEX
9b	Latissimus dorsi, inferior part	OPINIONS and SOL/PERF

The Muscles Marked on a Bodymap

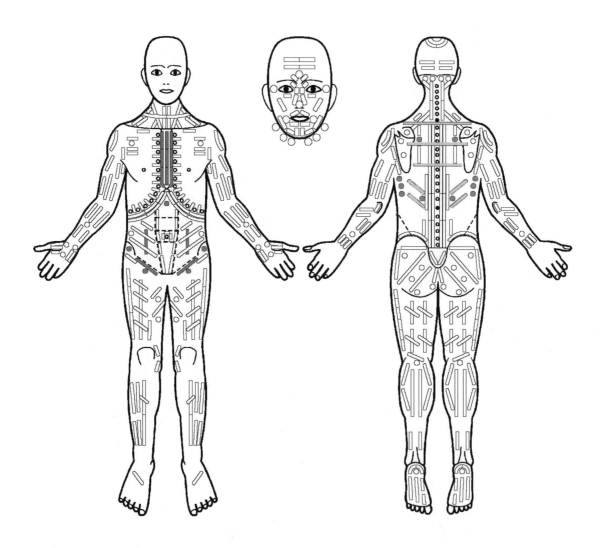

Each color represents a subfunction.

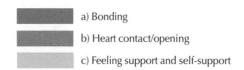

a) Bonding

b) Heart contact/opening

c) Feeling support and self-support

The Ego Function CONNECTEDNESS

The area around chest bone and between the shoulder blades, some of the deep muscles on the sides and on the back of the chest, and the big flat muscles on the back

Connectedness deals with the skills in connecting with other people, the degree of openness in experiencing contact, giving and receiving contact, receiving support and backup, as well as the integration of these skills. Integration means that you can experience that you are supported (by friends and family) if you activate these muscles even though none of the people are present in the situation.

Connectedness is divided into three subfunctions: (a) bonding, (b) heart contact/opening, (c) feeling support and self-support. The areas on the body that are empirically connected with this Ego Function and the subfunctions are:

(a) Bonding

- The connective tissue between the shoulder blades
- The deep muscles in the pelvis that connect the thigh and the lower part of the back (psoas major, iliacus)
- The origins on the breastbone and the fascia across the breastbone (origin of pectoralis major, sternal fascia)

(b) Heart contact/opening

- Some deep muscles in the back in the area behind the heart (serratus posterior superior)
- Muscles on the side of the chest (serratus anterior, reaching out)

(c) Feeling support and self-support

- The big flat muscles on the back (trapezius and latissimus dorsi)

The client can contact the heart area by moving these muscles, e.g., putting a hand in front of the heart or at the side of the chest. The therapist may put a hand on the same areas, while of course respecting the client's boundaries; this is a rule that always applies and which is taken for granted in the following.

The client can give herself backing and support by activating the big muscles in the back or by sensing the support from a chair, a wall, etc. Finally the therapist may give support with his or her hand followed by the words that the client missed in childhood (of course, the client's own words).

The bonding areas should only be activated if the therapist is qualified to do regressive therapy and if the client is ready for it.

II. The Ego Function POSITIONING

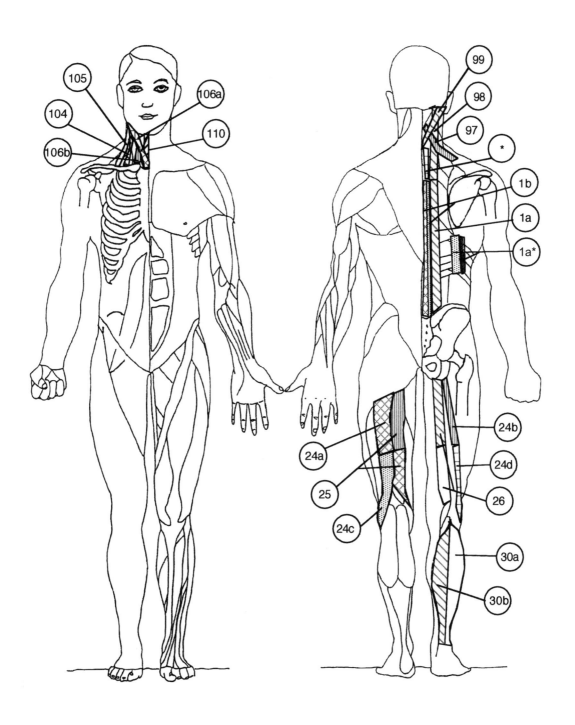

The Locations of Some of the Muscles and Connective Tissue in the Body

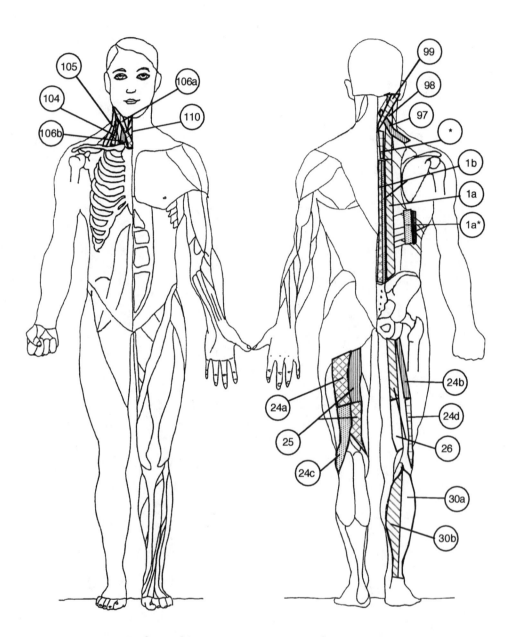

Each graphic pattern represents a Character Structure.

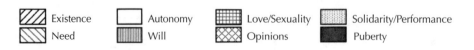

▨ Existence	☐ Autonomy	▦ Love/Sexuality	▨ Solidarity/Performance
▧ Need	▥ Will	▨ Opinions	■ Puberty

All the Muscles and Connective Tissue in Each Subfunction

(a) Stance toward life

110	Longus capitis and longus colli		EX
1a	Erector spinae		NEED
1a*	Erector spinae, lateral fibers level with thoracic vertebrae 8-12		SOL/PERF and PUB

(b) Staying power

26	Semimembranosus,	proximal part	NEED
		distal part	AUT
25	Semitendinosus,	proximal part	WILL
		distal part	OPINIONS
24d	Biceps femoris, short head		LOVE/SEX
	Biceps femoris,		
24a	long head, proximal part, superficial		OPINIONS
24b	long head, proximal part, deep		WILL
24c	long head, distal part, superficial		SOL/PERF

(c) Standing on one's own

30b	Soleus, medial part	NEED
30a	Soleus, lateral part	AUT

(d) Stance toward values and norms

1b	Erector spinae at spinous processes-rotators	OPINIONS and SOL/PERF

(e) Orienting (keeping or losing one's head)

110	Longus capitis and longus colli		EX
98	Semispinalis capitis		NEED
99	Splenius capitis		NEED
104	Scalenus anterior		NEED
105	Scalenus medius		AUT
97	Scalenus posterior		WILL
106b	Sternocleidomastoid, clavicular head		WILL
106a	Sternocleidomastoid, sternal head,	superior part	LOVE/SEX
		inferior part	OPINIONS
*	Splenius cervicis		LOVE/SEX

The Muscles Marked on a Bodymap

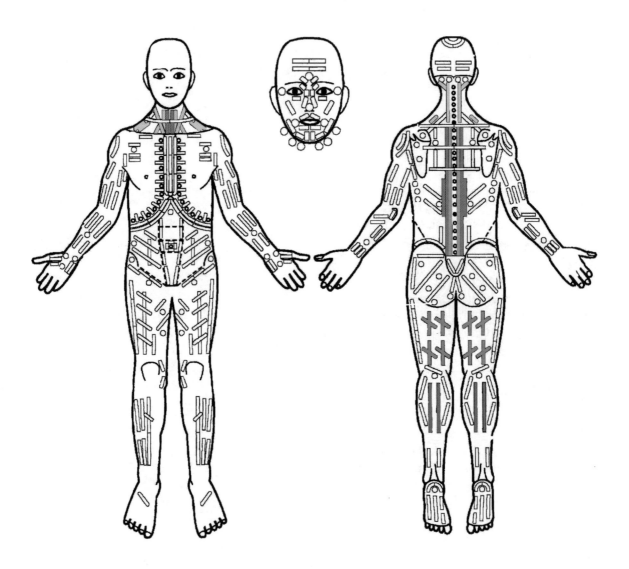

Each color represents a subfunction.

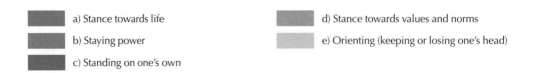

a) Stance towards life

b) Staying power

c) Standing on one's own

d) Stance towards values and norms

e) Orienting (keeping or losing one's head)

The Ego Function POSITIONING

The extensor muscles of the back, the neck, the back of the neck, the back of the thighs, and the calves

Positioning concerns the person's attitude to life. Literally, how does the person keep himself or herself in an upright position, and how does he or she meet the surrounding world—upright and open, or with a certain degree of reservation? In a figurative sense, how do you deal with the problems of life? For example, "Is the glass half full, or half empty?" How do you keep up your spirits even in a crisis or in sorrow and grief?

Positioning is divided into five different subfunctions: (a) stance toward life, (b) staying power, (c) standing on one's own, (d) stance toward values and norms, (e) orienting (keeping or losing one's head). The areas on the body that we have experienced to be empirically connected with this Ego Function and the subfunctions are:

(a) Stance toward life

· The extensors of the back, the long muscles of the back (erector spinae)
· A deep muscle in the neck (longus capitis)

(b) Staying power

· The muscles in the back of the thighs which are used in taking off (biceps femoris, semitendinosus, semimembranosus)

(c) Standing on one's own

· A deep muscle in the calf (soleus)

(d) Stance toward values and norms

· The small muscles close to the spinal column (rotators in the back)

(e) Orienting (keeping or losing one's head)

· The muscles in the neck and in the back of the neck whose function is to keep the head high and turn the head (semispinalis, splenius, scaleni, sternocleido-mastoid)

In practice, when dealing with this Ego Function, the therapist takes an interest in the client's attitude/position: the position of the head, both in standing and sitting, and the client's way of coming forward with or without taking off from the back of the thighs. It is possible to observe and make suggestions such as: What happens if you straighten yourself up a little bit? How would it feel if you looked up a bit instead of down?

Rigidity or flexibility, according to rules and norms, is often seen in the degree of rotation of the spinal column.

Skills in looking out and looking around (orienting) often show in the mobility of the neck and the back of the neck.

How is the client's outlook on life, attitude toward life, and spark of life influenced? Does the client hold the hope that there is possibility for contact?

III. The Ego Function CENTERING

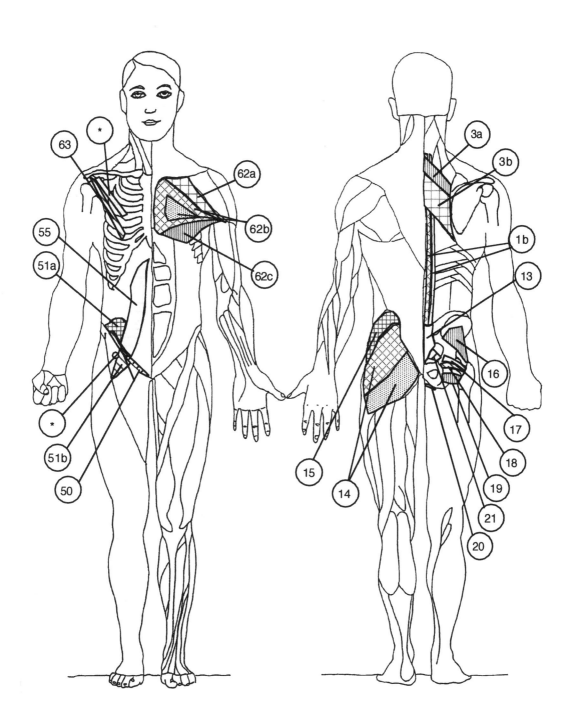

The Location of Some of the Muscles and Connective Tissue in the Body

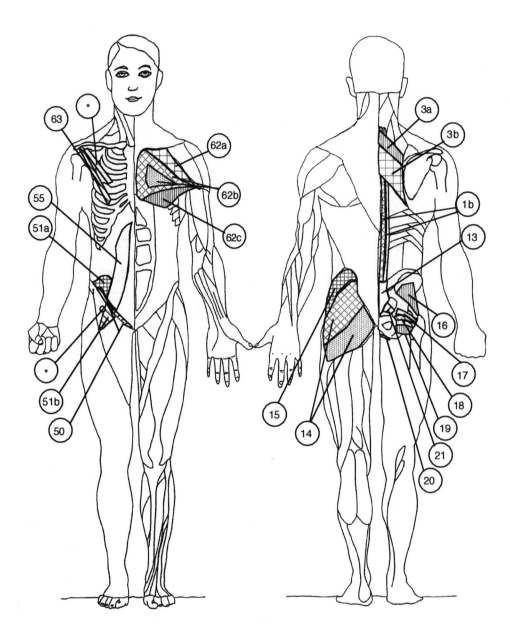

Each graphic pattern represents a Character Structure.

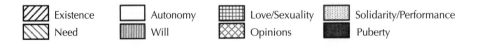

Pattern	Structure	Pattern	Structure	Pattern	Structure	Pattern	Structure
	Existence		Autonomy		Love/Sexuality		Solidarity/Performance
	Need		Will		Opinions		Puberty

All the Muscles and Connective Tissue in Each Subfunction

(a)   **Awareness of one's own center**

50	Inguinal ligament,	medial part	EX
		lateral part	NEED
*	Iliacus,	inferior part (ref. 51a)	EX
51b	Iliopsoas		NEED
55	Psoas major		AUT
51a	Iliacus, superior part		LOVE/SEX

(b)   **Filling out from the inside**

21	Sacrotuberous ligament		PERINATAL and EX
18	Gemelli and obturator internus		NEED
20	Obturator internus, near pelvic floor		AUT
17	Piriformis		AUT
19	Quadratus femoris		WILL
16	Gluteus minimus		WILL
15	Gluteus medius		LOVE/SEX
14	Gluteus maximus,	superior part	OPINIONS
		inferior part	SOL/PERF

(c)   **Being oneself in one's different roles**

3a	Rhomboid minor		WILL
3b	Rhomboid major		LOVE/SEX
1b	Erector spinae at spinous processes-rotators		OPINIONS and SOL/PERF

(d)   **Feelings of self-esteem**

13	Sacrum		PERINATAL
63	Pectoralis minor,	* superior part	NEED
		inferior/lateral part	AUT
62c	Pectoralis major,	abdominal part	WILL
62a	Pectoralis major,	clavicular part	LOVE/SEX
62b	Pectoralis major,	sternal part	OPINIONS and SOL/PERF

The Muscles Marked on a Bodymap

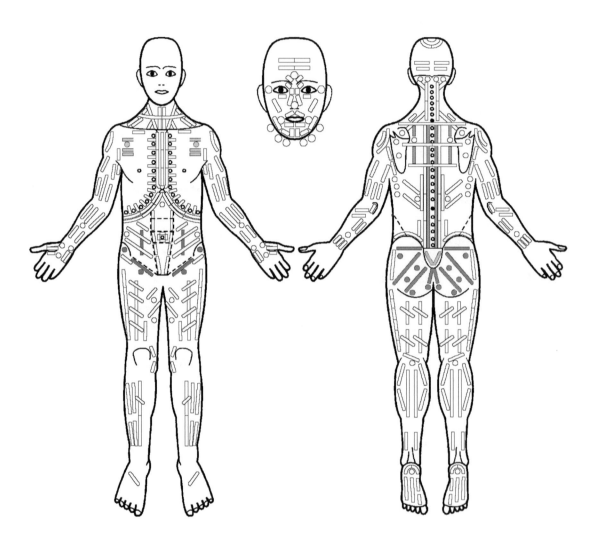

Each color represents a subfunction.

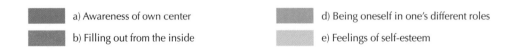

a) Awareness of own center

b) Filling out from the inside

d) Being oneself in one's different roles

e) Feelings of self-esteem

The Ego Function CENTERING

The deep muscles that have an influence on the lower back, the muscles close to the pelvic floor, the buttocks, the muscles between the shoulder blades, and the big chest muscles

Centering concerns the human skills of being in contact with oneself and the degree of self-esteem or valuing of one's own uniqueness.

Centering is divided in four subfunctions: (a) awareness of one's own center, (b) filling out from the inside, (c) being oneself in one's different roles, (d) feelings of self-esteem. The areas on the body that are empirically connected with this Ego Function and the subfunctions are:

(a) Awareness of one's own center

- The deep muscles of the pelvis that connect the thigh and the lower back (psoas major, iliacus)

(b) Filling out from the inside

- Some smaller muscles that are close to the pelvic floor (gemelli, obturator internus)
- The buttocks (sacrotuberous ligament, piriformis, gemelli, quadratus femoris)

(c) Being oneself in one's different roles

- A flat muscle between the shoulder blades that pulls these together (rhomboids)

(d) Feelings of self-esteem

- The sacrum
- The chest muscles (pectoralis major and minor)

Through training the sensing of one's center, the client's ability is increased in terms of sensing what he likes and dislikes, what he wants or takes an interest in, and what he needs.

It is possible to work with the client's centering by making the client take an interest in sensing the pelvic floor (rotate the thighs slightly outward, pull the lower part of the stomach in), the deep muscle of the pelvis (psoas), and the deep muscle of the lower back (quadratus lumborum)—in other words, the bodily container in the lower part of the torso. You can add more experiential and visual ways of working, such as, How does it feel in this center in the middle of pelvis? Are there colors? What forms or shapes are there? Many take pleasure in sensing a centering close to the spinal column, more like a vertical centerline than a point or center in the pelvis.

If you want to get closer to the connection from an inner experience of centering to a more outgoing energy, more centered around the roles one has in the world, then the muscles between the shoulder blades and the big chest muscles (and the way one "boasts," more or less) are obvious bodily areas to direct questions to and to do movement exercises with.

IV. The Ego Function BOUNDARIES

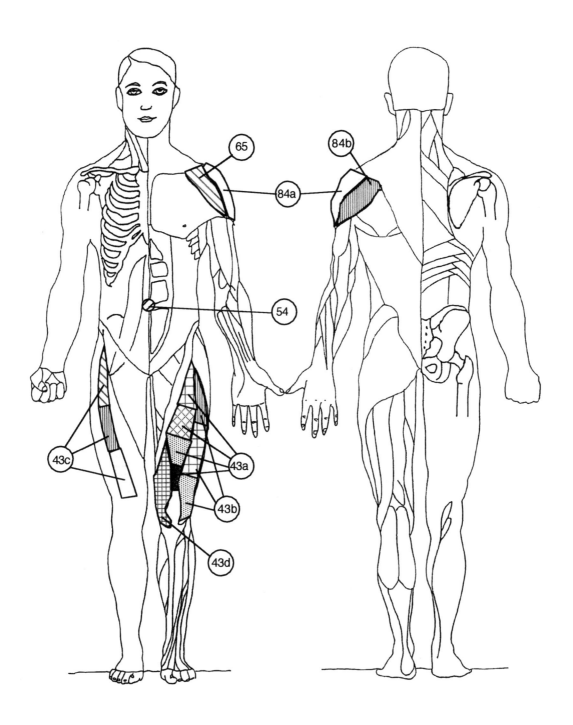

The Location of Some of the Muscles and Connective Tissue in the Body

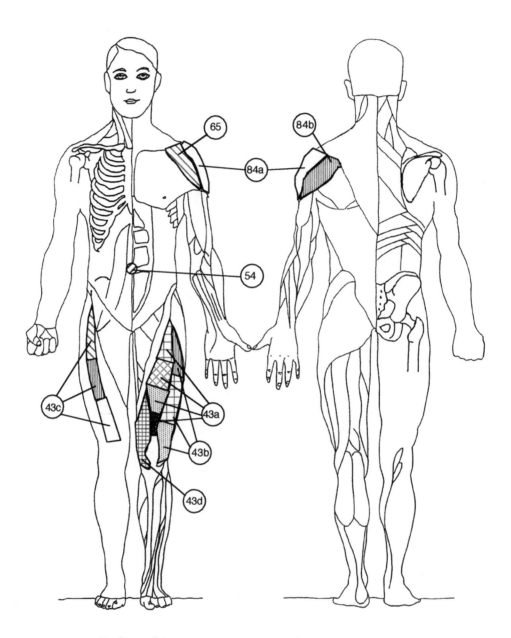

Each graphic pattern represents a Character Structure.

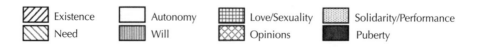

Existence
Need
Autonomy
Will
Love/Sexuality
Opinions
Solidarity/Performance
Puberty

All the Muscles and Connective Tissue in Each Subfunction

(a)	**The physical boundary**		
	The skin		EX and NEED
54	Umbilicus		PERINATAL and EX
(b)	**Boundaries of personal space (energetic boundaries)**		
	Quadriceps femoris,		
43c	Vastus intermedius,	proximal part	NEED
		middle part	WILL
		distal part	AUT
43d	Vastus medialis		LOVE/SEX and PUB
(c)	**Boundaries of territorial space**		
	Quadriceps femoris,		
43b	Vastus lateralis,	proximal part	WILL
		middle part	LOVE/SEX
		distal part	SOL/PERF
(d)	**Boundaries of social space**		
	Quadriceps femoris,		
43a	Rectus femoris,	1st part	LOVE/SEX
		2nd part	OPINIONS
		3rd part	SOL/PERF
		4th part	PUB
(e)	**Making space for oneself in social contact**		
65	Deltoid,	anterior part	NEED
84a	Deltoid,	middle part	AUT
84b	Deltoid,	posterior part	WILL

The Muscles Marked on a Bodymap

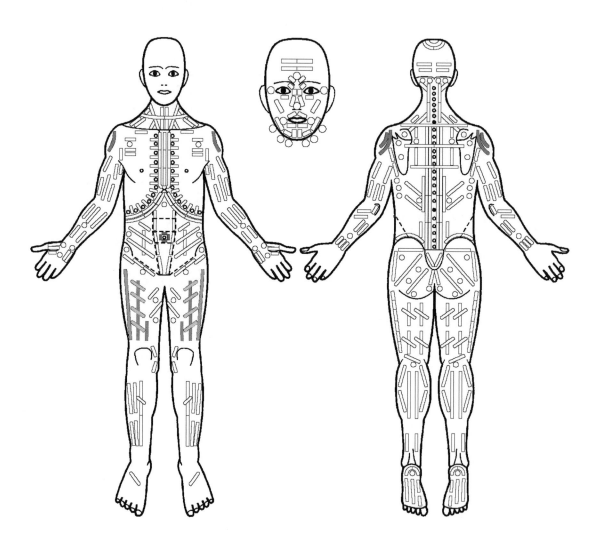

Each color represents a subfunction.

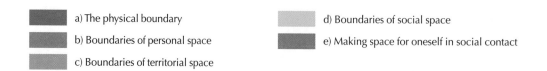

a) The physical boundary

b) Boundaries of personal space

c) Boundaries of territorial space

d) Boundaries of social space

e) Making space for oneself in social contact

The Ego Function BOUNDARIES

The skin, the front of the thighs, and the outside of the shoulders

Boundaries concerns the ability or the skills required in limiting oneself in relationship with others, and in a broader sense, to the surrounding world.

Boundaries is divided into five different subfunctions: (a) the physical boundary, (b) boundaries of personal space (energetic boundaries), (c) boundaries of territorial space, (d) boundaries of social space, (e) making space for oneself in social contact. The areas on the body that are empirically connected with this Ego Function and the subfunctions are:

(a) The physical boundary

· The skin

(b) Boundaries of personal space

· The middle and the inner muscles of the thigh (vastus intermedius and medialis)

(c) Boundaries of territorial space

· The outer deep muscle of the thigh (vastus lateralis)

(d) Boundaries of social space

· The front and outer muscle of the thigh (rectus femoris)

(e) Making space for oneself in social contact

· The outer muscles of the shoulder that lift the arms to the side (deltoids)

In addition, the following may be mentioned: the outside of the thighs and the hip, areas which normally belong to the subfunction: self-containment in the Ego Function Management of Energy, are also of importance to the boundaries (tensor fascia lata, iliotibial tract).

Boundaries is a common theme of personal work and often an important parallel theme in many forms of psychotherapy. For people who have boundary problems, it is often helpful to work with the sensation of the physical boundaries, i.e., the skin, possibly by touching it oneself, by sensing it from within, or possibly from another person's touch (except areas of the body where the person does not want to be touched).

You may work with the muscles of the thigh described above both in standing and sitting positions by activating them slightly or by touching them. These muscles of the thigh are used when you move (or step) forward to take your space, or to defend it, and when you move back to keep your space. The outer muscles of the shoulder start a "take more space" movement.

Besides these physical exercises, it may also be helpful to explore an experience of the boundaries of the "personal space" around the body, which for most people is approximately 1.5 to three feet. It is possible to make this more energetic space visible by talking about it, visualizing it, or by marking it with a piece of rope or string.

Having social boundaries deals with how we perceive the different groups we belong to and how we declare our membership in them, and if necessary defend them. This may be expressed as if we are holding or maintaining the space around the group (including oneself), even though the group is not physically present. Another way of putting it: you maintain your dignity by declaring the social network you belong to as part of your social system (or, of course, by how you do not declare it but back away from it).

Awareness of clothes, blankets, and of course the actual physical distance between the client and others, including the therapist, may be of help.

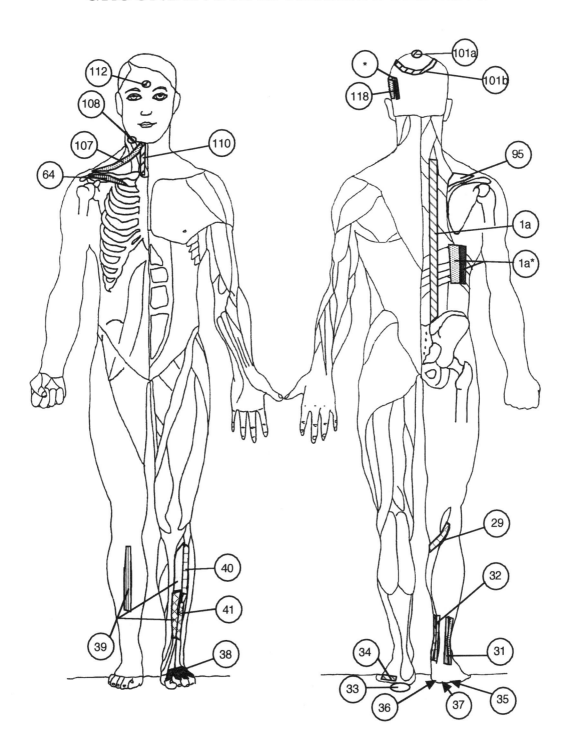

The Location of Some of the Muscles and Connective Tissue in the Body

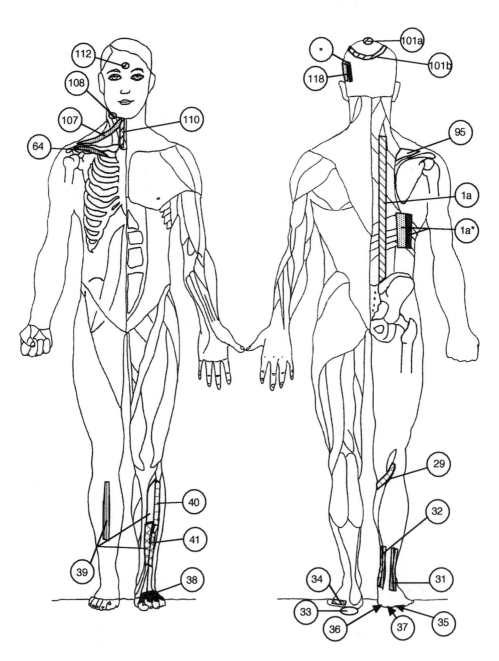

Each graphic pattern represents a Character Structure.

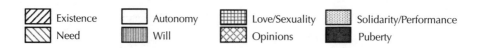

Existence   Autonomy   Love/Sexuality   Solidarity/Performance
Need   Will   Opinions   Puberty

All the Muscles and Connective Tissue in Each Subfunction

(a)   Ability to stand one's ground, feel rooted and supported by it

33	Plantar aponeurosis	PERINATAL
*	Insertions of abductor, flexors, and extensors on the proximal phalanx of the little toe	EX and NEED
34	Abductor digiti minimi	OPINIONS
*	Flexor digiti minimi brevis (34 and * are tested together)	NEED
35	Flexor digitorum brevis	NEED
37	Flexor hallucis brevis	AUT
32	Flexor digitorum longus	NEED and LOVE/SEX
31	Flexor hallucis longus	WILL and SOL/PERF
*	Quadratus plantae	LOVE/SEX
29	Popliteus	OPINIONS
36	Abductor hallucis	SOL/PERF

(b)   Relationship between reality and fantasy/imagination

39	Tibialis anterior, proximal part,	superficial	WILL
		deep	AUT
		distal part	OPINIONS
40	Extensor digitorum longus		LOVE/SEX
41	Extensor hallucis longus		OPINIONS
38	Extensor digitorum brevis and extensor hallucis brevis		PUB

(c)   Experience and grounding of extrasensory perceptions

101b	Galea aponeurotica (half circle around the top of the head)		PERINATAL
101a	Galea aponeurotica (a spot on top of the head)		EX
110	Longus capitis and longus colli		EX
112	"Third eye" (fascia)		EX
1a	Erector spinae		NEED
108	Mylohyoid		NEED
95	Supraspinatus		AUT
64	Subclavius		WILL
118	Temporalis	* insertion	EX
		muscle	SOL/PERF and PUB
107	Omohyoid		SOL/PERF
1a*	Erector spinae, lateral fibers level with thoracic vertebrae 8-12		SOL/PERF and PUB

The Muscles Marked on a Bodymap

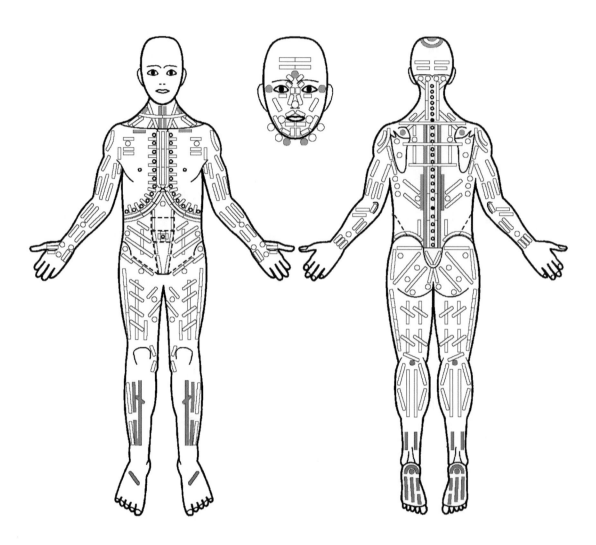

Each color represents a subfunction.

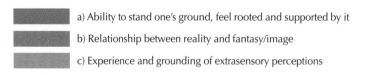

a) Ability to stand one's ground, feel rooted and supported by it

b) Relationship between reality and fantasy/image

c) Experience and grounding of extrasensory perceptions

The Ego Function GROUNDING AND REALITY TESTING

The toes, the feet and calves, the small deep shoulder muscles, the muscles in the neck, the back, the forehead, and the temples

Grounding and Reality Testing deals with the human ability to maintain connection to the floor or mat, and through this, contact with the earth—put simply, personal grounding. Psychologically it is a test of reality and the degree of contact we manage to have to outer reality and maintaining contact in communication. Finally, it is also the degree of openness toward extrasensory perception and experience, understanding this, and having the possibility of testing it.

Grounding and Reality Testing is divided into three different subfunctions: (a) ability to stand one's ground, feel rooted and supported by it, (b) relationship between reality and fantasy/imagination, (c) experience and grounding of extrasensory perceptions. The areas on the body that are empirically connected with this Ego Function and the subfunctions are:

(a) Ability to stand one's ground, feel rooted and supported by it

- The soles of the feet and the muscles that flex the toes (hold onto the floor/mat) (plantar aponeurosis, flexor digitorum brevis and longus, flexor hallucis)
- Muscles that spread the toes (abductor hallucis, abductor digiti minimi)
- A muscle on the back of the knee (popliteus)

(b) Relationship between reality and fantasy/imagination

- The front of the lower part of the leg, a muscle that lifts the forefoot (tibialis anterior)
- Muscles that extend/lift the toes (e.g., extensor digitorum longus)

(c) Experience and grounding of extrasensory perceptions

- The top of the head and the temples (e.g., temporalis)
- Some small muscles in the shoulders (supraspinatus, subclavius)
- Some deep muscles in the jaw and under the chin (omohyoid, mylohyoid)
- Muscles around the spinal column on the back (erector spinae and lateral fibers of erector spinae level with thoracic vertebrae 8-12)

The experience of grounding, of standing firm, of daring to be oneself, and so on may be strengthened by physically sensing the soles of the feet, the toes, the feet, and further up through the legs. It is also possible the work with "gripping the floor" with the toes, but it may be just as important to be able to alternate between gripping and letting go with the toes.

It is most obvious to work in a standing position (and in motion) and at the same time be aware of the connection from the floor or mat and the feet all the way up through the body, but it may also be done in a sitting position.

Contact and openness to, as well as embodiment and grounding of, extrasensory perception may be supported by working with the muscles of the shoulder girdle (subclavius, supraspinatus) described above. This work may help the client gain the experience of not "needing to"/"having to" dissociate.

VI. The Ego Function SOCIAL BALANCE

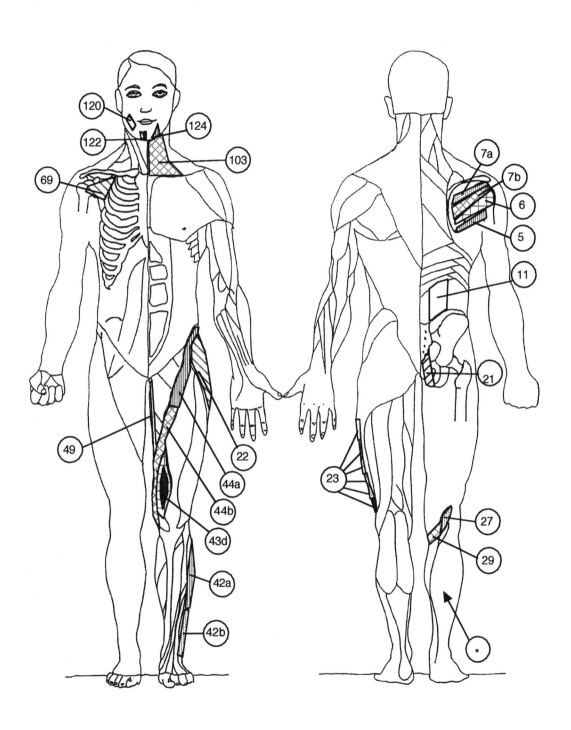

The Locations of Some of the Muscles and Connective Tissue in the Body

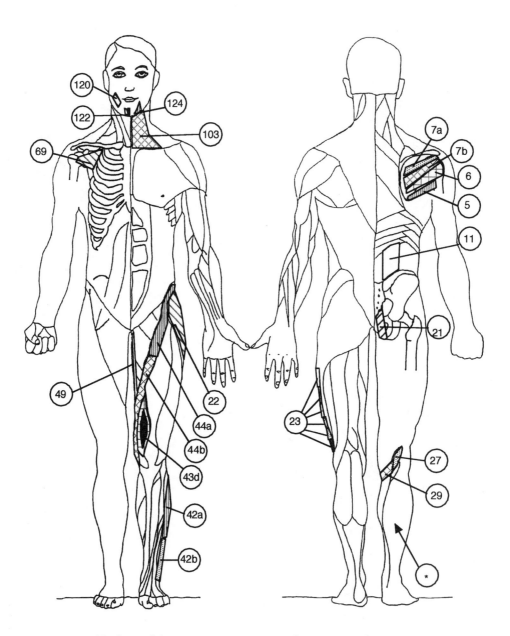

Each graphic pattern represents a Character Structure.

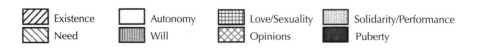

Pattern	Structure	Pattern	Structure	Pattern	Structure	Pattern	Structure
	Existence		Autonomy		Love/Sexuality		Solidarity/Performance
	Need		Will		Opinions		Puberty

All the Muscles and Connective Tissue in Each Subfunction

(a)	**Balancing one's own needs/feelings/desires against others' expectations**		
120	Buccinator		NEED
11	Quadratus lumborum		AUT

(b)	**Degree of pulling oneself together/letting go**		
22	Tensor fascia lata		NEED
23	Iliotibial tract	1st part	AUT
		2nd part	WILL
		3rd part	LOVE/SEX
		4th part	OPINIONS
		5th part	SOL/PERF
		at the knee, 6th part	PUB

(c)	**Degree of "facade" and maintaining one's front**		
69	Subscapularis		NEED
5	Teres major		WILL
6	Teres minor		LOVE/SEX
7b	Infraspinatus,	inferior part	OPINIONS
7a	Infraspinatus,	superior part	SOL/PERF
103	Platysma		OPINIONS
122	Mentalis		NEED and WILL
*	Risorius		LOVE/SEX
124	Depressor anguli oris		WILL
*	Depressor labii		OPINIONS

(d)	**Balancing a sense of personal identity against being a group member**		
*	Tibialis posterior		NEED and LOVE/SEX
42a	Peroneus longus		WILL
42b	Peroneus brevis		SOL/PERF
*	Lumbricals (foot)		SOL/PERF

(e)	**Balance of managing stress and resolving it**		
21	Sacrotuberous ligament		PERINATAL and EX
49	Gracilis		AUT
44a	Sartorius,	proximal part	WILL
44b	Sartorius,	distal part	OPINIONS
43d	Vastus medialis		LOVE/SEX and PUB
29	Popliteus		OPINIONS
27	Plantaris		SOL/PERF

The Muscles Marked on a Bodymap

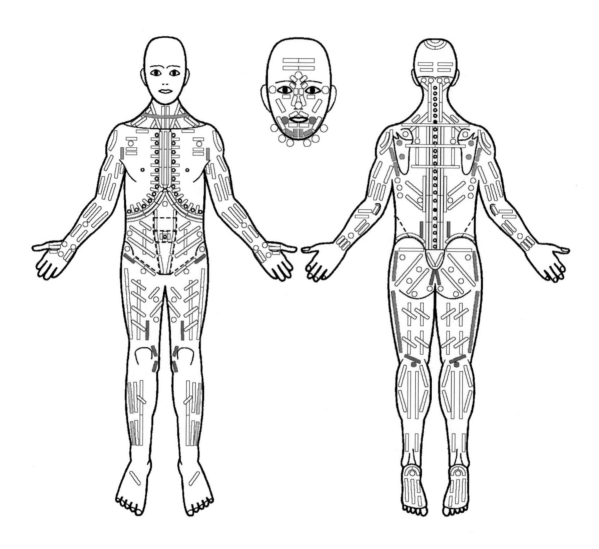

Each color represents a subfunction.

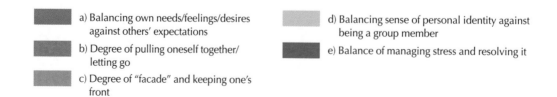

a) Balancing own needs/feelings/desires against others' expectations

b) Degree of pulling oneself together/ letting go

c) Degree of "facade" and keeping one's front

d) Balancing sense of personal identity against being a group member

e) Balance of managing stress and resolving it

The Ego Function SOCIAL BALANCE

A deep muscle in the lower back, outer side of the thighs, some shoulder, neck, and facial muscles, muscles in the calves and inner side of the thighs

Social Balance deals with different psychological and physical balances: the balance between being in contact with oneself and in contact with others—see (a), (c), and (d) below—and the balance between sensing and expressing one's emotions and the ability of containing and keeping them inside—see (b) and (e) below.

Social Balance is divided into five different subfunctions: (a) balancing one's own needs/feelings/desires against others' expectations, (b) degree of pulling oneself together/letting go, (c) degree of "facade" and maintaining one's front, (d) balancing a sense of personal identity against being a group member, (e) balance of managing stress and resolving it. The areas on the body that are empirically connected with this Ego Function and the subfunctions are:

(a) Balancing one's own needs/feelings/desires against others' expectations

- The deep muscle in the lower back (quadratus lumborum)

(b) Degree of pulling oneself together/letting go

- The outer side of the thighs and hips (tensor fascia lata, iliotibial tract)

(c) Degree of "facade" and maintaining one's front

- Muscles that rotate the shoulder joint (i.e., teres minor and major, infraspinatus)
- Some facial muscles (platysma, mentalis)

(d) Balancing a sense of personal identity against being a group member

- The front and the outer side of the lower leg (peroneus longus and brevis)

(e) Balance of managing stress and resolving it

- A ligament deep in the seat/buttocks (sacrotuberous ligament)
- Some muscles on the inner side of the thigh (e.g., gracilis, vastus medialis)
- Some small muscles deep in the knee (popliteus, plantaris)
- A muscle on the front of the thigh (sartorius)

Finding the balance between one's own needs/emotions and others' expectations is related in the body to the connection between the lower part and the upper part of the body. It is therefore important, among other things, to work with the lower back, especially the deep muscle, in relation to the movements that connect the lower and the upper parts of the body. This applies not only to the needs and emotions but also to the impulses of action that arise in interaction with others.

If you want to support the client in improving the ability to keep herself together, it may be efficient to teach her to slightly activate the muscles on the outer side of the thighs and hip.

The balance of maintaining the facade and being open may involve many areas in the body, but it might be especially helpful to work with some small muscles that rotate the upper arm in the shoulder joint (teres major and minor and infraspinatus).

The balance of being oneself and being part of the group is reflected in the tenseness of the muscles on the front and the outer side of the lower part of the leg/calf. Try out these movements: lift the forefoot and/or rock it from side to side with a focus on the outer side of the lower leg.

The balance in relation to being in stress and resolving stress may involve many different areas of the body, but empirically, the knees and inner side of the thighs secure the containment and management of stress.

VII. The Ego Function COGNITIVE SKILLS

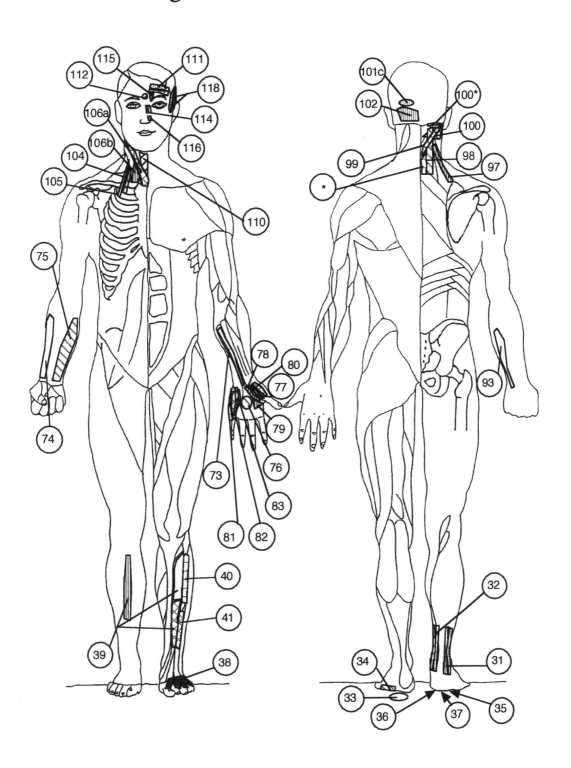

The Location of Some of the Muscles and Connective Tissue in the Body

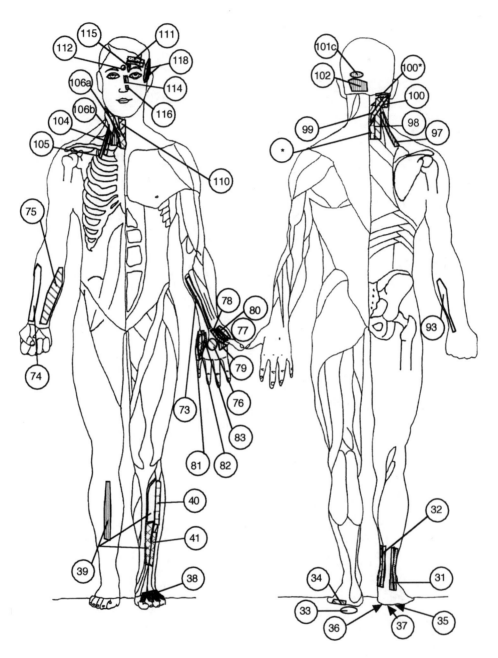

Each graphic pattern represents a Character Structure.

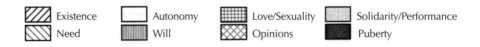

- Existence
- Need
- Autonomy
- Will
- Love/Sexuality
- Opinions
- Solidarity/Performance
- Puberty

All the Muscles and Connective Tissue in Each Subfunction

(a) Orienting

110	Longus capitis and longus colli		EX
100	Suboccipitals	*origins and insertions	EX
		muscle, medial part	PERINATAL
		lateral part	NEED
98	Semispinalis capitis		NEED
99	Splenius capitis		NEED
104	Scalenus anterior		NEED
105	Scalenus medius		AUT
97	Scalenus posterior		WILL
106b	Sternocleidomastoid, clavicular head		WILL
106a	Sternocleidomastoid, sternal head,	superior part	LOVE/SEX
		inferior part	OPINIONS
*	Splenius cervicis		LOVE/SEX

(b) Cognitive grasp

76	Palmar aponeurosis	NEED
82	Flexor digiti minimi brevis	NEED
75	Flexor digitorum profundus	NEED
73	Flexor digitorum superficialis	AUT
74	Flexor pollicis longus	AUT
93	Extensor indicis	AUT
78	Flexor pollicis brevis	WILL
79	Adductor pollicis	WILL
81	Abductor digiti minimi	LOVE/SEX
80	Opponens pollicis	OPINIONS
83	Opponens digiti minimi	OPINIONS
77	Abductor pollicis brevis	SOL/PERF
*	Lumbricals (hand)	SOL/PERF

(c) Understanding (getting something well enough to go forward with it)

33	Plantar aponeurosis	PERINATAL
*	Insertions of abductor, flexors, and extensors on the proximal phalanx of the little toe	EX and NEED
34	Abductor digiti minimi	OPINIONS
*	Flexor digiti minimi brevis	NEED
	(34 and * are tested together)	
35	Flexor digitorum brevis	NEED
32	Flexor digitorum longus	NEED and LOVE/SEX
37	Flexor hallucis brevis	AUT
31	Flexor hallucis longus	WILL and SOL/PERF
36	Abductor hallucis	SOL/PERF

The Location of Some of the Muscles and Connective Tissue in the Body

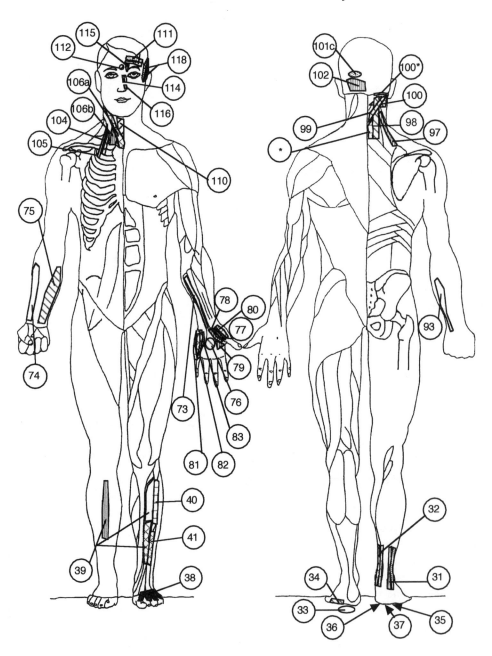

Each graphic pattern represents a Character Structure.

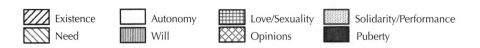

▨ Existence	☐ Autonomy	▦ Love/Sexuality	▨ Solidarity/Performance
▧ Need	▥ Will	▨ Opinions	■ Puberty

All the Muscles and Connective Tissue in Each Subfunction

(d)	**Grasp of reality (ability to apply cognitive understanding to different situations)**		
39	Tibialis anterior, proximal part,	superficial	WILL
		deep	AUT
		distal part	OPINIONS
40	Extensor digitorum longus		LOVE/SEX
41	Extensor hallucis longus		OPINIONS
38	Extensor digitorum brevis and extensor hallucis brevis		PUB
(e)	**Planning**		
102	Occipitofrontalis-venter occipitalis		WILL
101c	Galea aponeurotica		SOL/PERF
(f)	**Contemplation/consideration**		
112	"Third eye" (fascia)		EX
114	Procerus		NEED and AUT
115	Corrugator supercilii		WILL
111	Occipitofrontalis-venter frontalis,	superior part	SOL/PERF
		inferior part	OPINIONS
116	Nasalis		OPINIONS
118	Temporalis	* insertion	EX
		muscle	SOL/PERF and PUB

The Muscles Marked on a Bodymap

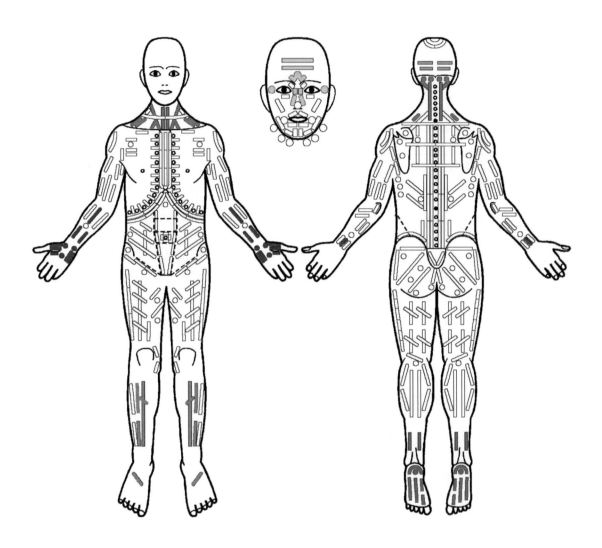

Each color represents a subfunction.

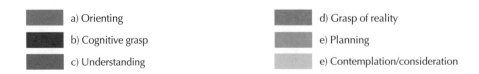

a) Orienting

b) Cognitive grasp

c) Understanding

d) Grasp of reality

e) Planning

e) Contemplation/consideration

The Ego Function COGNITIVE SKILLS

The neck, the back of the neck, the hands, the feet, and the muscles of the face and temples

Cognitive Skills deals psychologically with one's ability and skills in how to orient oneself, perceive and understand oneself and the world, as well as the bodily sensations corresponding to these issues.

How is it possible to think and speak from the different intellectual levels and switch or alternate between them? The levels are: *concrete, operative, general, symbolic, abstract,* and *philosophical.*

The areas of the body that are empirically connected with this Ego Function and the subfunctions are the neck and the back of the neck, which are literally connected to orienting, as well as the hands and feet. The hands are connected to getting hold of and forming an understanding or cognitive grasp (ideas), and the feet are connected to the way of "standing more or less" in the concrete, standing firm and standing by, as well as the willingness to release the concrete to enter into different degrees of abstraction and abstract thinking.

Cognitive Skills is divided in six different subfunctions: (a) orienting, (b) cognitive grasp, (c) understanding (getting something well enough to set out with it), (d) grasp of reality (ability to apply cognitive understanding to different situations), (e) planning, (f) contemplation/consideration. The areas on the body that are empirically connected with this Ego Function and the subfunctions are:

(a) Orienting

- Muscles of the neck and the back of the neck (e.g., semispinalis capitis)

(b) Cognitive grasp

- Muscles in the hands and lower part of the arm (e.g., flexor pollicis longus)

(c) Understanding (getting something well enough to go forward with it)

- Soles of the feet and the gripping muscles of the feet and lower part of the legs (e.g., flexor digitorum longus)

(d) Grasp of reality (ability to apply cognitive understanding to different situations)

- The muscle on the front of the lower part of the leg (e.g., tibialis anterior)
- The muscles that lift the toes (e.g., extensor digitorum longus)

(e) Planning

- The fascia on top of the head (galea aponeurotica)

(f) Contemplation/consideration

- Muscles of the forehead (occipitofrontalis, venter frontalis)
- A muscle of the nostrils (nasalis)
- The temples (temporalis)

Some may wonder what thinking has to do with the body. It is through a continuous confirmed experience that it is possible to observe and influence a human being's way of thinking through body movements.

It is difficult to have a sense of being able to orient in a flexible way if there is a lot of tension or despairing/looseness in the neck or in the back of the neck. Similarly, it is difficult to get hold of, examine, and let go of something without a certain amount of activity in the hands. And also, if you want to help yourself or others stand firmly, it actually helps to focus on the feet and toes, and if people are stuck in a very concrete way of thinking, it may be of help to work with walking around and lifting the feet from the floor or mat.

Another way of recognizing the embodiment of thinking may be to notice people's gestures and their body language: think for instance of how a physical "getting hold of" or "holding on to" motion is often followed by a persistent insisting argument or statement. Making these particular movements may also help when trying to understand something or trying to concretize the abstract. Also, think of how often people take hold of or touch the forehead or temples when they try to concentrate on a difficult matter.

The body areas and muscles described above are suggestions for areas you may be aware of within yourself, or as a therapist with your clients, when working with a particular attitude or when trying to think in different ways.

VIII. The Ego Function
MANAGEMENT OF ENERGY

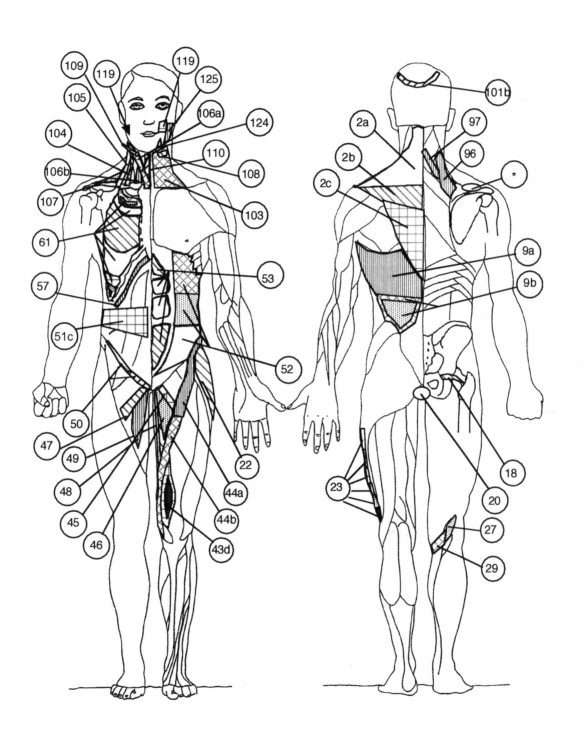

The Locations of Some of the Muscles and Connective Tissue in the Body

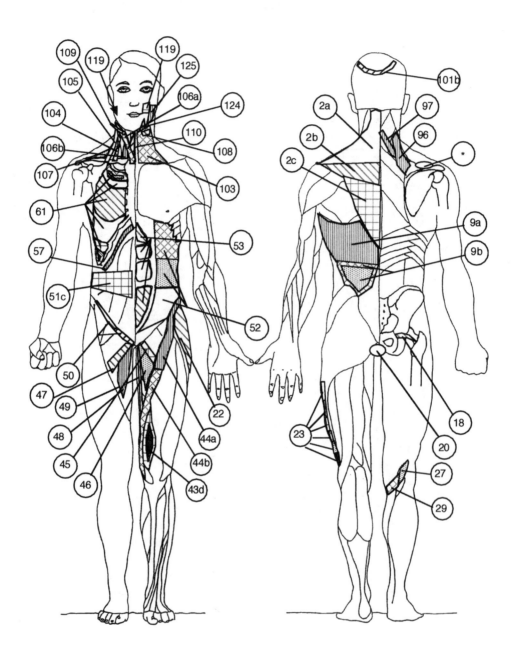

Each graphic pattern represents a Character Structure.

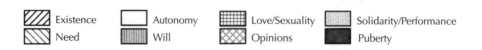

Existence	Autonomy	Love/Sexuality	Solidarity/Performance
Need	Will	Opinions	Puberty

All the Muscles and Connective Tissue in Each Subfunction

(a)   Containment of emotions

61	Intercostals,	between ribs 2-5	PERINATAL
		between ribs 3-7	NEED
		between ribs 6-9	AUT
		between ribs 9-10	LOVE/SEX
		between ribs 1-2 and 10-12	OPINIONS and SOL/PERF
57	Diaphragm		WILL
53	Rectus abdominis,	superior and inferior parts of 4	NEED
		two middle parts of 4	AUT
51c	Transversus abdominis		LOVE/SEX
52	Obliquus externus and internus,	superior part	OPINIONS
		middle part	SOL/PERF
		inferior part	AUT
50	Inguinal ligament,	medial part	EX
		lateral part	NEED
124	Depressor anguli oris		WILL

(b)   Containment of high-level energy
Head and neck:

*	Connective tissue on top of the shoulder (shoulder plexus)		PERINATAL
101b	Galea aponeurotica (half circle around the top of the head)		PERINATAL
109	Digastricus, posterior belly		EX
110	Longus capitis and longus colli		EX
108	Mylohyoid		NEED
104	Scalenus anterior		NEED
105	Scalenus medius		AUT
97	Scalenus posterior		WILL
96	Levator scapulae		WILL
125	Masseter		WILL
123	Medial pterygoid		AUT
106b	Sternocleidomastoid, clavicular head		WILL
106a	Sternocleidomastoid, sternal head	superior part	LOVE/SEX
		inferior part	OPINIONS
119	Zygomaticus		LOVE/SEX
103	Platysma		OPINIONS
*	Depressor labii		OPINIONS
107	Omohyoid		SOL/PERF

Trunk:

56	Costal curve,	medial one-third	LOVE/SEX
		middle one-third	OPINIONS
		lateral one-third	SOL/PERF
12	Iliac crest,	medial part	PERINATAL
		lateral part	PUB
20	Obturator internus, near pelvic floor		AUT

The Location of Some of the Muscles and Connective Tissue in the Body

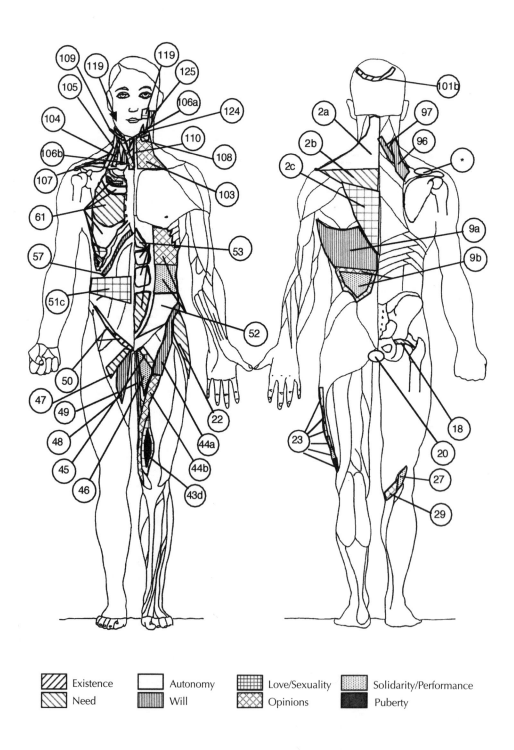

Existence   Autonomy   Love/Sexuality   Solidarity/Performance
Need   Will   Opinions   Puberty

All the Muscles and Connective Tissue in Each Subfunction

Trunk: (continued)

19	Quadratus femoris		WILL
*	Pelvic floor: pelvic diaphragm: coccygeus		NEED
		levator ani	AUT
	Sphincter ani externus		WILL
	Urogenital diaphragm		LOVE/SEX

Legs:

*	Connective tissue around knee and ankle		PERINATAL
*	Connective tissue of medial and lateral rotators of the hip joint		PERINATAL and EX
*	Connective tissue of medial and lateral rotators of the shoulder joint		PERINATAL
*	Connective tissue around elbow and wrist		PERINATAL
49	Gracilis		AUT
44a	Sartorius,	proximal part	WILL
44b	Sartorius,	distal part	OPINIONS
29	Popliteus		OPINIONS
27	Plantaris		SOL/PERF

(c) Self-containment

22	Tensor fascia lata		NEED
23	Iliotibial tract,	1st part	AUT
		2nd part	WILL
		3rd part	LOVE/SEX
		4th part	OPINIONS
		5th part	SOL/PERF
		at the knee, 6th part	PUB

(d) Self-containment—feeling "backed"

*	Connective tissue of the back level with thoracic vertebrae 3-5		EX
2b	Trapezius,	middle part	NEED
2a	Trapezius,	superior part	AUT
9a	Latissimus dorsi,	superior part	WILL
2c	Trapezius,	inferior part	LOVE/SEX
9b	Latissimus dorsi,	inferior part	OPINIONS and SOL/PERF

(e) Containment of sensuality

18	Gemelli and obturator internus		NEED
47	Adductor brevis		NEED
20	Obturatorius internus, near pelvic floor		AUT
48	Adductor magnus		WILL
45	Pectineus		LOVE/SEX
43d	Vastus medialis		LOVE/SEX and PUB
46	Adductor longus		SOL/PERF

The Muscles Marked on a Bodymap

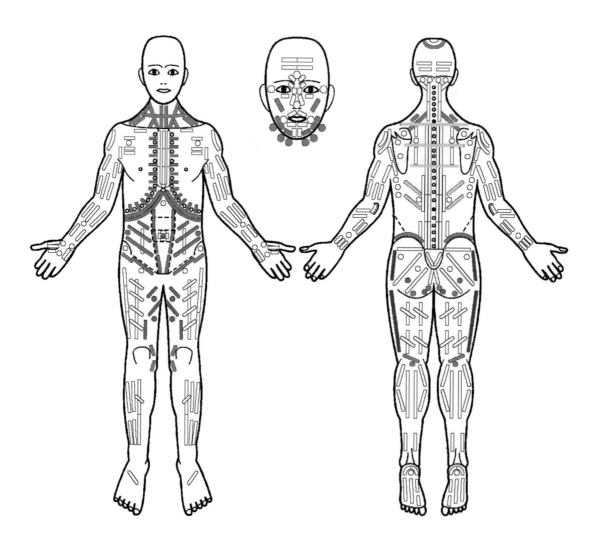

Each color represents a subfunction.

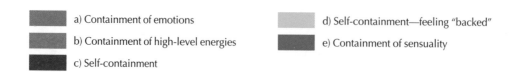

a) Containment of emotions

b) Containment of high-level energies

c) Self-containment

d) Self-containment—feeling "backed"

e) Containment of sensuality

The Ego Function MANAGEMENT OF ENERGY

The midriff, the muscles between the ribs and the stomach muscles, the muscles in the neck, the pelvic floor, and the inner thigh, and the big flat muscles of the back

Management of Energy deals with one's ability and skills in building up and containing powerful energy inside oneself, both emotional energy and stress energy. The areas of the body that are empirically connected with this Ego Function are in some degree centered around the primary and secondary muscles of respiration or the muscles in or around the torso.

Management of Energy is divided into five different subfunctions: (a) containment of emotions, (b) containment of high-level energy, (c) self-containment, (d) self-containment—feeling "backed," (e) containment of sensuality. The areas on the body that are empirically connected with this Ego Function and the subfunctions are:

(a) Containment of emotions (muscles of respiration)
- The small muscles between the ribs (intercostals)
- The midriff muscle (diaphragm)
- The muscles of the stomach (e.g., transversus abdominis)

(b) Containment of high-level energy
- Some muscles in the neck (digastricus, longus capitis, mylohyoid, scaleni, sternocleidomastoid)
- A muscle that pulls the shoulder blade upward (levator scapulae)
- Muscles close to the pelvic floor (piriformis, obturator internus, gemelli, quadratus femoris)
- The pelvic floor
- The inner side of the thighs (gracilis, sartorius) and the knees (popliteus, plantaris)

(c) Self-containment
- The outer side of the hip and thigh (tensor fascia lata, iliotibial tract)

(d) Self-containment—feeling "backed"
- Connective tissue between the shoulder blades (thoracic vertebrae 3-5) and the big flat superficial muscles of the back (trapezius, latissimus dorsi)

(e) Containment of sensuality
- A muscle close to the pelvic floor (obturator internus)
- The inner side of the thigh (e.g., pectineus)

There are lots of muscles connected to this Ego Function, many of them part of respiration. It is obvious that a deepened respiration may be followed by a more powerful emotional experience. Therefore if people speak of strong emotions with feeble or held-back respiration, the message is "I experience, but I hold back."

If you work on helping yourself or others with the containment of powerful emotions, an awareness of the physical space in the chest and torso may be helpful; do not forget the neck, the back of the neck, or the pelvic floor, and also the legs—a good grounding often supports the containment of emotions.

Alternatively, if you are working with letting go of or deepening emotions, loosening up in the chest and the stomach (torso) will be helpful. It may also help to loosen the neck and the back of the neck as well as to move the legs. Often the client has to express a sound to release the muscles in all these places. Besides energy moving up and out, it also needs to move downward and become grounded, and it may be moved out through a stamping motion.

IX. The Ego Function SELF-ASSERTION

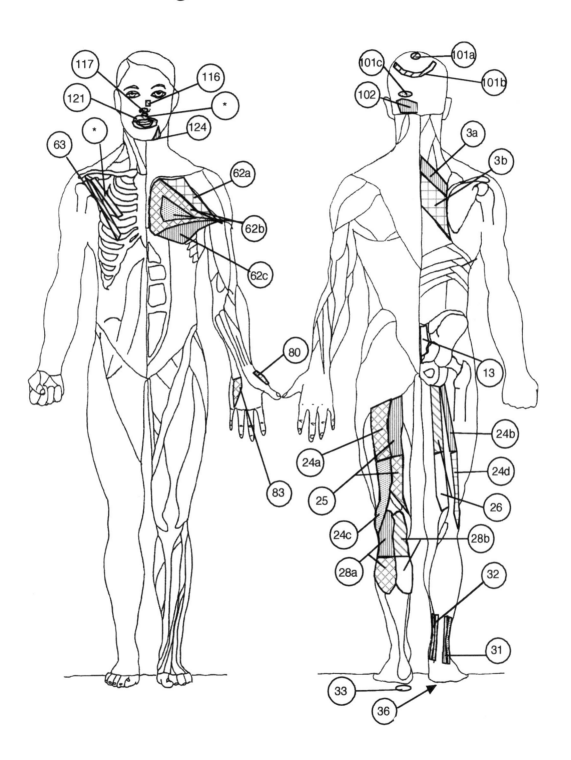

The Location of Some of the Muscles and Connective Tissue in the Body

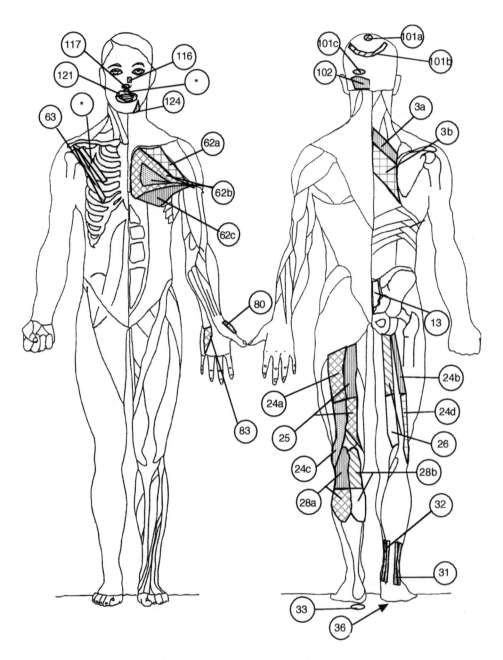

Each graphic pattern represents a Character Structure.

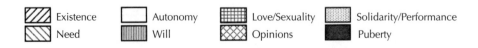

▨ Existence	☐ Autonomy	▦ Love/Sexuality	▨ Solidarity/Performance
▧ Need	▥ Will	▨ Opinions	■ Puberty

All the Muscles and Connective Tissue in Each Subfunction

(a)	Self-assertion (manifesting one's power)		
*	Connective tissue around knee and ankle		PERINATAL
*	Connective tissue of medial and lateral rotators of the hip joint		PERINATAL and EX
*	Connective tissue of medial and lateral rotators of the shoulder joint		PERINATAL
*	Connective tissue around elbow and wrist		PERINATAL
121	Orbicularis oris		NEED
28b	Gastrocnemius, medial head,	proximal part	NEED
		distal part	AUT
28a	Gastrocnemius, lateral head,	proximal part	WILL
		distal part	OPINIONS
117	Tip of the nose		WILL
32	Flexor digitorum longus		NEED and LOVE/SEX
31	Flexor hallucis longus		WILL and SOL/PERF
80	Opponens pollicis		OPINIONS
83	Opponens digiti minimi		OPINIONS
*	Depressor septi		OPINIONS

(b)	Asserting oneself in one's roles		
63	Pectoralis minor,	* superior part	NEED
		inferior/lateral part	AUT
62c	Pectoralis major,	abdominal part	WILL
62a	Pectoralis major,	clavicular part	LOVE/SEX
62b	Pectoralis major,	sternal part	OPINIONS and SOL/PERF
124	Depressor anguli oris		WILL
3a	Rhomboid minor		WILL
3b	Rhomboid major		LOVE/SEX
116	Nasalis		OPINIONS

(c)	Forward momentum and sense of direction		
13	Sacrum		PERINATAL
33	Plantar aponeurosis		PERINATAL
101b	Galea aponeurotica (half circle around the top of the head)		PERINATAL
101a	Galea aponeurotica (a spot on top of the head)		EX
24d	Biceps femoris, short head		LOVE/SEX
	Biceps femoris,		
24a	long head,	proximal part, superficial	OPINIONS
24b	long head,	proximal part, deep	WILL
24c	long head,	distal part, superficial	SOL/PERF
26	Semimembranosus,	proximal part	NEED
		distal part	AUT
25	Semitendinosus,	proximal part	WILL
		distal part	OPINIONS
36	Abductor hallucis		SOL/PERF
101c	Galea aponeurotica		SOL/PERF
102	Occipitofrontalis-venter occipitalis		WILL

The Muscles Marked on a Bodymap

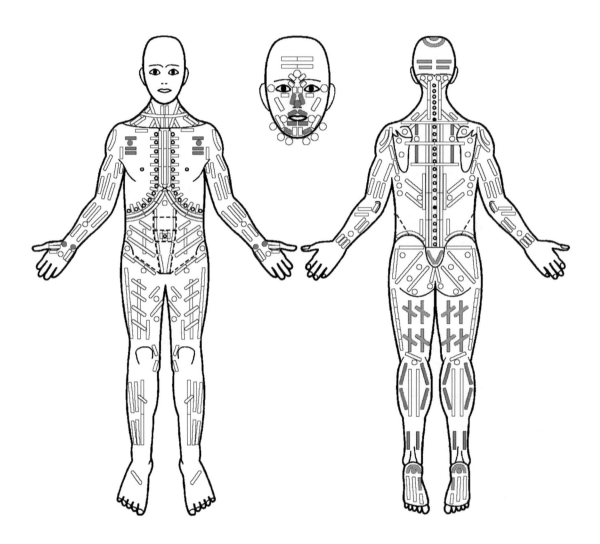

Each color represents a subfunction.

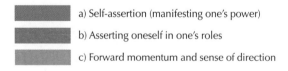

a) Self-assertion (manifesting one's power)

b) Asserting oneself in one's roles

c) Forward momentum and sense of direction

The Ego Function SELF-ASSERTION

The eyes, the mouth, the hands, the calves, the large chest muscles, and the backs of the thighs

Self-Assertion psychologically deals with the position and attitude the person has in relation to his or her surroundings, or in other words, how he or she approaches the outside world. What expression of the eyes and face does the individual meet the world with? Which position of the body–upright and forward-looking, or slightly cowered and timid/cautious–does he or she go forward and move in the world with?

Self-Assertion is divided into three different subfunctions: (a) self-assertion (manifesting one's power), (b) asserting oneself in one's roles, (c) forward momentum and sense of direction. The areas on the body that are empirically connected with this Ego Function and the subfunctions are:

(a) Self-assertion

- A muscle around the mouth (orbicularis oris)
- The big outer muscles of the calf (gastrocnemius)
- The muscles that move the thumb toward the little finger (opponens pollicis and opponens digiti minimi)

(b) Asserting oneself in one's roles

- The big chest muscles (pectoralis major and minor)
- The muscles between the shoulder blades (rhomboid major and minor)
- The muscle of the wings of the nose (nasalis)

(c) Forward momentum and sense of direction

- The sacrum
- The back of the thighs (pushing off) (biceps femoris, semitendinosus, semimembranosus)
- The muscle that pulls the big toe to the side (abductor hallucis)

Some suggestions for awareness and intervention: it is obvious that you have to include eye contact if you want to work with revealing yourself (bringing yourself forward). In the same way, having an awareness of the large muscles of the chest–and daring to push the chest forward–may support a felt sense of self-assertion. Or vice versa; it may make you or the client anxious for what might happen and lead to a specific piece of personal work with what might prevent you from stepping forward into confrontation.

The expression "to step forward" has a bodily analogue that is not accidental. If you want to work with "stepping forward," it can be quite helpful to physically take the step forward while you are speaking about the issue (speaking from your heart).

X. The Ego Function
PATTERNS OF INTERPERSONAL SKILLS

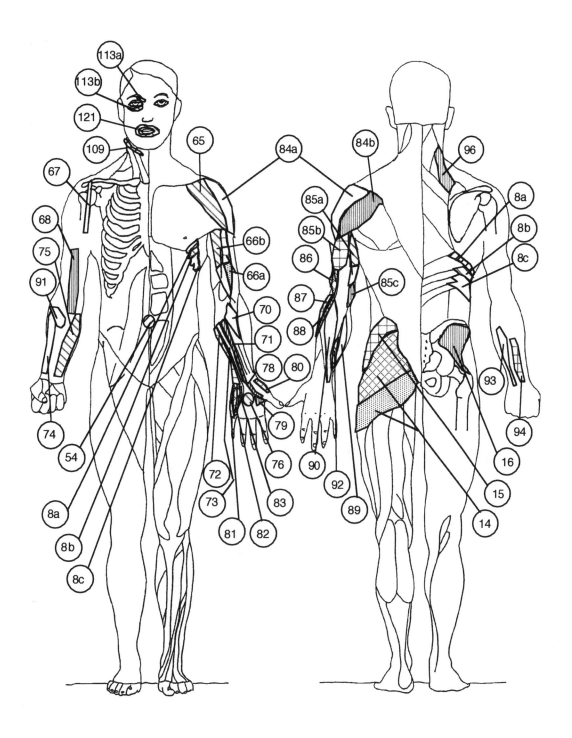

The Location of Some of the Muscles and Connective Tissue in the Body

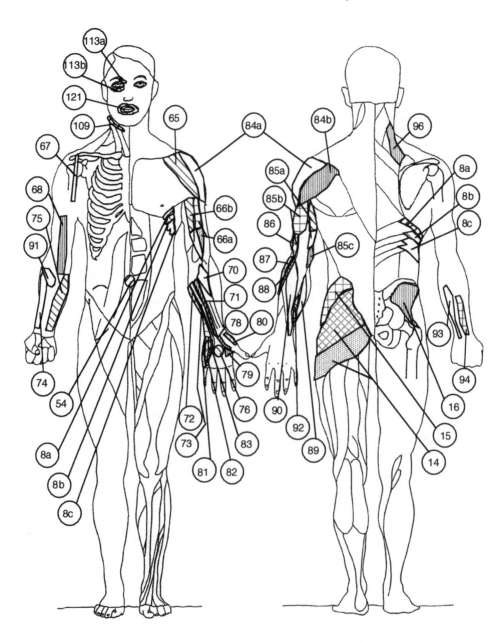

Each graphic pattern represents a Character Structure.

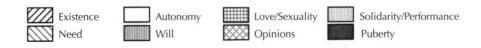

▨ Existence	▢ Autonomy	▦ Love/Sexuality	▨ Solidarity/Performance
▨ Need	▥ Will	▧ Opinions	■ Puberty

All the Muscles and Connective Tissue in Each Subfunction

(a)	**Reaching out**		
8a	Serratus anterior,	superior part	EX
8b	Serratus anterior,	medial part	NEED
65	Deltoid,	anterior part	NEED
8c	Serratus anterior,	inferior part	AUT
67	Coracobrachialis		AUT

(b)	**Gripping and holding on**	
*	Insertions of flexors and extensors on the proximal phalanx of the little finger	EX and NEED
76	Palmar aponeurosis	NEED
82	Flexor digiti minimi brevis	NEED
75	Flexor digitorum profundus	NEED
73	Flexor digitorum superficialis	AUT
74	Flexor pollicis longus	AUT
78	Flexor pollicis brevis	WILL
79	Adductor pollicis	WILL
80	Opponens pollicis	OPINIONS
83	Opponens digiti minimi	OPINIONS

(c)	**Drawing toward oneself and holding on closely**		
66b	Biceps brachii, short head,	proximal part	NEED
		distal part	AUT
67	Coracobrachialis		AUT
68	Brachialis		WILL
71	Flexor carpi radialis		WILL
72	Flexor carpi ulnaris		LOVE/SEX
87	Brachioradialis		LOVE/SEX
66a	Biceps brachii, long head,	proximal part	LOVE/SEX
		distal part	SOL/PERF

(d)	**Receiving and giving from one's core**	
54	Umbilicus (take in-keep out)	PERINATAL and EX
109	Digastricus, posterior belly	EX
113a	Orbicularis oculi, in the corner above the eye	NEED
113b	Orbicularis oculi, beneath the eye	NEED
121	Orbicularis oris	NEED
91	Supinator (receive)	AUT
70	Pronator teres (give out)	AUT

The Location of Some of the Muscles and Connective Tissue in the Body

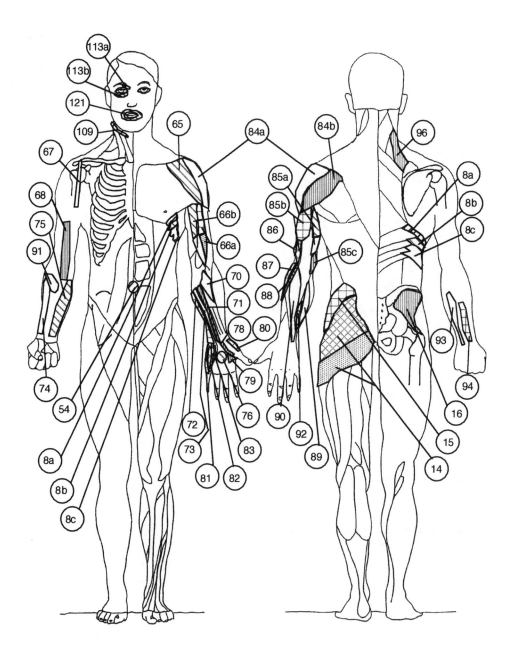

Each graphic pattern represents a Character Structure.

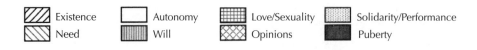

▨ Existence	☐ Autonomy	▦ Love/Sexuality
▧ Need	▥ Will	▨ Opinions

Solidarity/Performance

Puberty

All the Muscles and Connective Tissue in Each Subfunction

(e)	**Pushing away and holding at a distance**		
85a	Triceps brachii, long head,	proximal part	NEED
		distal part	AUT
89	Extensor carpi ulnaris		AUT
85c	Triceps brachii, medial head		WILL
88	Extensor carpi radialis longus and brevis		WILL
85b	Triceps brachii, lateral head,	proximal part	LOVE/SEX
		distal part	OPINIONS
86	Anconeus		SOL/PERF
(f)	**Releasing, letting go**		
*	Insertions of flexors and extensors on the proximal phalanx of the little finger		EX and NEED
92	Extensor digiti minimi		NEED
90	Extensor digitorum		AUT
93	Extensor indicis		AUT
94	Extensor pollicis brevis and abductor pollicis longus		LOVE/SEX
81	Abductor digiti minimi		LOVE/SEX
(g)	**Taking on chores (assignments)**		
84a	Deltoid,	middle part	AUT
84b	Deltoid,	posterior part	WILL
96	Levator scapulae		WILL
16	Gluteus minimus		WILL
15	Gluteus medius		LOVE/SEX
14	Gluteus maximus,	superior part	OPINIONS
		inferior part	SOL/PERF

The Muscles Marked on a Bodymap

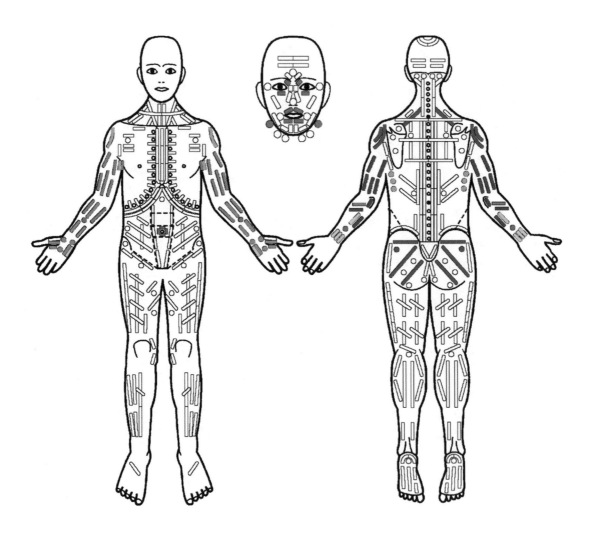

Each color represents a subfunction.

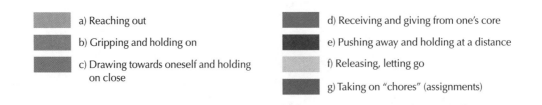

a) Reaching out

b) Gripping and holding on

c) Drawing towards oneself and holding on close

d) Receiving and giving from one's core

e) Pushing away and holding at a distance

f) Releasing, letting go

g) Taking on "chores" (assignments)

The Ego Function PATTERNS OF INTERPERSONAL SKILLS

The hands, the lower part of the arms, the upper part of the arms, and the shoulders

Patterns of Interpersonal Skills deals with how a person interacts with his or her surroundings. Tasks of taking hold of, holding on to, letting go, insisting, creating space for oneself, receiving or taking in, giving away, taking on, and carrying are all issues that may be understood psychologically, as interactions, and in a concrete bodily way.

Patterns of Interpersonal Skills is divided into seven subfunctions: (a) reaching out, (b) gripping and holding on, (c) drawing toward oneself and holding on closely, (d) receiving and giving from one's core, (e) pushing away and holding at a distance, (f) releasing, letting go, (g) taking on chores (assignments). The areas of the body that are empirically connected with this Ego Function and the subfunctions are:

(a) Reaching out
- Muscles on the side of the chest (serratus anterior)
- Front part of the superficial shoulder muscle (anterior deltoid)

(b) Gripping and holding on
- Muscles that allow the hands to hold (e.g., flexor pollicis brevis)

(c) Drawing toward oneself and holding on closely
- Muscles in the lower and upper arm that draw toward oneself (e.g., biceps brachii)

(d) Receiving and giving from one's core
- The area around the navel
- The area around the eyes
- The muscles that rotate the lower arm (supinator and pronator)

(e) Pushing away and holding at a distance
- The back of the upper arm (push away) (triceps brachii)
- The extensor muscles in the lower arm (extensor carpi radialis and ulnaris)

(f) Releasing, letting go
- Muscles in the hands and the lower arms that make "letting go" motions (e.g., extensor digitorum)

(g) Taking on chores (assignments)
- The outer shoulder muscle, the middle and back parts (deltoids)
- A muscle that lifts the shoulder blade and the shoulder girdle (levator scapulae)
- The muscles of the seat/buttocks (gluteus maximus, minimus, and medius)

It may sound like an awful lot of subfunctions, but in the overall view it is not at all complicated in practice. Think of using the hands and arms and follow the words: hold on, let go, receive, etc. Doing the action while talking about it, saying for instance, "let go," is a most effective way to internalize the action, and it is a good way to concretize the therapeutic work.

A few more nuances: the motion of reaching out may be deepened if you reach out all the way from the side of the chest at the same time as breathing in.

The experience of receiving and giving contact may be deepened if you are aware of the degree of letting go and controlling eye movement as well as the experience of opening and closing the eyes along with the degree of focus.

People who have difficulties with boundaries in contact may find it is helpful to hold a hand over their navel (an indication that boundaries in a very early contact have been difficult to keep).

When people talk about having taken on a task, or being weighed down by a task or assignment, it may often be helpful to be aware of how the "task" is carried in regard to the tension in the shoulder muscles. As when carrying a yoke, you take on a weight that you lift and that you will put down again as soon as possible. A task or burden is often experienced as a yoke—something you have to do (or carry). If you have taken on a task without having consciously chosen it, it is often experienced as a yoke. It may feel extraordinarily heavy if you haven't looked at the consequences of the choice such as time, economy, and so on.

XI. The Ego Function GENDER SKILLS

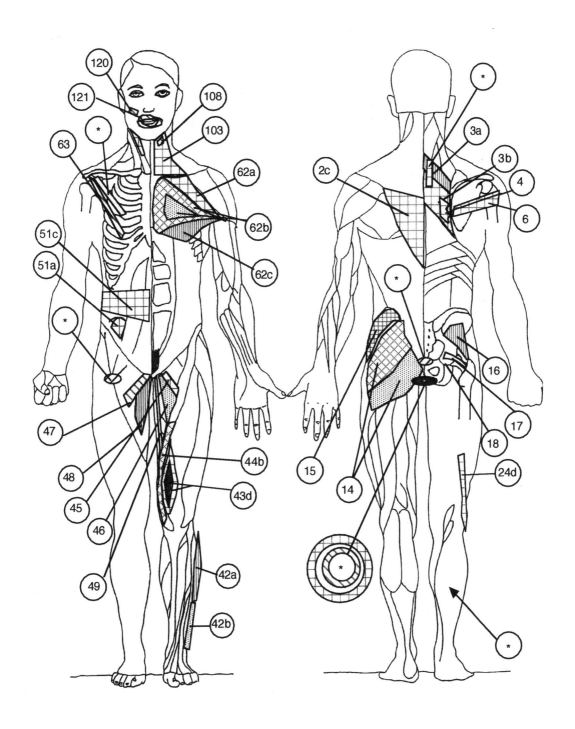

The Location of Some of the Muscles and Connective Tissue in the Body

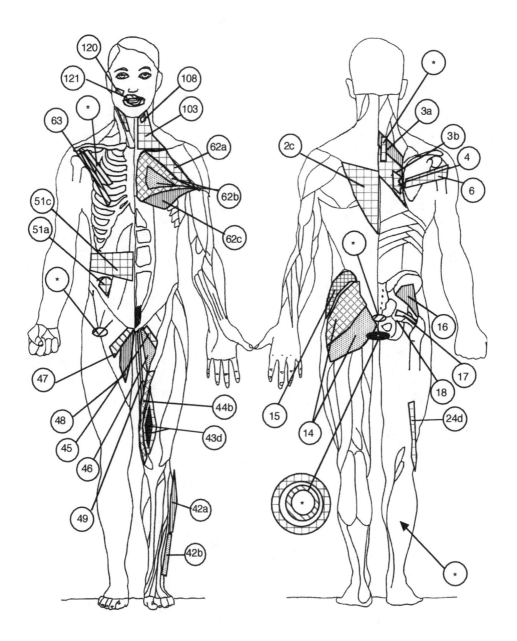

Each graphic pattern represents a Character Structure.

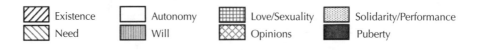

▨ Existence	☐ Autonomy	▦ Love/Sexuality	▩ Solidarity/Performance
▧ Need	▥ Will	▨ Opinions	▨ Puberty

All the Muscles and Connective Tissue in Each Subfunction

(a)   Awareness of gender

*	Origin of iliacus (ref. 51a)	PERINATAL
	Cellular level	
	Primary gender characteristics:	
	Inner and outer gender organs	
	Secondary gender characteristics:	

	Females:	Males:
	Little higher heart-rhythm	Little lower heart-rhythm
	Less height and weight	More height and weight
	Slighter bone structure	Stronger bone structure
	Less muscle mass (with more fat)	More muscle mass
	More and different subcutaneous fat	Less subcutaneous fat
	Less hairy	More hairy
	Broader pelvis (esp. inner pelvis)	More narrow pelvis
	Smaller throat, lighter voice	Broader throat, deeper voice
Gender hormones:	Estrogen	Testosterone

(b)   Experience of gender

*	Connective tissue at coccyx (not described in this book)		
*	Pelvic floor: pelvic diaphragm: coccygeus		NEED
		levator ani	AUT
	Sphincter ani externus		WILL
	Urogenital diaphragm		LOVE/SEX
17	Piriformis		AUT
16	Gluteus minimus		WILL
51a	Iliacus,	superior part	LOVE/SEX
15	Gluteus medius		LOVE/SEX

(c)   Experience of gender role

62c	Pectoralis major,	abdominal part	WILL
3a	Rhomboid minor		WILL
3b	Rhomboid major		LOVE/SEX
4	Serratus posterior superior,	caudal part	LOVE/SEX
2c	Trapezius,	inferior part	LOVE/SEX
15	Gluteus medius		LOVE/SEX
*	Splenius cervicis		LOVE/SEX
62a	Pectoralis major,	clavicular part	LOVE/SEX
62b	Pectoralis major,	sternal part	OPINIONS and SOL/PERF

The Location of Some of the Muscles and Connective Tissue in the Body

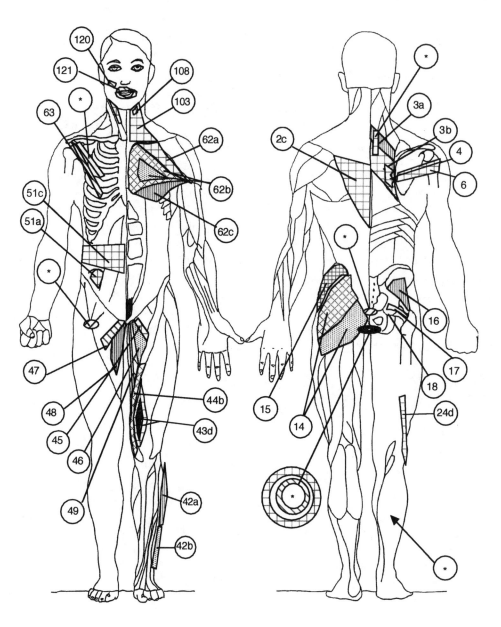

Each graphic pattern represents a Character Structure.

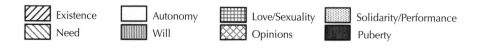

Pattern	Character Structure		Pattern	Character Structure
	Existence			Love/Sexuality
	Need			Opinions
	Autonomy			Solidarity/Performance
	Will			Puberty

All the Muscles and Connective Tissue in Each Subfunction

(d)	Containment of sensuality and sexuality		
108	Mylohyoid		NEED
120	Buccinator		NEED
18	Gemelli and obturator internus		NEED
47	Adductor brevis		NEED
49	Gracilis		AUT
48	Adductor magnus		WILL
51c	Transversus abdominis		LOVE/SEX
45	Pectineus		LOVE/SEX
43d	Vastus medialis		LOVE/SEX and PUB
44b	Sartorius,	distal part	OPINIONS
46	Adductor longus		SOL/PERF

(e)	Manifestation of sensuality and sexuality		
	Upper part of body:		
121	Orbicularis oris		NEED
2c	Trapezius,	inferior part	LOVE/SEX
106a	Sternocleidomastoid, sternal head,	superior part	LOVE/SEX
6	Teres minor		LOVE/SEX
81	Abductor digiti minimi		LOVE/SEX
62a	Pectoralis major,	clavicular part	LOVE/SEX
62b	Pectoralis major,	sternal part	OPINIONS and SOL/PERF
103	Platysma		OPINIONS
	Lower part of body:		
*	Tibialis posterior		NEED and LOVE/SEX
42a	Peroneus longus		WILL
24d	Biceps femoris, short head		LOVE/SEX
15	Gluteus medius		LOVE/SEX
51a	Iliacus,	superior part	LOVE/SEX
14	Gluteus maximus,	superior part	OPINIONS
		inferior part	SOL/PERF
44b	Sartorius,	distal part	OPINIONS
42b	Peroneus brevis		SOL/PERF
*	Pyramidalis (ref. 53)		PUB

The Muscles Marked on a Bodymap

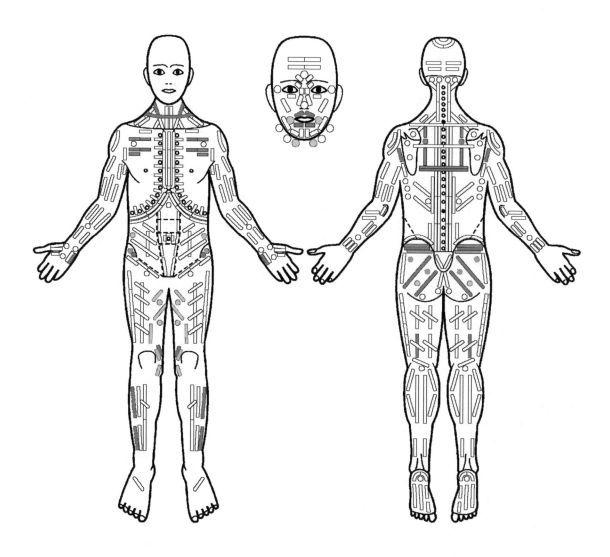

Each color represents a subfunction.

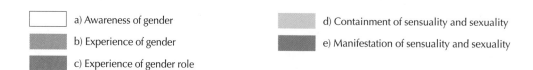

a) Awareness of gender

b) Experience of gender

c) Experience of gender role

d) Containment of sensuality and sexuality

e) Manifestation of sensuality and sexuality

The Ego Function GENDER SKILLS

The primary and secondary sexual characters, the pelvic floor and the pelvis, the muscles in the neck, the chest muscles, shoulders, and the back of the neck

Gender Skills deals with how human beings experience, carry, and show gender, gender role, sexuality, and sensuality in interaction with the surroundings. In the Bodynamic way of thinking, an inner experience of the gender skills and interacting with them in the outside world will be connected to Tenseness Systems and position/posture patterns of the body.

Gender Skills will automatically mirror itself in an individual's primary and secondary sexual character, not least in how the individual carries and shows or does not show these features in the culture or subculture with which he or she interacts.

The areas of the body that are empirically connected with this Ego Function are the shoulders and the back of the neck and the chest, muscles in the back, muscles around the pelvis, and the inner thighs. Gender Skills is divided into five different subfunctions: (a) awareness of gender, (b) experience of gender, (c) experience of gender role, (d) containment of sensuality and sexuality, (e) manifestation of sensuality and sexuality. The areas of the body that are empirically connected with this Ego Function and the subfunctions are:

(a) Awareness of gender

- The primary and secondary sexual characters

(b) Experience of gender

- The pelvic floor and some deep muscles in the seat/buttocks (e.g., piriformis)

(c) Experience of gender role

- The chest muscles (pectoralis major)
- The muscles between the shoulder blades (rhomboid major and minor)
- The superficial muscle of the back (trapezius)
- A deep muscle in the back of the neck (splenius cervicis, not tested)

(d) Containment of sensuality and sexuality

- The deepest muscle in the stomach (transversus abdominis)
- The muscle of the inner thighs (pectineus, gracilis, adductor brevis and magnus)

(e) Manifestation of sensuality and sexuality

- The expression of the eyes and the area around the mouth (orbicularis oris)
- The muscles of the neck (sternocleidomastoid, platysma)
- The muscles of the chest (pectoralis major)
- A muscle in the little finger (abductor digiti minimi)

Women and men both experience and carry their gender (or to be specific, their private parts, sex organs, and genitals) in ways that mirror or reflect their gender in Tenseness Systems in and around the pelvis, which may be kept more or less drawn back or pushed forward. People carry their shoulders, chest, and breasts in a way that mirrors or reflects their gender in Tenseness in the back, neck, back of neck, and the chest.

When you work with yourself or others around awareness of gender (more inward) and awareness of gender role (more about how you carry yourself out in the world) it may be a concrete way of getting closer to the problem or theme if you are aware of the body's posture, the expression of the eyes, etc. In any case, seeing how people relate to their gender and gender role becomes more available, more concrete, and clearer if you ask them to feel these and demonstrate them rather than if you just talk about them.

It is important, though, to remember that there are very big differences in how different cultures and subcultures have formed their gender roles, how they show their sexual character, flirt, or show attraction or lack of atttaction to the other person.

By giving workshops and training in different places around the world, we have experienced that this particular gender skill shows the largest variations of action. But it is also obvious that the complexity of problems is still connected to the same groups of muscles and individual muscles. In this regard it is also worth mentioning an obvious fact that is not always paid due attention in the psychotherapeutic context and is not directly but indirectly related to the body: the way people dress. Even small nuances in clothing, makeup, and choice of jewelry tell an awful lot about how people deal with their gender and gender role and with their sensuality and sexuality. The surface, or the facade, is a powerful approach to working with gender, consciousness of gender, and gender role. This also applies to the Ego Function Positioning and Self-Assertion.

Indications of Shock and
Post-Traumatic Stress Disorder (PTSD)

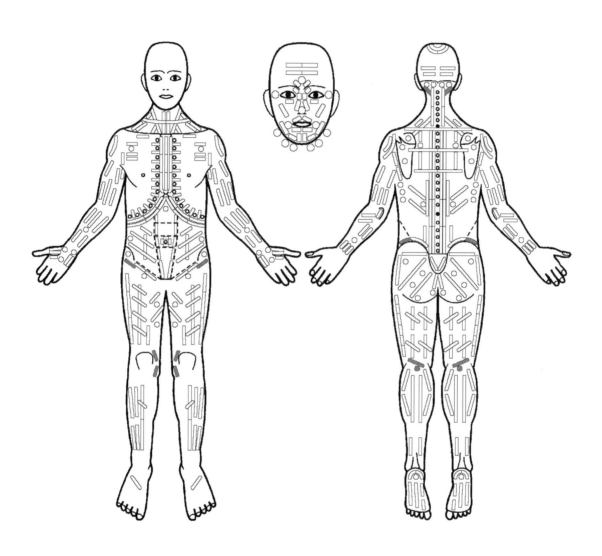

The Muscles Marked on a Bodymap

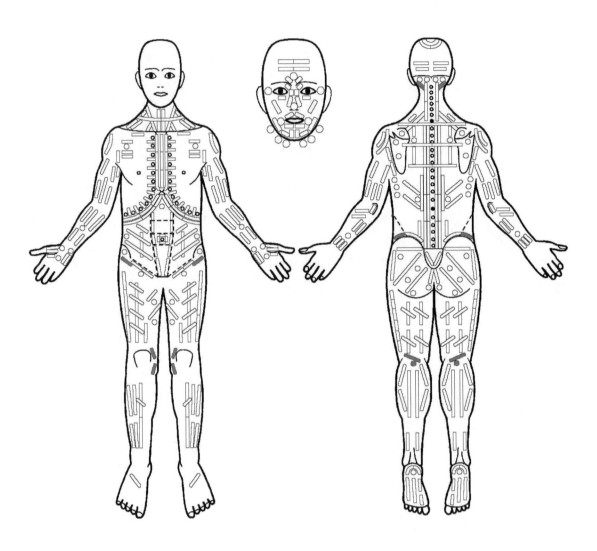

All the Muscles in Shock and PTSD

99	Splenius capitis		NEED
*	Pelvic floor: pelvic diaphragm: levator ani		AUT
49	Gracilis		AUT
44a	Sartorius,	proximal part	WILL
44b	Sartorius,	distal part	OPINIONS
29	Popliteus		OPINIONS
27	Plantaris		SOL/PERF
12	Iliac crest,	lateral part	PUB

When you evaluate whether a client has PTSD, it is also relevant to examine the muscles in other Ego Functions and subfunctions:

· VIII. Management of Energy, (b) containment of high-level energy
· VI. Social Balance, (e) balance of managing stress and resolving it

Also note:

1. What is the level of the client's body awareness or relationship to the body?
2. How does the client use the body at both work and in leisure?
3. How does the client react to emotions?
4. How does the client remember:
   · kinesthetic (motor)
   · visual
   · auditory
   · gustatory (taste)
   · olfactory
   · tactile

5. How is the development of the client's language seen in relation to life around him or her?
6. How does the client use language?:
   A lot
   · as a defense
   · in contact with himself or herself/embodied
   A little
   · holding back
   · missing language

7. How are the client's creative abilities?

Bibliography

Andreasen, E., and F. Bojsen-Møller. 1988. *Bevægeapparatet Anatomi I, 8. udgave (The anatomy of the motion apparatus/system, 8th edition).* Copenhagen: Gyldendal.

Argyle, M. 1988. *Bodily communication.* London and New York: Methuen.

Arnfred, A. 1992. *Uvante ord om kropsterapi og psyke (Unaccustomed Words about Body Therapy and Mind).* Copenhagen: LEV.

Ayres, J. A. 1979. *Sensory integration and the child.* Los Angeles: Western Psychological Services.

Bentsen, B. S. 1972. *Børnemotorik. Småbørns bevægelsesudvikling (Children's Motion: Small Children's Motoric Development).* Copenhagen: Gyldendal's Pedagogical Library.

Bentsen, B. S. 1975. *Spædbarnet bevæger sig—gi det en hånd. (The Baby Is Moving—Give It a Hand).* Copenhagen: Gyldendal's Pedagogical Library.

Bentzen, M., P. Bernhardt, and J. Isaacs. 1997. *Waking the Body Ego I and II.* Copenhagen: Kreatik.

Birdwhistel, R. L. 1972. *Kinesics and Context.* New York: Ballantine.

Boadella, D. 1974. Stress and character structure: A synthesis of concepts. *Energy & Character* 5:2.

Braatøy, T. 1947. *De Nervøse Sinn—medicinsk psykologi og psykoterapi (The Nervous Minds—Medical Psychology and Psychotherapy).* Copenhagen: Einar Munksgaard.

Brantbjerg, M. H., D. Marcher, and M. Kristiansen. 2006. *Resources in Coping with Shock: A Pathway to a Resource-Oriented Perspective on Shock Trauma.* Copenhagen: Kreatik.

Brantbjerg, M. H., and L. Ollars. 2006. *Musklernes intelligens. Om 11 Bodynamic Jeg-funktioner. (The Intelligence of the Muscles: About the 11 Bodynamic Ego Functions).* Copenhagen: Kreatik.

Bratt, N. 1972. *Den tidlige jeg-udvikling (The Early Ego-Development).* Copenhagen: Gyldendal's Pedagogical Library.

Bruun, U. B. 1977. *Førskolealderens psykologi (Psychology of the Preschool Age).* Copenhagen: Gyldendal's Pedagogical Library.

Burgoon, J. K. 1985. Nonverbal signals. In *Handbook of Interpersonal Communication,* ed. M. L. Knapp and G. R. Miller. Beverly Hills, CA: Sage.

Burgoon, J. K., D. B. Buller, and W. G. Woodall. 1989. *Nonverbal Communication: The Unspoken Dialogue.* New York: Harper & Row.

Candland, K. C. 1993. *Feral Children and Clever Animals: Reflections on Human Nature.* New York: Oxford University Press.

Chamberlain, D. 1988. *Babies Remember Birth.* Los Angeles: Jeremy P. Tarcher.

Darwin, C. 1872. *The Expression of the Emotions in Man and Animal.* Repr. London: University of Chicago Press, 1965.

Downing, G. 1997. *Kroppen og ordet. Om en europæisk form for kropspsykoterapi som også inkluderer verbalt arbejde på psykodynamisk grundlag (The Body and the Word: About a European Kind of Body Psychotherapy That Also Includes Verbal Work on a Psychodynamic Foundation).* Borås, Sweden: Nature and Culture. (Contains a good introduction and chapters (Part 5) about the roots of the body psychotherapy).

Dreyfus, H., S. Dreyfus, and T. Athanasiou. 1986. *Mind over Machine.* Rev. ed., New York: Free Press, 1988.

Ekman, P., W. V. Friesen, and P. Ellsworth. 1972. *Emotion in the Human Face.* Elmsford, NY: Pergamon.

Erikson, E. 1968. *Childhood and Society.* New York: W. W. Norton.

Feneis, H. 1989. *Anatomisk billedordbog (Anatomical Picture Dictionary).* Copenhagen: Munksgaard. Original title: *Anatomisches Bildwörterbuch,* Stuttgart, Germany: Thieme, 1967.

Ferner, H., and J. Staubesand. 1982. *Sobotta Atlas of Human Anatomy, Vols. 1 and 2.* Munich: Urban & Schwartzenberg.

Fich, S. 1997a. *A Manual with the Muscles Included in the Ego Functions and Their Different Subfunctions.* Copenhagen: Kreatik.

Fich, S. 1997b. *Testmanual–Bodymap. 2. udgave (Test Manual and Bodymap, 2nd ed.).* Copenhagen: Kreatik.

Fich, S., and L. Marcher. 1997. *Psykologi og Anatomi. En manual om barnets udviklingsfaser og deres muskulære forankring (Psychology and Anatomy: A Manual about the Child's Developmental Stages and Their Muscular Rooting).* Copenhagen: Kreatik.

Gardner, H. 2004. *Frames of Mind.* New York: Basic.

Gjesing, G. 2004. *Nysgerrige børn i bevægelse og aktivitet–i dagpleje, børneinstitution (Curious Children in Motion and Activity in Day Care and Child Care Institutions).* Copenhagen: Krogh's.

Goleman, D. 1995. *Emotional Intelligence.* New York: Bantam.

Gray, H. 2005. *Gray's Anatomy, 39th ed.* London: Elsevier Churchill Livingstone.

Hall, E. T. 1966. *The Hidden Dimension.* New York: Doubleday.

Holle, B. 1981. *Motor Development in Children.* Copenhagen: Munksgaard.

Hougaard, E. 1996. *Psykoterapi–teori og forskning (Psychotherapy: Theory and Research).* Copenhagen: Danish Psychological Publishing Co.

Hvid, T. 1990. *Kroppens fortællinger. Om en dansk kropspsykoterapeutisk teori/ Bodynamic Analyse. (Stories of the Body: About a Danish Body-Psychotherapeutic Theory/Bodynamic Analysis).* Aarhus, Denmark: Modtryk.

Hvid, T. 1992. *Kroppens fortællinger i billeder. Om nuanceret kropslæsning af personlighedstræk (Stories of the Body in Pictures: About Nuanced Body-Reading of Personality Features).* Aarhus, Denmark: Modtryk.

Jacobsen, C. 2005. *Sundhed i pædagogisk praksis (Health in Educational Praxis).* Aarhus, Denmark: Systime.

Jarlnaes, E. 1995. *Betydningen af at høre sammen (The Significance of Mutual Connectedness).* Copenhagen: Kreatik Publishers.

Joergensen, S. 1990. *3 artikler om kropssprog og kropslæsning (Three Articles about Body Language and Body Reading).* Copenhagen: Bodynamic Institute.

Joergensen, S., and L. Marcher. 1997. "Fortolkning af Bodymap—Bodynamic Analyses Personlighedstest." Trykt i *Testmanual—Bodymap, 2. udgave* ("Interpretation of Bodymap: Bodynamic Analysis—Personality Test." In *Test Manual—Bodymap, 2nd ed.).* Copenhagen: Kreatik.

Joergensen, S., and L. Ollars. 2000. "Kropslig forankring i psykoterapeutisk arbejde" ("Body Rooting in the Psychotherapeutic Work"). *Psykologisk Set* 18:42 (September 2000).

Johnsen, L. 1970. *Integrated Respiration Therapy.* Oslo: Sem & Stenersen.

Johnsen, L. 1975. *Integrert respirasjons terapi. En nøkkel til livsgledens skjulte kilde (Integrated Respiration Therapy: A Key to the Hidden Source of Cheerfulness).* Oslo: University Publishing Co.

Jydebjerg, U. C., and C. Fonsmark. 1970. *Nogle personlighedsteorier (Some Theories about Character).* Brønderslev, Denmark: Marko.

Katzenelson. 1994. *Homo socius.* Copenhagen: Gyldendal.

Kendall, H. O., F. P. Kendall, and G. E. Wadsworth. 1971. *Muscle Testing and Function.* Baltimore and London: Williams & Wilkins.

Krarup, F. C. 1906. *Hvad vi kan lære af Ritschl (What We Can Learn from Ritschl).* Copenhagen: V. Pio's Bookshop.

Lake, F. 1966. *Clinical Theology.* London: Darton Longman & Todd.

Lier, L. and N. Michelsen. 1978. *Fumlere og tumlere, nogle studier om kluntede skolebørn (Children with Motor Difficulties: Studies of "Clumsy" Schoolchildren).* Copenhagen: University of Copenhagen Institute of Social Medicine.

Lisina, M. 1985. *Child-Adults-Peers.* London: Progress.

Lisina, M. 1989. *Kommunikation og psykisk udvikling fra fødslen til skolealderen (Communication and Psychological Development from Birth to School Age).* Copenhagen: Sputnik.

Lorenz, K. 1977. *Behind the Mirror.* New York: Harvest/HBJ.

Lorenz, K. 1997. *King Solomon's Ring: New Light on Animal Ways.* London: Penguin.

Lowen, A. 1975. *Bioenergetics.* New York: Coward, McCann & Geoghegan.

Macnaughton, I. 2004. *Body, Breath, and Consciousness: A Somatics Anthology.* Berkeley: North Atlantic Books.

Maley, M. (n.d.). *Training Manual for the First Year of Training in Bioenergetic Analysis* (unpublished manuscript from Minnesota Institute for Bioenergetic Analysis).

Marcher, L., and L. Ollars. 1989. *Kropsdynamisk Analytisk arbejde med refødselsterapi (Body-Dynamic Analytic Work in Rebirth Therapy).* Copenhagen: Kreatik.

Mirdal, G. M. 1976. *Det ufødte barn, det nyfødte barn (The Unborn Baby, the Newborn Baby).* Copenhagen: Munksgaard.

Morris, D. 1984. *Menneskers adfærd (Human Behavior).* Copenhagen: Gyldendal.

Mossige, H., and E. Seeland. 1984. *Fra menneskekryb til gående barn (From Human Creepy-Crawly to Walking Child).* Oslo: University Publishing Co.

Norretranders, T. 1999. *The User Illusion: Cutting Consciousness Down to Size.* New York: Penguin.

Ollars, L. 1990. *Muskelpalpationstests pålidelighed (The Reliability of the Muscle Palpation Test).* Copenhagen: personal publication.

Olson, T. R. 1996. *ADAM Student Atlas of Anatomy.* Baltimore: Williams & Wilkins.

Scheflen, A. E. 1972. *Body Language and Social Order: Communication.* Englewood Cliffs, NJ: Prentice Hall.

Sobotta-Becker. 1975. *Atlas of Human Anatomy, 9th. ed.* Munich, Berlin, and Vienna: Urban and Schwarzenberg.

Stern, D. 2004. *The Present Moment.* New York: Norton.

Stone, R. J., and J. A. Stone 1997. *Atlas of Skeletal Muscles.* Dubuque, IA: Wm. C. Brown.

Theilgaard, A. 2000. "Den negligerede krop. Argumentation for at inddrage kroppen i psykoterapi" ("The Neglected Body: Argument for Involving the Body in Psychotherapy"). *Matrix* 17 (2000): 2, 137-151.

Vygotsky, L. S. 1978. *Mind in Society.* Cambridge, MA: Harvard University Press.

Vygotsky, L. S. 1986. *Thought and Language, 2nd ed.* Cambridge, MA: MIT Press.

Vygotsky, L. S. 1998. *The Collected Works of L. S. Vygotsky.* New York: Plenum.

Watzlawick, P., J. H. Beavin, and D. D. Jackson. 1998. *Pragmatics of Human Communication.* London: Faber.

Willert, S. 2000. "Bevidsthedsfunktionen—biologiske og psykologiske perspektiver" ("The Function of Consciousness: Biological and Psychological Perspectives"). *Bulletin for Anthropological Psychology* 7.

List of Muscles and Connective Tissue

A

81   abductor digiti minimi, 34-35, 236, 238, 240, 242, 246, **247-248**, 250, 419, 421, 429, 433, 483, 485, 495, 519, 527, 529

34   abductor digiti minimi and flexor digiti minimi brevis, 116, **120-121**, 122, 124, 126

36   abductor hallucis, 35, 116, 120, 122, **124-125**, 126, 439, 443, 483, 495, 511

77   abductor pollicis brevis, 34, 236-**237**, 238, 240, 242, 246, 248, 250, 266, 270, 272, 439, 441, 495

47   adductor brevis, 34, 152, 154-**155**, 156, 385, 505, 527, 529

46   adductor longus, 34, 150, 152-**153**, 154-159, 439, 505, 527

48   adductor magnus, 34, 150, 152-154, 156-**157**, 158, 407, 505, 527

79   adductor pollicis, 34, 236, 238, 240-**241**, 242, 246, 248, 250, 407, 409, 495, 517

86   anconeus, 35, 252, 254, 256-**257**, 439, 441, 519

B

66a, b   biceps brachii, **209**

24a, b, c, d   biceps femoris, 21, **93**, **95**

68   brachialis, 34, 208, 210, 212-**213**, 214, 407, 517

87   brachioradialis, 35, 258-**259**, 260-262, 264, 266-268, 270, 272, 419, 421, 517

120   buccinator, 34, 332, 334-**335**, 338, 340, 344, 350, 383, 489, 527

C

*   connective tissue of the back level with thoracic vertebrae 3-5, **37**, 373, 375, 459, 505

*   connective tissue around elbow and wrist, **219**, 365, 505, 511

*   connective tissue of medial and lateral rotators of hip joint, 365, 367, 373, 505, 511

*   connective tissue around knee and ankle, 365, 429, 505, 511

*   connective tissue of medial and lateral rotators of shoulder joint, **217**, 365, 373, 505, 511

*   connective tissue on top of the shoulder (shoulder plexus), 365, 503

67   coracobrachialis, 34, 208, 210-**211**, 212, 214, 395, 517

115   corrugator supercilii, 34, 324-**325**, 326, 407, 497

56   costal curve, 34, **187**

D

65	deltoid, anterior, 24, 198, 202, 204, 206-**207**, 383, 387, 477, 517
84a, b	deltoid, middle and posterior, 35, 252-**253**, 254, 256, 395, 397, 477, 519
124	depressor anguli oris, 34, 332, 334, 338, 340, 344-**345**, 350, 407, 489, 503, 511
*	depressor labii, **347**, 429, 431, 489, 503
*	depressor septi, **349**, 429, 431, 511
57	diaphragm, 34, 177, 186-**189**, 190, 192, 194, 196, 200, 279, 402, 407, 411, 503, 507
109	digastricus, posterior belly, 34, 308, 310, 312-**313**, 373, 375, 503, 517

E

1a	erector spinae, 35, 37-**39**, 40-42, 67, 69, 367, 383, 387, 429, 431, 465, 483, 485
1a*	erector spinae, lateral fibers on level with thoracic vertebrae 8-12, 439, 447, 465, 483
1b	erector spinae at spinous processes–rotators, 38, 40, 42
88	extensor carpi radialis longus and brevis, **261**, 519
89	extensor carpi ulnaris, 35, **263**, 395, 519
92	extensor digiti minimi, 35, **269**, 383, 519
90	extensor digitorum, 35, 258, 260, 262, 264-**265**, 268, 395, 519
38	extensor digitorum brevis and extensor hallucis brevis, **129**, 447, 483, 497
40	extensor digitorum longus, 34, 128, 130, 132-**133**, 134-135, 138, 419, 483, 497
41	extensor hallucis longus, 34, 128, 130, 132, 134-**135**, 138, 429, 483, 497
93	extensor indicis, 35, **271**, 395, 495, 519
94	extensor pollicis brevis and abductor pollicis longus, **273**, 419, 519

F

71	flexor carpi radialis, 220, 222-**223**, 224, 226, 228-230, 407, 517
72	flexor carpi ulnaris, 220, 222, 224-**225**, 226, 228, 230, 419, 421, 517
82	flexor digiti minimi brevis, 34, 116, 120-122, 124, 126, **249**, 383, 385, 387, 389, 483, 495, 517
*	flexor digiti minimi brevis (ref. 34), 34, 116, 120-122, 124, 126, **249**, 383, 385, 387, 389, 483, 495, 517
35	flexor digitorum brevis, 35, 116, 120, 122-**123**, 124, 126, 385, 483, 485, 495
32	flexor digitorum longus, 35, **111**, 113, 115, 137, 385, 419, 483, 495, 511
75	flexor digitorum profundus, 34, **231**, 233, 383, 495, 517
73	flexor digitorum superficialis, 34, 220, 222, 224, 226-**227**, 228, 230, 395, 495, 517

37	flexor hallucis brevis, 35, 116, 120, 122, 124, 126-**127**, 395, 399, 483, 495
31	flexor hallucis longus, 35, 104, 106, 108-**109**, 110, 407, 439, 483, 495, 511
78	flexor pollicis brevis, 34, 236, 238-**239**, 240, 242, 246, 248, 250, 407, 495, 517
74	flexor pollicis longus, 34, **229**, 395, 495, 517

G

101a	galea aponeurotica (a spot on top of the head), 35, **291**, 373, 483, 511
101b	galea aponeurotica (half circle around the top of the head), 35, 365, 503, 511
101c	galea aponeurotica, 35, 290, 292, 294-**295**, 296, 317, 439, 497, 511
28a, b	gastrocnemius, 101, **103**, 105, 107
18	gemelli and obturator internus, 35, 74, 76, 78-**79**, 80, 385, 471, 505, 527
14	gluteus maximus, **71**, 73, 75, 77, 79, 89, 91
15	gluteus medius, 35, 66, 70, 72-**73**, 75, 419, 423, 471, 519, 525, 527
16	gluteus minimus, 35, 66, 70, 72, 74-**75**, 76-78, 80, 407, 411, 471, 519, 525
49	gracilis, 34, 150, 152-154, 156-**159**, 395, 489, 491, 505, 507, 527, 529, 533

I

12	iliac crest, 35, 65, **67**, 73, 91, 167, 171, 177
51a	iliacus, 34, 164, 170-**171**, 172-173, 184, 373, 419, 423, 461, 471, 473, 527
51b	iliopsoas, 34, 164, 170-**173**, 184, 385, 389, 471
23	iliotibial tract, 35, 71, 89, **91**, 143, 489
7a, b	infraspinatus, 35, 52, 54-**57**, 429, 431, 439, 441, 489, 491
50	inguinal ligament, 34, 164-**165**, 170, 172-173, 184
*	insertion of iliopsoas (ref. 51b), **169**, 365, 367, 459
*	insertions of abductor, flexors, and extensors on the proximal phalanx of the little toe, **119**, 373, 377, 385, 483, 495
*	insertions of flexors and extensors on the proximal phalanx of the little finger, **245**, 375, 517, 519
61	intercostals, 34, 186, 188, 190, 192, 194, 196-**197**, 200, 365, 367, 383, 389, 395, 419, 429, 439, 503, 507

L

9a, b	latissimus dorsi, 53, **61**, 63
96	levator scapulae, 35, 276, 278-**279**, 281-282, 284, 303, 407, 409, 503, 519

110	longus capitis and longus colli, 34, **315**, 373, 375, 465, 483, 495, 503
*	lumbricals (foot), 489
*	lumbricals (hand), 495

M

125	masseter, 34, 332, 334, 337, 338, 340, 343-344, 350-**351**, 407, 409, 503
123	medial pterygoid, 330, 342-**343**, 395, 503
122	mentalis, 34, 332, 334, 338, 340-**341**, 344, 350, 383, 407, 489, 491
108	mylohyoid, 34, 308, 310-**311**, 312, 383, 483, 503, 507, 527

N

116	nasalis, 34, 324, 326-**327**, 429, 431, 497, 499, 511, 513

O

52	obliquus externus and internus, 34, 175, **177**, 187
20	obturator internus, near pelvic floor, 35, 395, 471, 503
111	occipitofrontalis—venter frontalis, **317**
102	occipitofrontalis—venter occipitalis, 35, 290, 292, 294, 296-**297**, 407, 497, 511
107	omohyoid, 34, 308-**309**, 310, 312, 439, 483, 503
83	opponens digiti minimi, 25-26, 236, 238, 240, 242, 246, 248, 250-**251**, 429, 431, 495, 511, 517
80	opponens pollicis, 34, 236, 238, 240, 242-**243**, 246, 248, 250, 429, 431, 495, 511, 513, 517
113a, b	orbicularis oculi, 34, 298, 316, 318, 320-**321**, 322, 328, 383
121	orbicularis oris, 34, 332-334, 338-**339**, 340, 344, 350, 383, 511, 517, 527
*	origin of iliacus (ref. 51a), **167**, 365, 459, 525
59	origin of pectoralis major—sternal head, 34, **193**

P

76	palmar aponeurosis, 34, 234-**235**, 383, 495, 517
45	pectineus, 34, 150-**151**, 152-156, 158, 419, 423, 505, 507, 527, 529
62 a,b,c	pectoralis major, 59, 195, **199**, 201, 203, 211, 473, 513
63	pectoralis minor
*	pelvic floor, **203**
42a, b	peroneus longus and brevis, 137, **139**
17	piriformis, 35, 74, 76-**77**, 78-80, 395, 399, 471, 473, 507, 525, 529
33	plantar aponeurosis, 35, 116-**117**, 120, 122-124, 126, 133, 135, 365, 367, 483, 495, 511
27	plantaris, 35, 100-**101**, 102, 104, 106, 108, 110, 133, 439, 489, 491, 505, 507, 533

103	platysma, 34, 298-**299**, 316, 318, 320, 322, 328, 332, 334, 338, 340, 344, 347, 350, 429, 431, 489, 491, 503, 527, 529
29	popliteus, 35, 100, 102, 104-**105**, 106, 108, 110, 429, 433, 483, 485, 489, 491, 505, 507, 533
114	procerus, 34, 298, 316, 318, 320, 322-**323**, 328, 383, 395, 497
70	pronator teres, 34, 220-**221**, 222-224, 226, 228, 230, 267, 395, 397, 517
55	psoas major, 34, 164, 170-172, 184-**185**, 395, 399, 459, 471
*	pyramidalis, **181**, 447, 449, 527

Q

19	quadratus femoris, 35, 74, 76, 78, 80-**81**, 407, 411, 471, 505
11	quadratus lumborum, 35, 60, 62, 64-**65**, 67-68, 395, 397, 489
*	quadratus plantae, **115**, 419, 483
43	quadriceps femoris, 141, 143, 145, 147, 423, 449

R

53	rectus abdominis, 34, 177, **179**
43a	rectus femoris, 34, 141, 145, 147, 149, 173
3a, b	rhomboids minor and major, **49**
*	risorius, **337**, 419, 489

S

21	sacrotuberous ligament, 71, 85, **87**, 365, 367, 373, 377, 471, 489
13	sacrum, 35, 39, 60, 62, 64, 68-**69**, 71, 77, 87, 365, 367, 471, 473, 511, 513
44a, b	sartorius, 18, 20, 34, 140, 142, 146-**149**, 151, 157, 159,173, 407, 429, 489, 491, 505, 507, 527, 533
104	scalenus anterior, 280, 300-**301**, 302, 314, 383, 387, 465, 495, 503
105	scalenus medius, 34, 280-281, 300, 302-**303**, 314, 395, 397, 465, 495, 503
97	scalenus posterior, 35, 280-281, 300, 302, 314, 407, 465, 495, 503
26	semimembranosus, **99**
98	semispinalis capitis, 35, 276, 278, 282-**283**, 284, 383, 387, 465, 495
25	semitendinosus, 21, 35, 82, 86, 92, 94, 96-**97**, 98-99, 157, 159, 402, 407, 411, 429, 433, 465, 511, 513
8a, b, c	serratus anterior, **59**
10	serratus posterior inferior, 39, **63**
4	serratus posterior superior, **51**, 421
30a, b	soleus, 105, **107**, 109, 111
99	splenius capitis, 35, 276, 278, 282, 284-**285**, 383, 465, 533
*	splenius cervicis, **287**, 419, 465, 495, 525
60	sternal fascia, 34, 186, 188, 190, 192, 194-**195**, 196, 200, 365, 373, 459

106a, b	sternocleidomastoid, 34, 279, 281, 285, 301, 303-**305**, 306-307, 313, 315, 407, 419, 421, 429, 431, 465, 467, 495, 503, 507, 527, 529
64	subclavius, 34 198, 202, 204-**205**, 206-207, 483, 485
100	suboccipitals, 35, 288-**289**, 365, 367, 373, 375, 383, 495
69	subscapularis, 34, 208, 210, 212, 214-**215**, 383, 387, 489
91	supinator, 35, 266-**267**, 270, 272, 395, 397, 517, 521
95	supraspinatus, 35, 252, 254, 256, 275-**277**, 278, 282, 284, 395, 397, 483, 485

T

118	temporalis, 34, 330-**331**, 342-343, 373, 439, 447, 449, 483, 485, 497, 499
22	tensor fascia lata, 35, 71, 88-**89**, 90-91, 140, 142, 146, 148, 385, 389, 489, 505
5	teres major, 35, 44, 46, 48, 52-**53**, 54-56, 407, 409, 489, 491
6	teres minor, 35, 52, 54-**55**, 56, 419, 489, 491, 527
112	"third eye," 34, 298, 316, 318-**319**, 320, 322. 328, 332, 334, 338, 340, 344, 350, 373, 483, 497
39	tibialis anterior, **131**, 133, 135
*	tibialis posterior, **137**, 385, 419, 489, 527
117	tip of the nose, 298, 316, 318, 320, 322, 328-**329**, 349, 407, 511
51c	transversus abdominis, 34, 174-**175**, 176, 178, 182, 419, 421, 503, 527
58	transversus thoracis, 34, 186, 188, 190-**191**, 192, 194, 196, 200
2a, b, c	trapezius, 35, 39, 43-**45**, 46-48, 51, 61, 275, 277, 279, 281, 283, 285, 287, 301, 303, 383, 387, 395, 397, 419, 421, 459, 461, 505, 507, 525, 527, 529
85a, b, c	triceps brachii, **255**

U

54	umbilicus, 34, 179, **183**, 365, 367, 373, 375, 477, 517

V

43c	vastus intermedius, 34, **145**, 479
43b	vastus lateralis, 34, 95, **143**
43d	vastus medialis, 34, 140, 142, 146-**147**, 148-149, 419, 423, 447, 449, 477, 489, 505, 527

Z

119	zygomaticus (major and minor), 34, 332-**333**, 334, 338, 340, 344, 350, 419, 503

About the Authors

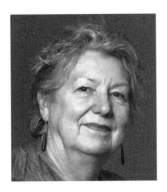

Lisbeth Marcher is one of the founders of the Bodynamic Institute, a worldwide organization that offers Bodynamic Analysis and psychotherapy training and services. A carefully researched and constructed somatic developmental psychology, Bodynamic Analysis developed over a period of forty years as Marcher and other researchers studied a combination of psychomotor development and psychotherapy. They have presented their material at conferences and lectures throughout the world. The president of the European Association for Body-Psychotherapy (EABP) since 2008 and a board member since 2004, Marcher currently provides workshops and training in Bodynamic Analysis in Europe, Asia, and the USA.

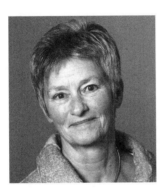

A psychotherapist, bodynamic analyst, and psychomotor educator, Sonja Fich is a founding member of the Bodynamic Institute, a codeveloper of the Bodynamic System, and the institute's anatomy specialist. As a bodynamic psychotherapist, Fich has undergone a two-year training program in "Loss and Trauma," and has researched how Bodynamic Analysis is helpful for treating autism in children under the supervision of Axel Arnfred, one of Denmark's most well-known pediatric psychiatrists. She also participated in a research project regarding the outcome and methods of psychotherapy systems that was organized by the Institute of Sociology at the University of Copenhagen. Fich is a member of the Danish Association for Psychotherapists.